TRANSVAGINAL SONOGRAPHY
Second Edition

D1560830

TRANSVAGINAL SONOGRAPHY

Second Edition

Edited by

Ilan E. Timor-Tritsch, MD

Professor of Clinical Obstetrics and Gynecology
College of Physicians and Surgeons of Columbia University, New York
Director of Obstetrical and Gynecological Ultrasound
The Sloane Hospital for Women of the Presbyterian Hospital,
New York City

Shraga Rottem, MD, DSc

Department of Obstetrics and Gynecology
Rambam Medical Center
Haifa, Israel

Elsevier

New York • Amsterdam • London • Tokyo

Elsevier Science Publishing Co., Inc.
655 Avenue of the Americas, New York, New York 10010

Distributors outside the United States and Canada:
Elsevier Science Publishers B.V.
P.O. Box 211, 1000 AE Amsterdam, The Netherlands

©1991 by Elsevier Science Publishing Co., Inc.

Library of Congress Cataloging-in-Publication Data

Transvaginal sonography / edited by Ilan E. Timor-Tritsch, Shraga
    Rottem. – 2nd ed.
        p.   cm.
    Includes bibliographical references and index.
    ISBN 0-444-01577-9 (hardcover : alk. paper)
    1. Ultrasonics in obstetrics. 2. Generative organs. Female-
Diseases – Diagnosis. 3. Obstetrics – Diagnosis. I. Timor-Tritsch,
Ilan E. II. Rottem, Shraga.
    [DNLM: 1. Genital Diseases, Female – ultrasonography. 2. Prenatal
Diagnosis – methods. WP 141 T772]
RG527.5.U48T73 1991
618′.047543 – dc20
DNLM/DLC
for Library of Congress   91-6500
                                                              CIP

This book is printed on acid-free paper.

Current printing (last digit):
10 9 8 7 6 5 4 3 2

Manufactured in the United States of America

We dedicate this book to our understanding wives
Hava and Dalia
and to our children
Daphna, Orna, and Nadav.

We also dedicate this compendium
to the constantly decreasing number of fetuses
who are still denied the benefit
of routine antenatal sonography.

Contents

Foreword

Once again the authors bring to the practitioners of women's health care advances that place them in the vanguard of transvaginal ultrasonography. Reviewing the rapid changes in this field since the last edition leaves me wondering how far and how rapidly the use of this new diagnostic (and therapeutic) tool will change our medical view.

The evolution of early sonoembryology is as exciting and as well detailed as materials once seen in morphologic embryology texts. Indeed in this edition we see the developing brain and body as effectively as once seen in the classic embryology textbooks. The next sonographic steps may take us into the area of gene therapy in the embryologic stage—now a distinct possibility.

The transvaginal route provides a new diagnostic pathway for early as well as later fetal development and fetal blood flow. The potential of color Doppler flow becomes even more exciting. In charting new areas, one needs to consider the potential use of this modality for women in their postreproductive years. In the text you will find illustrations of blood flow in placental lakes which predict obstetrical emergencies such as the placenta accreta. For the past 25 years minimal progress has been made in lowering mortality rates following the earlier diagnosis of ovarian malignancy. Can the color flow probe document the earlier presence of ovarian neoplasms? This area needs exploration.

The co-existence and vital importance of transvaginal sonography in follicular sizing, *in vitro* fertilization, and ectopic pregnancy identification (and possible treatment) is obvious to all. The formation of the urinary tract may foreshadow fetal surgery. As we stated in the first edition, remaining unclear and still on the horizon is where it will all end. Perhaps that is rhetorical. Will the value of this device remain limited to the hands of the specialist in sonography, or will it become part of the clinician's diagnostic and therapeutic armament at patient office visits? To reach this latter plateau (if it should be reached), we must educate more clinicians to use transvaginal sonography well, and to actively study whether the clinician's hands and judgment can be improved by the vaginal probe. The reader of this monograph will benefit from the writings of excellent clinicians who, once again, present a compendium of good data and good illustrations.

Mortimer G. Rosen, M.D.
Willard C. Rappleye Professor of
Obstetrics and Gynecology and
Chairman of the Department
College of Physicians and Surgeons of
Columbia University and
The Presbyterian Hospital
in the City of New York

Preface to the Second Edition

The compilation of this second edition brought home with vivid clarity the overwhelming amount of data that has been accumulated and published over the relatively short period following publication of the first edition of *Transvaginal Sonography*. Over 80 original articles involving the vaginal scanning route appeared in the English and German literature as opposed to the five (5!) cited in the first edition. This fact alone attests to the importance of transvaginal scanning in every field of obstetrics and gynecology. The great demand for information generated by this new technique resulted in one or two day courses mushrooming everyplace in the world, drawing record numbers of participants. Two major imaging journals published special editions covering the subject. Our first edition proved to be in great demand despite the fact that it was only descriptive without any clinical research data.

In view of the enormous amount of material gathered for this edition, in retrospect we would like to have subtitled the first edition "Look what we can see!". Throughout the 19 chapters this second edition has over 370 illustrations, citing over 730 references to support data generated in the last three years. This edition might rightfully be subtitled "Look what was found!".

In this second edition we strengthened and practically rewrote the chapters from the first edition. We expanded the book significantly by adding 10 new chapters. Among the new subjects are those dealing with placenta previa, the lower urinary tract, early fetal malformations, and the fetal brain in the second and third trimester. Some special applications, such as Doppler flow measurements and color coded Doppler sonography, were also added. Last but not least, the fascinating and new office and emergency room use of transvaginal sonography is presented.

Our congratulations go to all the skeptics who over the past three years "converted" and jumped on the bandwagon after years of previous disbelief. They provided excellent patient care. For those who are still untouched and shielded by an armor of disbelief we hope this book provides the convincing data apparently lacking in previous publications they have read.

We also pay tribute to the manufacturing companies who most of the time *listened* to our suggestions and desires in terms of technology, but do not always *hear* our plea for wider imaging angle, better magnification and zooming, straight probe handle (for the gynecologists!), simple but powerful and fast software, and international keyboard labeling.

The authors have no doubts about the future of transvaginal sonography. This was expressed by us in the preface to the first edition; almost all that was written by us there is still true today. Transvaginal sonography will be an integral part of teaching programs; the equipment will be present in every examining room of all ob/gyn and emergency departments; the probe will hang around the neck or lie in the pocket of the person doing the imaging as the good old stethoscope and the ophthalmoscope have through the years.

Ilan E. Timor-Tritsch
Shraga Rottem

Preface to the First Edition

The use of a relatively high-frequency probe through the vaginal vault for pelvic organ imaging was the product of some basic knowledge in the physics of ultrasound and the frustration of a gynecologist facing a diagnostic dilemma in a slightly obese patient suffering from a gynecological disease.

Through the last decade, the obstetrician/gynecologist has experienced a Janus-like personality. On the one hand, the "obstetrician" side of practice possessed the ability to detect intricate fetal malformations, and, lately, even to direct needles into the fetal vascular system. But the gynecology "face" was confronted with inconclusive ultrasound reports and experienced the frustration of inadequate equipment to guide the diagnostic ability available to the obstetrician.

Immediately after the ultrasonic engineers turned over to us the prototype of the first 6.5-MHz vaginal probe, we could not contain our excitement at the clarity of the pictures. They were amazingly sharp, and it was clear to all of us that we were seeing and working with something very important. Suddenly, there was no doubt about a fetal heartbeat at the end of five completed weeks from the last menstrual period in an obese patient. The developing ovarian follicles could be followed through a cycle as clearly as seeing the inside of a fruit cut through with a sharp knife. The early unruptured tubal pregnancy sprang into view and could easily be diagnosed.

Because the authors feel that these achievements are of tremendous importance to the profession, we have turned our attention to this book in order to share our techniques and results. Some of the material contained in the following pages has never before appeared in print, and we are certain that the reader will find the data as exciting as we did during the discovery. We believe that the material contained in this book represents the state of the art as we now know it, and we feel duty-bound to share this information with our colleagues.

If the diagnostic domains of early normal and abnormal pregnancy are regarded as part of the practice of gynecology rather than obstetrics, then we are rightfully entitled to consider transvaginal sonography as a major addition to gynecology. Obstetrics had its turn several years ago with the introduction of linear real-time sonography. At that time, the greatest leap forward in progress was made since the introduction of electronic and biochemical fetal monitoring. Now it is the gynecologists who are receiving attention with their new sonographic methods for diagnostic and therapeutic decision making.

The pertinent chapters will speak for themselves, but the reader must forgive us our biases when we discuss several areas we consider the "icing on the cake."

Undoubtedly, a closer and better look at ovarian tumors, with the potential opportunity to develop a generally used screening program for their earlier detection, may provide high-frequency transvaginal sonography with its most important role in our specialty.

Diagnosis of tubal pathology in general and early detection of tubal pregnancy in particular constitute another area in which this method has produced exciting images. If the semi-invasive transvaginal approach of treating early unruptured tubal pregnancies—saving the patient abdominal surgery and even laparoscopy (see Chapter 4)—proves to be clinically useful, we shall regard this as another outstanding achievement of transvaginal sonography.

The imaging of details of the very early pregnancy should also be mentioned here for its clinical merits as well as the potential for early recognition of the pathological pregnancy. Monitoring of follicular growth and transvaginally guided transvaginal ovum aspiration are appreciated by an increasing number of centers.

Many obstetrics and gynecology residency programs throughout the world require formal training periods in obstetrical and gynecological sonography. We speculate that within a relatively short time all departments dealing with resident training will recognize the importance of formal, hands-on training in obstetrical and gynecological ultrasonography in general, and vaginal sonography in particular. This projected rise in knowledge, together with practical experience in handling different types of transducer probes by the new generation of obstetricians and gynecologists, will necessarily bring about new methods in medical practice. If the medicolegal atmosphere can be improved by such means as excellence in practice, patient education, and education of the public at large, we envision the presence of modestly priced but clinically efficient ultrasound equipment, with its various probes, and its extensive use in each and every practice of obstetrics and gynecology. We project that the vaginal probe will be used on the spot, without much ado, as routinely as the classical vaginal speculum.

Ilan E. Timor-Tritsch
Shraga Rottem

Acknowledgments

The authors express their thanks to all those who made this publication possible: our secretaries Annette Kirschner and Britt F. Minott for preparing the manuscript from the endless flow of tapes and illegible handwriting; Reba Nosoff, for reviewing, correcting, and editing the manuscript; and the staff at Elsevier Science Publishing Company, for their professional help and support. The sonographers of our departments must be commended for their observations and help in creating a vast data base. We are also thankful to the Kerenyi Perinatal Fund, Rambam Research Fund, and Columbia University for their generous support.

Finally, special thanks are given to Dr. Mortimer G. Rosen, who created a scientific ambiance, conducive to creative clinical research. This research led to valuable results, and finally to the compilation of this book.

Contributors

Carol B. Benson, MD
Brigham & Women's Hospital, Department of Radiology, Boston, Massachusetts

Zeev Blumenfeld, MD
Reproductive Endocrinology Unit, Department of Obstetrics and Gynecology, Rambam Medical Center, Haifa, Israel

Joseph Brandes, MD
Professor, Obstetric and Gynecology Technion Medical School; Director, Department of Obstetrics and Gynecology, Rambam Medical Center, Haifa, Israel

Moshe Bronshtein, MD
Department of Obstetrics and Gynecology, Rambam Medical Center, Haifa, Israel

Avraham Bruck, PhD
Chief Scientist, Department of Ultrasound, Elscint Limited, Haifa, Israel

Arie Drugan, MD
In Vitro Fertilization Unit, Department of Obstetrics and Gynecology, Rambam Medical Center, Haifa, Israel

Stephen S. Entman, MD
Associate Professor and Vice Chairman, Department of Obstetrics and Gynecology, Vanderbilt University, Nashville, Tennessee

Dan Farine, MD
Assistant Professor of Obstetrics and Gynecology, Director of Perinatology, Department of Obstetrics and Gynecology, Mount Sinai Hospital, Toronto, Canada

Arthur C. Fleischer, MD
Professor of Radiology and Chief, Diagnostic Sonography, Vanderbilt University, Nashville, Tennessee

Joseph Itskovitz, MD, DSc
Associate Professor of Obstetrics and Gynecology, Technion Medical School;
In Vitro Fertilization, Department of Obstetrics and Gynecology, Rambam Medical
Center, Haifa, Israel

Donna M. Kepple, RDMS
Chief, Sonographer, Obstetrics and Gynecology Ultrasound, Vanderbilt University,
Nashville, Tennessee

Asim Kurjak, MD, PhD
Professor of Obstetrics and Gynecology, University of Zagreb, Head of Ultrasonic
Institute, Department of Obstetrics and Gynecology, Kajfes Hospital, Zagreb,
Yugoslavia

Marcia J. Lavery, RDMS
Ultrasonographer, Park Health Care Services, Brookline, Massachusetts

Nathan Lewit, MD
Department of Obstetrics and Gynecology, Rambam Medical Center, Haifa, Israel

Dorit Manor, MD
Department of Obstetrics and Gynecology, Rambam Medical Center, Haifa, Israel

Ana Monteagudo, MD
Assistant Professor of Obstetrics and Gynecology, Department of Obstetrics and
Gynecology, Columbia Presbyterian Medical Center, New York, New York

Lawrence W. Oppenheimer, MD, MRCOG
Clinical Fellow in Maternal Fetal Medicine, Department of Obstetrics and Gynecology,
Mt. Sinai Hospital, Toronto, Canada

David B. Peisner, MD
Assistant Professor of Obstetrics and Gynecology, Department of Obstetrics and
Gynecology, Columbia Presbyterian Medical Center, New York, New York

Martin Quinn, MD
Research Fellow, University of Bristol, Department of Obstetrics and Gynecology, Bristol
Maternity Hospital, Bristol, England

M. Lynne Reuss, MD
Assistant Professor of Obstetrics and Gynecology, Department of Obstetrics and
Gynecology, Columbia Presbyterian Medical Center, New York, New York

Mortimer G. Rosen, MD
Willard C. Rappleye Professor of Obstetrics and Gynecology and Chairman,
Department of Obstetrics and Gynecology, Columbia Presbyterian Medical Center,
New York, New York

Shraga Rottem, MD, DSc
Department of Obstetrics and Gynecology, Rambam Medical Center, Haifa, Israel

Israel Thaler, MD
Department of Obstetrics and Gynecology, Rambam Medical Center, Haifa, Israel

Ilan E. Timor-Tritsch, MD
Professor of Clinical Obstetrics and Gynecology, Director of Obstetrical Service and of
Obstetrical and Gynecological Ultrasound, Columbia Presbyterian Medical Center, New
York, New York

Zeev Wiener, MD
Department of Obstetrics and Gynecology, Rambam Medical Center, Haifa, Israel

Ivica Zalud, MD
Department of Obstetrics and Gynecology, Kajfes Hospital, Zagreb, Yugoslavia

Etan Zimmer, MD
Department of Obstetrics and Gynecology, Rambam Medical Center, Haifa, Israel

CHAPTER 1

Transvaginal Sonography and Doppler Measurements— Physical Considerations

Israel Thaler, MD
Avraham Bruck, PhD

Ultrasound is used in medical diagnosis to produce images of tissue structures from which the size and nature of the structures can be determined. For example, information concerning many types of soft-tissue organs and lesions is gathered, and the interaction of transmitted ultrasound with tissue structures gives rise to information that can be visually displayed. This information is, therefore, directly related to the acoustic, ie, ultrasonic, properties of the tissues, and is essentially different from that supplied by other diagnostic tools such as x-rays or isotope scanning.

The imaging process consists of sending short *pulses* of ultrasound into the body and using the *reflections* received from various tissues and organs to produce an image of internal structures.

Ultrasound is the term applied to mechanical pressure waves transmitted as *mechanical vibrations* through the medium. These vibrations are not random, but orderly oscillatory vibrations generated by an external source. A typical source is a crystal, electrically driven to vibrate, that is placed in contact with the outside surface of the medium. Interactions occur between the source and the particles of the surface of the medium, causing them to vibrate. These particles, in turn, cause their adjacent neighbors to start oscillating, and in a similar manner the mechanical vibrations pass very quickly through the material.

A *particle* is a small portion of the medium through which the sound travels. If the motion of a particle in a medium transmitting ultrasound is examined in detail, the particle is seen to be moving slightly back and forth parallel to the direction of wave travel. This motion is similar to that of the weight on the end of a pendulum, although the distances actually moved are microscopic (in the range of one-millionth of a centimeter). Simple harmonic motion, or sinusoidal motion, is the term used here (Fig 1.1).

THE PROPERTIES OF SOUND WAVES AND IMAGE QUALITY

Like all waves, sound is described by several parameters: frequency, wavelength, propagation speed, amplitude, intensity.

Frequency is the number of complete oscillations a particle performs per second. Sound with a frequency of 20 kHz or higher is termed ultrasound, because it

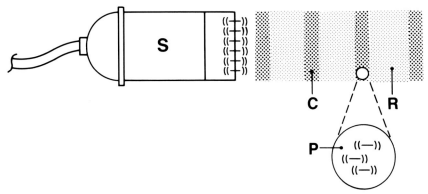

Figure 1.1 Formation of longitudinal waves. The vibratory motion of the source (S) forms compressions (C) and rarefactions (R). The vibrating particles (P) are similar to the weight on the end of a pendulum and vibrate along the same direction as the source motion.

is beyond the frequency range of the human ear. In medical imaging, frequencies in the range 2–10 MHz are employed. The frequency of ultrasound has great influence on the image quality.

Wavelength is the length of space over which one cycle occurs, ie, the distance between any two identical points on the waveform (Fig 1.2). It plays an important role in determining ultrasonic beam widths and pulse lengths and so influences the detail (ie, resolution) obtainable in an image.

Propagation speed is the velocity of the sound wave moving through a medium. Wavelength frequency and velocity are related by

$$velocity = frequency \times wavelength$$
$$V = f \times \lambda \tag{1.1}$$

In general, the higher the stiffness of an object, the higher the propagation speed (Table 1.1).

Propagation speed is important because imaging instruments make use of it in generating the display. If the velocity of sound in the medium is known, it is possible to calculate the wavelength using Eq. 1.1. If the average velocity of sound in tissue is assumed to be 1540 m per second and its frequency 1 MHz, then

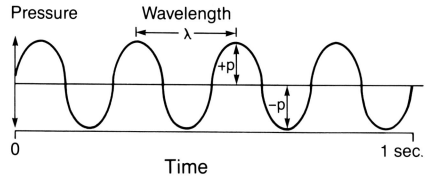

Figure 1.2 Wavelength (λ) and amplitude (p) of a wave. The frequency is four complete cycles per second, or 4 Hz.

TABLE 1.1 The Velocity of Ultrasound in Certain Tissues and Materials

Material	Propagation Speed (m/s)
Fat	1,450
Brain	1,540
Liver	1,550
Muscle	1,570
Soft-tissue average	1,540
Water (20°C)	1,480
Bone	4,080
Air	330

$$1540 = 1 \times 10^6 \times \lambda$$

Therefore

$$\lambda = 0.00154 \text{ m} = 1.54 \text{ mm}$$

Similarly, at

$$\begin{array}{ll} 2 \text{ MHz} & \lambda = 0.77 \text{ mm} \\ 5 \text{ MHz} & \lambda = 0.31 \text{ mm} \\ 7 \text{ MHz} & \lambda = 0.22 \text{ mm} \\ 10 \text{ MHz} & \lambda = 0.1 \ \text{ mm} \end{array}$$

This demonstrates that the higher the frequency the smaller the wavelength, and the result is better image detail.

Amplitude of an ultrasonic wave is the maximum change in pressure caused by the wave itself and is related to the intensity of the ultrasonic radiation (Fig 1.2). The greater the intensity, the greater the amplitude. The term *amplitude* is also used to describe the pulse magnitude of echoes.

Intensity is the rate at which energy flows through the unit area. This energy passes from the source to the tissue. Intensity is also defined as the power in a wave divided by the area over which the power is applied:

$$\text{intensity (W/cm}^2) = \frac{\text{power (W)}}{\text{area (cm}^2)} \tag{1.2}$$

Intensity is expressed as watts per centimeter squared (W/cm²).

During ultrasonic scanning, the output intensity of many instruments plays a prime role in determining the sensitivity of the instrument, that is, in determining the number and size of echoes recorded. Studies on the safety of ultrasonic techniques also require accurate knowledge of the intensities involved.

Power is the energy flow rate through the whole cross section of the beam. The power is expressed in watts. For imaging of structures in close proximity to the transducer, relatively low intensities are sufficient to obtain a good-quality picture. On most instruments the intensity settings can be controlled by the user.

THE BEHAVIOR OF ULTRASONIC WAVES IN TISSUES

Diagnosis through ultrasound is accomplished by interpreting the *reflections* occurring at tissue interfaces. Short ultrasound pulses are transmitted into the region of interest, and a returning pulse or echo is generated at organ boundaries or tissue interfaces. These echoes provide rich sources of diagnostic information. An echo is generated at an interface between tissues with different acoustic properties. These properties are described as *acoustic impedance*, which is determined by the density of the tissue and the velocity of sound in that tissue:

$$\text{acoustic impedance} = \text{density} \times \text{velocity of sound}$$

$$\text{AI} = p \times v \tag{1.3}$$

The echo size, or intensity, is determined by the difference between the acoustic impedances of the two tissue forming the interface. The acoustic impedances of most biological tissues are so similar that only a fraction of the ultrasound is returned at each interface, most of the energy being transmitted to deeper levels. As a result, echoes from more distant (deeper) structures are also returned. This makes it possible to analyze many successive interfaces for diagnostic purposes. A notable exception is the soft tissue–bone interface. Bone has a much higher impedance than soft tissue (Table 1.2); therefore, a very strong echo is produced. The energy reflected is so large that it greatly attenuates the transmitted beam. Imaging of structures lying behind bones, therefore, becomes difficult as an *acoustic shadow* is created. Even more marked is the reflection of a gas–soft tissue interface. This makes scanning through lung or gas in the bowel impossible. In practice, gas is regarded as an impenetrable barrier that gives rise to huge echoes. When an ultrasound transducer is applied to the skin, a very thin film of air would cause a very strong attenuation of the ultrasonic beam before it even entered the body. For this reason, a coupling medium (an oil or gel) is used to provide a good sound path from the source to the skin.

As transmitted ultrasound and echoes pass through tissue, they are reduced in intensity and amplitude. This reduction in amplitude and intensity is called *attenuation*. It is due to *reflection* (described earlier), *absorption* (conversion of sound to heat), *refraction*, and *scattering*.

One result of attenuation is that echoes from structures deep within the body are much weaker than those from superficial regions. This limits the depth at

TABLE 1.2 Acoustic Impedances of Ultrasound in Certain Materials

Material	Acoustic Impedance (g/cm^2 s)
Fat	1.38×10^5
Liver	1.65×10^5
Kidney	1.62×10^5
Soft-tissue average	1.63×10^5
Water (20°C)	1.48×10^5
Bone	7.80×10^5
Air	0.0004×10^5

TABLE 1.3 Half-Intensity Depths of Various Materials in Different Frequency Ranges

Material	Half-Intensity Depth (cm)		
	2 MHz	5 MHz	10 MHz
Soft-tissue average	1.5	0.5	0.3
Blood	8.5	3	2
Water	340	54	14
Bone	0.1	0.04	—
Air	0.06	0.01	—

which images can be obtained. Ultrasound-detecting systems used for diagnostic imaging are manipulated to correct this imbalance to a certain extent.

Attenuation is amplified by an increase in frequency, mainly because of a larger absorption. To give some appreciation of the role of attenuation in practice, reference is made to the thickness of tissues required to reduce intensity by half, called the *half-intensity depth*. The latter correlates with the attainable imaging depth. Half-intensity depth decreases with increased frequency and, for a given frequency, is dependent on the characteristics of the medium (Table 1.3). It can be seen from Table 1.3 that air and bone strongly attenuate the intensity of sound, whereas fluids within the body are only weakly absorbing. These fluids are often referred to as *transonic* or *translucent*. Another factor that determines echo intensity is the angle at which the ultrasonic beam strikes the reflecting surface. Because tissue interfaces are not flat, smooth reflectors, but are irregular in shape, echoes are returned even from oblique interfaces. These echoes are weaker than those reflected from perpendicular surfaces, and some may not reach the transducer face at all (Fig 1.3). In practice, complete images are obtained by varying the scanning beam direction and picking up as many reflectors (or echoes) as possible.

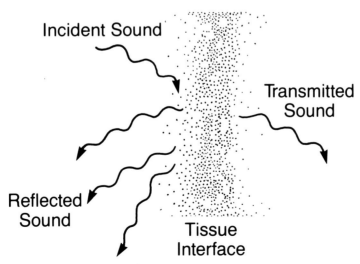

Figure 1.3 Reflection at a rough interface.

GENERATION OF ULTRASONIC BEAMS

An essential feature of ultrasonic instruments is the ability to produce narrow *ultrasound beams* that are highly directional. The *ultrasonic field* is a geometric description of the region encompassed by the ultrasound beam. At the high frequencies used in diagnostic ultrasound, well-directed beams can be readily generated by simple devices called *ultrasonic transducers* or *probes*. Ultrasonic transducers operate on the *piezoelectricity* principle, which states that some materials (eg, ceramics, quartz) produce a voltage when deformed by an applied pressure. Piezoelectricity also results in production of a pressure when these materials are deformed by an applied voltage. As a result of both these effects, a single crystal element can be used both as a transmitter and as a receiver of ultrasonic waves. The term *transducer element* (or piezoelectric element) refers to the piece of piezoelectric material that converts electricity to ultrasound and vice versa. Typical diagnostic ultrasound transducer elements are 6–19 mm in diameter and 0.2–2 mm thick. The element and its associated case and damping and matching materials constitute the *transducer assembly or probe* (Fig 1.4). The damping material reduces pulse duration by damping down the vibrations. This improves axial resolution (discussed later). The matching layer facilitates sound transmission into the tissue. Each transducer operates at a particular frequency determined by the thickness of the transducer element and by the propagation speed of the transducer material. Source transducers can operate in two modes. The *continuous mode* is obtained by driving the transducer with a continuous alternating voltage; this produces alternating pressure that propagates as continuous sound waves. The *pulsed mode* is obtained by driving the transducer with voltage pulses; this produces ultrasound pulses. These transducers also convert received reflections into voltage pulses. This mode is commonly used for diagnostic ultrasound imaging.

Increasing the frequency or decreasing the number of cycles of the pulse would result in shorter spatial pulse length and, thus, better axial resolution. Damping material in the transducer probe decreases the spatial pulse length by reducing the number of cycles in each pulse.

FOCUSING OF ULTRASONIC BEAMS

Ultrasonic transducers produce narrow ultrasound beams. The shape of the beam depends primarily on the frequency and the crystal diameter for flat, unfocused

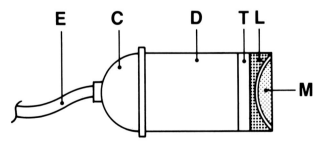

Figure 1.4 Structure of a basic transducer for generating pulsed ultrasound. C = case, D = damping material, E = electric cable, L = matching layer, T = transducer element, M = filler material.

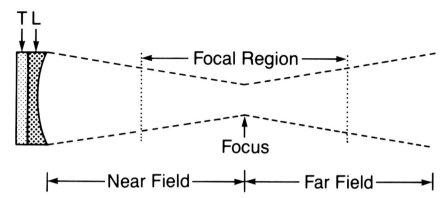

Figure 1.5 Focusing transducer (T) with lens (L). The focus comes closer to the transducer as the lens curvature increases, thereby shortening the near field.

transducers. The ultrasonic beam consists of two main parts: the *near zone* (or near field), which is located between the transducer and the natural focus, and the *far zone* (or far field), which is the region beyond a distance of one near-zone length (Fig 1.5). The lateral boundary of the sound field is not sharp, for the beam intensity falls off gradually with distance from the central beam axis. For improved lateral resolution (discussed later), beam diameter can be reduced by *focusing* the sound. This is accomplished by employing a curved (rather than flat) transducer element, a curved reflector, a lens, or a phased array in the probe. Focusing always occurs in the near zone. The beam diameter is decreased in the *focal region* between it and the transducer. It is widened in the region beyond. *Focal length* is the distance from the transducer to the center of the focal region. Most diagnostic imaging transducers are focused to some extent.

AXIAL AND LATERAL RESOLUTION

In discussing the quality of ultrasonic images, it is important to consider the fine details of the display. The basic issue is related to the minimum separation between two surfaces that gives rise to two identifiable signals. This determines the resolution attainable.

In ultrasound imaging there are two resolutions of importance: *axial* (or linear) and *lateral* (azimuthal). *Axial resolution* is the minimum reflector separation required along the direction of sound travel so that separate reflections will be produced. The important parameter in determining axial resolution is the ultrasonic pulse length (spatial pulse length):

$$\text{axial resolution} = \text{spatial pulse length}/2 \qquad (1.4)$$

Spatial pulse length can be decreased by increasing the frequency and/or reducing the number of cycles in each pulse. The latter is achieved by increasing the transducer *damping*. When damping is reduced to a minimum (ie, 2–3 cycles per pulse), the only way to improve axial resolution further is to increase frequency. Unfortunately, this possibility is also limited because attenuation increases concomitantly with frequency (see Table 1.3). The useful frequency range in medical imaging is 2 to 10 MHz because of this limitation. The closer the object of interest, the higher the frequency that can be utilized and, therefore, the better the axial resolution.

Lateral resolution is the minimum separation in the direction perpendicular to the direction of the ultrasonic beam. This is the minimal distance between two reflectors that will produce two separate reflections when the beam is scanned across them. Lateral resolution is directly proportional to the beam diameter (or width). It may be improved by reducing beam diameter, which is achieved by increasing the frequency; however, the primary means for reducing beam diameter is focusing.

THE VAGINAL ULTRASOUND PROBE

Optimal ultrasound imaging of the female pelvic organs is difficult to achieve. This is due to the pelvis being "crowded" with various structures of similar acoustic impedance (and which are, therefore, poor reflectors). The distance from the abdominal probe to these organs is relatively large, precluding the use of frequencies higher than 5 MHz. This limits both axial and lateral resolution. One method of improving image quality is by taking pelvic scans while the bladder is full. By introduction of a fluid-filled space, it is possible to observe more clearly some of the pelvic organs. Nevertheless, the problems discussed before are still present, so many fine details are missed. The concept of the vaginal probe solved many of these problems and made it possible to obtain high-quality images of the pelvic anatomy.

The main improvement is achieved by placing the ultrasonic probe closer to the pelvic structures. Most of the relevant anatomy for transvaginal imaging is within 9 cm of the vaginal fornices. This makes it possible to increase the transducer frequency up to 7 MHz while attenuation is still acceptable. Axial resolution is improved by 40–50% compared with the resolutions obtained with the conventional 3.5 to 5 MHz transducers used in abdominal scanning. Lateral resolution is also improved with the use of higher frequency, and stronger focusing is enabled by the proximity of the scanning head to the pelvic tissues.

IMAGE FORMATION

After an ultrasonic pulse has been emitted, the transducer serves as a "listening" device by detecting echoes from reflectors and scatterers. Echo signals picked up by the transducer are sent to a receiver where *amplification* and *signal processing* are performed. The next stage is perhaps the most important one from the operator's point of view—the display of information. There are several ways in which the information carried by the reflected echoes can be presented. The common ones are the *A-mode*, the *M-mode*, and the *B-mode*. The B-mode, or brightness mode display, is used for most clinical imaging studies and will be discussed here. In the B-mode, the echo signals are electronically converted to intensity modulated dots on the display. This causes a bright spot to be displayed each time an echo is returned to the transducer (Fig 1.6). In *gray-scale* processing the relative brightness of the dot is related to the amplitude of the reflected echo. If the reflector is nonstationary (ie, is moving back and forth) the bright spot will be seen moving back and forth on the display. An ultrasound image (B-scan) may be obtained by moving the transducer over the organs of interest. Echo signals are positioned on the display in a location that corresponds to the reflector position in the body. The

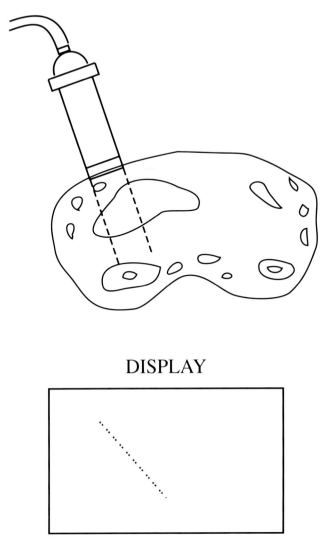

DISPLAY

Figure 1.6 Production of the B-mode image. The reflections (generated at tissue interfaces) produce bright spots on the display. As the ultrasound beam is swept over the region of interest, the starting position and the orientation of the B-mode line on the display (bottom) tracks the position and orientation of the transducer (top). By manually placing the transducer in many locations and orientations, a complete image (B-scan) of the object is built up on the display (this stage requires a memory).

location of each reflector is determined by the position and orientation of the sound beam axis and the go–return time of the ultrasonic pulse. Storing echo information is mandatory in B-mode scanning, where a static (or single frame) imaging is obtained. The memory that stores the echo information is referred to as a *scan converter* as it sends the stored image to a video display unit (eg, television monitor, multiformat camera, and video cassette recorder). In most modern instruments the memory is *digital*. In this system voltages produced by the reflected echoes (analog echo signals) are converted into a digital form by an *analog-to-digital converter*. The digital numbers thus obtained are stored in the scan converter memory, which is a *matrix* of individual addressable cells (Fig 1.7).

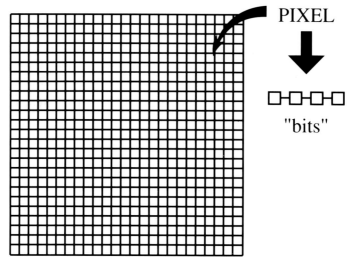

Figure 1.7 Scheme of a digital scan converter memory consisting of pixels, each of which is made up of storage units called bits.

A square matrix (eg, 512 × 512) or rectangular matrix (512 × 640) is typically used. Each cell in the matrix forms a picture element or *pixel* (Fig 1.7). Each pixel consists of basic binary storage units called *bits* (Fig 1.7). The number of bits at each pixel location determines the number of amplitude levels, or shades of gray, that can be stored in each memory location. For example, in a two-bit system (ie, binary digits) each pixel could store one of two numbers, zero or one, and represent only two conditions: on or off. This would only permit a *bistable* or black and white image. In order to display a gray-scale image, each pixel location should have a larger number of bits. The relationship between the number of bits and the number of shades that can be obtained is shown in Table 1.4. Larger numbers of shades (ie, gray-scale resolution) improve spatial resolution. The number of bits and the size of the image memory are therefore important parameters that determine image quality.

The practical approach for storing the information required for display of the two-dimensional cross-sectional image will be described for a manual scanning instrument. In these instruments a single element transducer is attached to an

TABLE 1.4 The Relationship Between the Number of Bits of the Digital Memory and the Number of Shades Obtained in an Ultrasound System

Number of Bits	Number of Shades
4	16
5	32
6	64
7	128
8	256

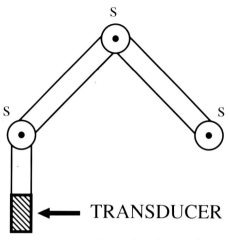

Figure 1.8 An articulated scanning arm for B-scan imaging (static scanner). Potentiometers or optical encoders (S) send information regarding transducer location and orientation to the memory or display.

articulated scanning arm (Fig 1.8). The transducer is scanned manually over the surface of the patient (eg, abdomen) so that the sound beam cuts through the tissue in cross section. Echoes reflected from all tissue interfaces on this cross section are converted to digital numbers, which are stored in the corresponding locations in the digital memory. The scan arm contains sensors that allow the transducer position and orientation to be tracked during the scan. This arrangement enables the instrument to place echo signals in their proper location in the memory (or image). As the transducer is moved through many locations and orientations, the final image of the scanned object is built up. The stored information of the cross-sectional image can then be displayed on a video display unit with the appropriate brightness (or gray-scaling) as described.

Signal processing refers to the conditioning of the echo signals by electronic or digital systems. This procedure is aimed at improving image quality. Generally there are two steps in signal processing: preprocessing and postprocessing. *Preprocessing* is the processing of echo intensities (voltages) before they are stored in the instrument's memory. It is frequently used to emphasize specific echo amplitude range. For example, it is possible to decrease the difference between the smallest and the largest amplitudes. This is accomplished by logarithmic amplifiers that amplify weak signals more than stronger signals, a process termed *compression* (Fig 1.9). As previously discussed, weak signals may arise when echoes are reflected from tissue interfaces where the acoustic impedance of the bordering tissues is similar (Table 1.2). By preprocessing, this echoes are amplified to an extent where the diagnostic information is not lost. In a similar manner other regions of the echo signal range may be emphasized. In this context the term *dynamic range* should be defined. This is the ratio of the largest power to the smallest power that the system is capable of handling properly. Different components of an instrument have different dynamic range capabilities. The input amplifier of a pulse-echo machine can handle a much greater dynamic range than the scan converter. It is generally desirable to display echo signals that extend over at

COMPRESSION

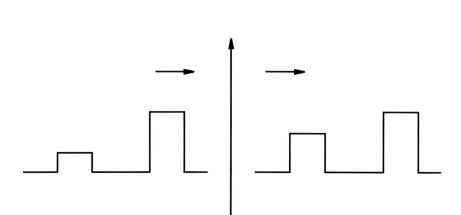

Figure 1.9 Compression decreases the difference between the smallest and the largest voltages (ie, size of echo reflections).

least 40 dB dynamic range (or a 100-fold signal amplitude range). Most display devices cannot handle such large signal level variation. Moreover, the human eye can handle an even smaller dynamic range of brightness than most scan converters are capable of storing. By applying signal compression in the preprocessing stage, the display equipment can handle a wider variation in echo signal amplitude. Following compression, a 40 dB dynamic range (100-fold difference between the largest and smallest signal) can be "squeezed" into a 20 dB dynamic range (10-fold difference). It is also desirable in many instances to remove low-level signals arising from electronic or acoustic "noise." Such noise does not carry useful information and may interfere with the observation of diagnostic information. Such noise may be eliminated to a great extent by using a *threshold suppression* (all signals below a given threshold are rejected).

Postprocessing is the conditioning of signals already stored in memory, just before they are directed to the display. Generally speaking it can be defined as the assignment of specific display brightnesses to numbers coming out of specific pixel locations in memory. In this manner the user can control the brightness of specific echo levels on the ultrasound image. This stage does not provide new data but simply allows the same echo signals to be displayed differently, either during the scanning process or after the image was obtained and "frozen" on the screen. A diagram of all stages involved in image formation is shown in Fig 1.10. Briefly, the pulser generates electric pulses that drive the transducer—T. It also transmits pulses to the receiver and memory to synchronize them each time the transducer has been excited. The transducer (acting as a source) generates ultrasound pulses for each electric pulse that has been applied to it. For each echo reflection received from a tissue interface, an electric voltage is produced by the transducer (acting as a receiving transducer). The voltages so produced are transmitted to the receiver where they are processed to a form suitable for driving the memory. Information on transducer position and orientation is transferred to the memory (dashed lines). Electric information from the memory is sent to the display (after appropriate digital conversion), which produces a visual image.

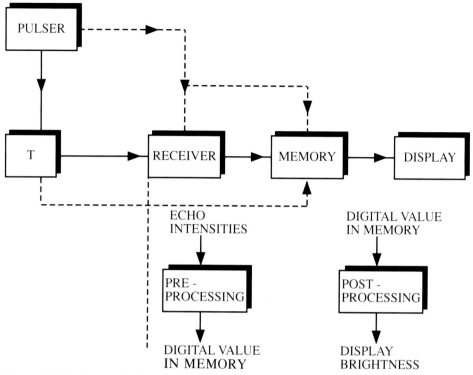

Figure 1.10 A diagram displaying the components of a pulsed-echo imaging system. Pre- and postprocessing are also illustrated. T is the transducer, which acts both as a source (generating ultrasound pulses for each electric pulse applied by the pulser) and as a receiver (for each echo reflection received from the tissues an electric voltage is produced by the transducer).

DYNAMIC IMAGING

So far we have confined our discussion to a single-element transducer. In order to obtain a two-dimensional B-scan image, the operator has to scan the transducer in various planes over the object. With such manual static scanning, it is not possible to generate images rapidly enough to produce a ''real-time'' display that continuously images moving structures. A real-time or *dynamic imaging* scanner must produce several cross-sectional images per second. This is accomplished by automatically scanned transducer assemblies. These transducers can generate up to several dozen images per second. As the transducer is moved over the body surface the display continuously changes, so that the desired image can be obtained more rapidly and more conveniently than with the static B-mode scanners. It also enables two-dimensional imaging of the motion of moving structures.

A dynamic B-mode display can be obtained by either *mechanical scanners* or *electronic scanners*. Both methods provide means for sweeping the sound beam through the tissues rapidly and repeatedly. Mechanical scanning transducer assemblies sweep the beam from a single oscillating transducer (Fig 1.11), from a rotating group of transducers (Fig 1.12), or from a stationary transducer with oscillating mirror. The rotating or oscillating components are immersed in a coupling liquid within the transducer assembly so that the sound beam is swept at a

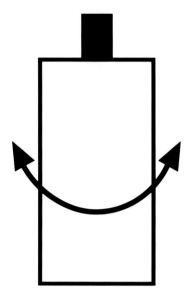

Figure 1.11 A mechanical real-time oscillating transducer.

rapid rate without moving the entire assembly. Electronic scanning is performed with *transducer arrays*. Transducer arrays are a group of piezoelectric elements, each of which can be excited individually and whose echo signals can be detected and amplified separately. The elements are rectangular in shape and arranged in a line—*linear arrays*—(Fig 1.13) or ring-shaped and arranged concentrically—*annular arrays*—(Fig 1.14). A linear array is operated by applying voltage pulses to a subgroup or cluster of elements and displaying echo signal using the B-mode display. Another cluster is then excited which contains all the elements of the previous cluster except the first, and to which a new adjacent element is added.

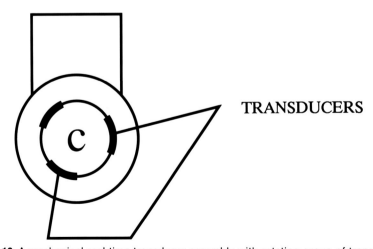

Figure 1.12 A mechanical real-time transducer assembly with rotating group of transducers.

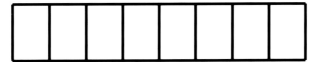

Figure 1.13 A linear array transducer consisting of rectangular elements (typically 64–256 elements are assembled).

This process is continued down the array until a complete image is formed. The cycle is then repeated from the beginning. The generated sound beam is the sum of individual beams from each of the elements. Thirty or more scans per second can be generated in this manner—rapid enough for a real-time presentation of the information. The image may also be "frozen" in a scan converter memory. The transmitted beam from an array may be focused by introducing a short delay to the excitation pulses applied to individual elements (Fig 1.15). The resulting beam appears as if a curved element or a focusing lens had been used. By selecting a different delay sequence for pulses applied to individual elements, the focal distance (ie, the distance between the surface of the transducer and the focal region) can be varied. The user can select the transmit focal distance or the instrument can automatically provide multiple transmit focal distances while scanning, optimizing the resolution throughout the depth range of the scan. Since an individual sound pulse may only be focused at a single depth, individual acoustic pulses must be transmitted for each transmit focal distance in order to provide for variable focusing. Simultaneous multiple transmit focal zones are therefore obtained at the expense of increased scanning times for a single image, with an inevitable decrease in the frame rate.

Array transducers also allow focusing of received echo signals. When an array is receiving reflections, following the transmission of a sound pulse, its electrical outputs can be timed, so that the array "listens," focused at a particular depth. As the transmitted pulse travels through the tissues (or the time duration after the pulse was transmitted increases) the receiver focus is increased automatically,

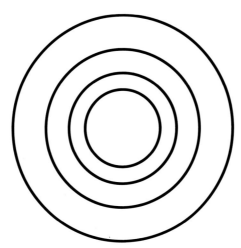

Figure 1.14 Annular array transducer with four elements.

ELECTRONIC DELAY

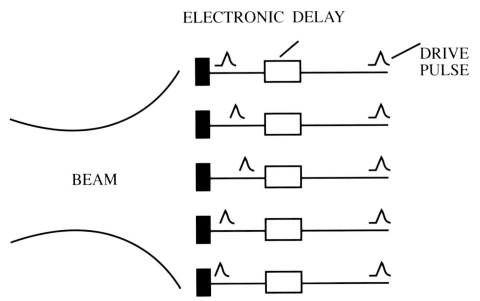

Figure 1.15 A linear phased array. By applying voltage pulses to the upper and lower elements (black rectangles) earlier than the middle elements, the beam is focused. This is achieved by introducing time delays in the excitation pulse sequence for the elements. View is from the side with the beam traveling to the left.

tracking the position of the sound pulse as it encounters deeper reflections. This process is termed *dynamic focusing* and results in an extended focal region. Electronic focusing of the transmitted beam and dynamic focusing of the received echoes are used to enhance spatial resolution throughout the image.

A *phased array* scanner is an array of transducer elements whose sound beam can be "steered" by introducing small time delays between pulses emitted by individual elements. When all elements of the array are excited simultaneously, the resulting sound beam is perpendicular to the center of the transducer assembly (Fig 1.16**A**). By introducing the delay, the array may be steered at an angle (Fig 1.16**B**,**C**). The longer the delay, the sharper the angle and vice versa. The time delays are controlled electronically and can be varied with each successive repetition of element excitation, so that the beam direction (or steering) can be changed continually. In this manner an electronic sector scanner is obtained. Electronic techniques such as dynamic focusing, which enhance image resolution as was previously described, can also be applied to phased arrays. An advantage of phased arrays over sequential linear arrays is the smaller size of transducer assembly, enabling the operator to maneuver in "difficult" anatomical regions. While a linear phased array can focus or steer only in the scan plane, *annular phased arrays* can focus in various planes but cannot provide beam steering. By integrating an oscillating mirror to these arrays it is also possible to steer the beam.

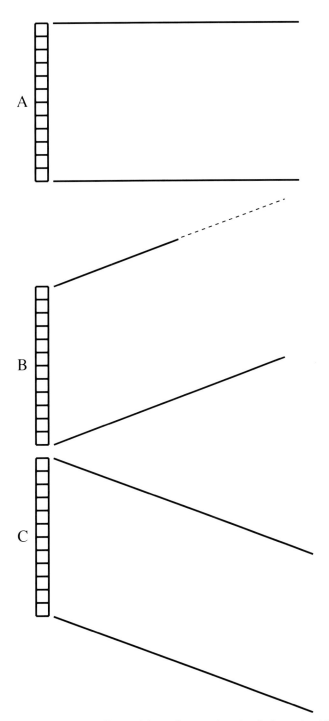

Figure 1.16 A linear phased array. By applying voltage pulses to all elements at the same time, an unfocused, nonsteered beam is produced (**A**). By applying voltage pulses to the lower elements earlier than to the upper elements, the beam can be steered up (**B**). With the opposite excitation sequence the beam is steered down (**C**).

REAL-TIME DISPLAYS

In all instruments employing a real-time transducer of any kind, each complete scan of the sound beam produces an image on the screen that is called a *frame*. Each frame is made of scan lines—one for each time the transducer is pulsed. The number of lines per frame is directly proportional then, to the *pulse repetition frequency*. This relationship is given in the following equation:

$$PRF = LPF \times FR \tag{1.5}$$

Where PRF = pulse repetition frequency
LPF = lines per frame
FR = frame rate

The highest speed with which a real-time instrument can form an image is limited by the travel time of sound pulses in tissue. After the transducer emits an acoustic pulse, it must wait to detect all the reflected echoes along the scan line. The time delay required between pulses depends on the speed of sound in tissue and the maximum visualization depth. If the maximum visualization depth in Fig 1.17 is d, the delay time t_d required to acquire all echoes from a single line is given by:

$$t_d = 2d/c \tag{1.6}$$

where c is the speed of sound in tissue.
   The minimum time required to complete an image consisting of N scan lines is:

$$T_{\min} = Nt_d = 2Nd/c \tag{1.7}$$

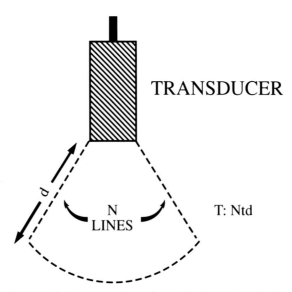

Figure 1.17 Scanning speed and frame rate are limited by the pulse-echo travel time required to obtain an echo from a distance, *d*. *T* is the time required for a single complete scan and *t* is the time required for a single line. *N* is the number of acoustic lines making up a scan. If *c* is the speed of sound in tissue, the equation *T* = 2*Nd*/*c* may also be employed.

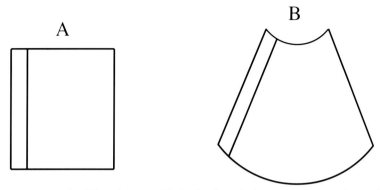

Figure 1.18 Rectangular (**A**) and sector (**B**) display formats in a dynamic-imaging system.

The maximum frame rate (R) possible in a given situation is given by:

$$R = 1/T_{min} \text{ (frames per second)} \tag{1.8}$$

The size of the field of view may therefore limit the scanning speed of the instrument. When increasing the field of view, the instrument has to decrease either the line density (this creates larger gaps between scan lines which decreases image quality) or the frame rate. In contrast, reduced fields of view allow substantially higher frame rates to be employed.

The scanning method dictates the display format for a given instrument. Linear array transducers produce a rectangular display (Fig 1.18**A**). Mechanical sector scanners (rotating or oscillating) and electronic phased arrays produce a sector display format (Fig 1.18**B**). The *line density* is the ratio of the number of lines per frame to the width (in centimeters) of the display for rectangular displays, and for sector scan format it is the ratio of the number of lines per frame to the total sector angle.

DOPPLER ULTRASONOGRAPHY

Basic Principles and Terms

When an emitted ultrasonic pulse is echoed back to its source from a reflecting surface which is moving relative to the transmitted pulse, the frequency of the echo is different from that of the transmitted pulse. The magnitude of the change in frequency is directly proportional to the velocity of the moving surface, and is also known as the *Doppler shift*. In blood flow studies, the Doppler equation allows calculation of the velocity of red blood cells (which are termed scatterers)—v—when the other variables are known:

$$Fd = v(2f \cos \theta)/c \tag{1.9}$$

where Fd represents the frequency (or Doppler) shift, f represents the frequency of the emitted pulses (ie, the frequency of the transducer), θ represents the angle between the direction of the incident sound wave and the direction of the scatterers, and c is the speed of sound in tissue (1540 m/s) (Fig 1.19). The Doppler shift is

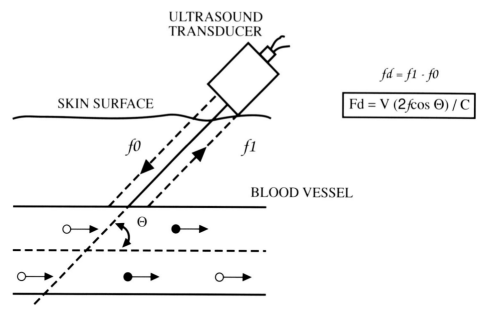

ULTRASOUND
TRANSDUCER

$fd = f1 - f0$

$Fd = V (2 f \cos \Theta) / C$

SKIN SURFACE

$f0$ $f1$

BLOOD VESSEL

Θ

Figure 1.19 The Doppler effect when reflectors (ie, blood corpuscles) are moving at an angle θ with respect to the ultrasound beam. The equation for the Doppler shift is also shown.

calculated by a spectrum analyzer using the fast Fourier transform (FFT) technique. This instrument, which is used on most duplex systems, is capable of determining the relative powers of the various frequency components that are present in a signal at a given time. Short periods of the signal (1–10 msec) are digitized and analyzed mathematically for their frequency components. The spectrum is then displayed as a *sonogram*, in which a single spectrum is depicted as a vertical line, on whose axis lies frequency brightness, modulated at each point to represent amplitude. Subsequent spectra are displayed as vertical lines at a fixed distance apart, creating an image that scrolls from left to right with time. The three variables—time, frequency, and amplitude—are thus shown in real time. Since velocity is directly proportional to frequency, the sonogram is also commonly termed *time-velocity profile* and in case of pulsatile flow—it demonstrates the time velocity waveforms. As the display is two-dimensional, the amplitude of the signal at any given time is represented as a gray-scale (or color code) display and reflects the number of red cells traveling at a given velocity at any particular time. It is a fortunate coincidence that the Doppler shift frequencies in most medical applications happen to lie in the audible range, so the operator can hear the signals as the sonogram is displayed on the video display unit. In this way, audible and visual recognition can greatly assist the operator to obtain optimal signals for analysis. A diagram showing the principles of a pulsed Doppler instrument is shown in Fig 1.20.

The main types of Doppler devices that are commonly used for clinical measurements are the *continuous wave* and the *pulsed wave* systems. The former consists of a simple transducer that continuously sends ultrasonic sound waves and is attached to a second transducer that continuously receives the reflected echoes returning from the sound's beam path. The main advantages of this system are its ease of operation, portability, low output sound intensity (less than 25 mW/

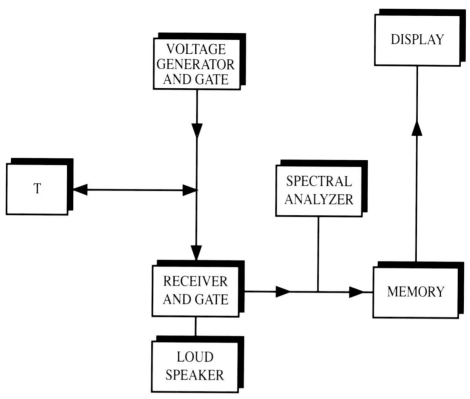

Figure 1.20 A diagram of an image-directed pulsed Doppler instrument. T is the transducer which is used both for imaging and for Doppler. The Doppler receiver gate depth can be located visually inside the vessel under study. The loudspeaker produces audible Doppler shift signals. The spectral analyzer generates the sonogram (ie, flow velocity waveforms) which are displayed on the screen with the two dimensional image.

cm^2), and relatively low price. In addition, it permits very high frequency shifts (ie, high blood flow velocities) to be measured, even in deep vessels lying far from the transducer. However, it does not permit visualization of the sound beam as it crosses the tissues, or of the blood vessels themselves. Moreover, it is not range-specific and the rather large volume of overlap between the two probes' crystals may contribute to the Doppler shift that is displayed after spectrum analysis. In fact, any vessel that happens to lie across the sound's beam path will be sampled and "contaminate" the sonogram obtained. These limitations preclude the use of a continuous-wave Doppler in many applications, and for these reasons it is also unsuitable for blood flow measurements in reproductive studies, as will be described later.

In pulsed Doppler systems, the transducer sends short pulses of high frequency sound waves repetitively. The same transducer is used to receive the reflected echoes in the intervals between sending the pulses. In such pulse-echo systems the range (or depth) of the target can be estimated from the corresponding time delay in the reception of echoes following the transmission of the ultrasonic pulse, assuming a constant value for the speed of ultrasound (1540 cm/sec). This *range-gated* detection permits the selection of Doppler frequency shift signals from moving targets according to their distance from the ultrasonic probe. This principle is implemented in *duplex scanning*, where a pulsed wave Doppler transducer is integrated into a two-dimensional ultrasound imaging unit to permit accurate identification of the volume in space from which Doppler shifted frequencies are to be received. This volume is commonly termed the *sample volume*, and both its width and distance from the transducer can be controlled by the user (Fig 1.21). This orientation in space and the depth selectivity make the pulsed duplex systems so much superior to the continuous-wave Doppler systems. Practically, the duplex systems are categorized according to whether they employ mechanical or electronic systems for real-time imaging. In order to sample Doppler signals, the Doppler beam should be virtually stationary in the desired direction for a sufficiently long time during each acquisition period, to allow adequate sampling of the moving targets (ie, red blood cells). In most mechanical systems, the imaging transducer is also used for Doppler studies. The duplex transducer probe arrangement is such that it can be servo-controlled to the desired stationary position for Doppler measurements. This arrangement provides for a line representing the desired eventual servo-controlled direction of the ultrasonic Doppler beam to be superimposed on the real-time image to allow appropriate orientation and positioning of the sample volume. Once this is obtained, the operator switches to the Doppler mode (using a foot or handheld switch) and the stationary image is continually displayed while the Doppler signals are collected. The system can be reverted to the imaging mode (interrupting the Doppler signal acquisition) by activating the switch again, so the user can check the position of the sample volume. This problem of switching between Doppler and imaging modes can be avoided by using separate transducers for imaging and for Doppler operation. In

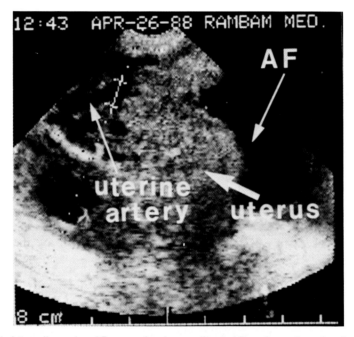

Figure 1.21 A two-dimensional B-scan of an image-directed Doppler system showing a segment of the uterine artery. The sample volume is placed over the vessel and the angle of insonation is determined by aligning the visible unbroken line parallel to the long axis of the vessel. The dotted line represents the line of insonation of the Doppler beam.

electronic duplex systems, typically employing phased array transducers, the Doppler beam can be formed electronically at any desired angle. Pulsed Doppler operation can then be interpolated among the imaging pulses, allowing simultaneous duplex scanning. One significant limitation when using pulsed Doppler systems is the maximum range limitation or the *range–velocity limitation*. Analog signals (such as Doppler shift signals) can only be unambiguously represented by samples if they are sampled at a rate that exceeds twice the highest frequency in the signal itself (also known as the Nyquist limit). This means that when high flow velocities are encountered, the pulse repetition frequency has to be increased sufficiently to accommodate for this limitation. If the vessel is situated far from the transducer (eg, when performing Doppler studies on deep pelvic vessels using an abdominal probe), the potential increase in pulse repetition frequency is limited by the pulse–echo round-trip delay time. Under such conditions false signals are displayed, a phenomenon termed *aliasing*. One way to partially overcome this problem is to use a lower frequency transducer when operating in the Doppler mode on duplex systems. The Doppler shift frequency would then be lower for any given velocity of the target and the range-velocity ambiguity problem would be less likely to arise. More extensive reviews on the physical principles of pulsed Doppler duplex systems are given in the reference section.

Interpretation of the Doppler Spectrum

The information that is provided by the pelvic duplex examination can be analyzed in three different ways.

Qualitative Methods

The characteristics of waveform shape and spectral distribution reflect the hemodynamic factors in a particular vessel. Thus, with some experience, the operator can identify the origin of flow as coming from the uterine artery, from spectral display and the aural quality of the sound.

Semiquantitative Methods

The pulsatility of an arterial waveform can be influenced by the impedance of the distal vascular bed. This is of great significance for the clinical application of Doppler ultrasound: it means that vessels that control organ and tissue perfusion, but are too small to be interrogated directly with Doppler ultrasound, are capable of influencing flow characteristics upstream. Organ systems that are supplied by major vessels that can be examined using Doppler scanning methods (but whose downstream vasculature is inaccessible to direct scanning) are the uterus and ovaries. Another typical example is the umbilical artery supplying the fetal placental circulation.

Numerous indices have been proposed to describe such waveforms. Each of these indices is a ratio of Doppler shift frequencies and so independent of Doppler angle. Because of this independency, pulsatility can be assessed in vessels that are too small or too tortuous to be imaged (eg, the intraovarian arterioles). The most common indices in use are (Fig 1.22):

$$\text{Pulsatility Index } (PI){:} = (A - B)/\text{mean} \qquad (1.10)$$

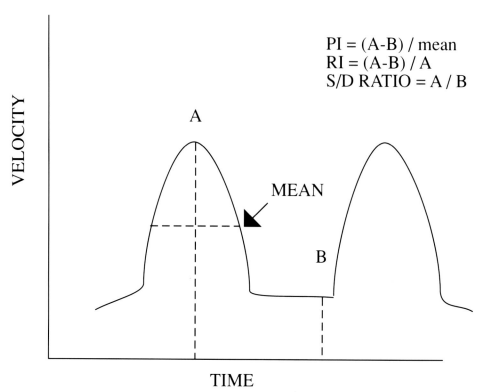

Figure 1.22 Doppler indices calculated from the maximum frequency shift envelope.

where *A* is the maximal Doppler shift frequency (*Fd*) in the cardiac cycle, *B* is the minimum *Fd*, and the "mean" is the time average of the maximum *Fd* over the cardiac cycle. This index has the advantage of remaining determinable even when the least *Fd* takes on a negative value (reverse flow) and it is relatively insensitive to changes in heart rate. However, it requires a computer program capable of doing an on-line area-under-the-curve calculation.

$$\text{Resistance Index } (RI){:} = (A - B)/A \qquad (1.11)$$

$$\text{S/D Ratio: } = A/B \qquad (1.12)$$

For any measurement reflecting the shape of the Doppler waveform, the index should be calculated for each of several cardiac cycles and the average value taken.

Quantitative Methods

1. *Velocity of Blood Flow.* When the angle between the Doppler beam and the long axis of the scanned vessel is known, the Doppler frequency shift can be converted into an actual velocity using the Doppler equation as previously described. The maximal Doppler shift at any given time in the sonogram represents the maximum velocity and can be automatically calculated and presented by most duplex machines. The mean Doppler shift (or mean velocity) can also be calculated from the three-dimensional data in the sonogram (ie, based on the amplitude

or intensity of the signal at any given moment). In estimating velocity the magnitude of potential errors induced by an uncertainty in the angle measurement should be born in mind. These errors increase rapidly with increasing angle. For example, at 45°, a 5° uncertainty in angle measurement would result in a 9% error in velocity. At 70°, the same level of uncertainty would result in a 25% error. At angles less than 20° these errors are insignificant. Generally, if substantial errors are to be avoided, the angle should not exceed 55°.

2. *Volume Flow Measurements.* By multiplying the mean flow velocity by the cross-sectional area of the vessel, the instantaneous flow rate is obtained. This product is then integrated over the cardiac cycle to yield the time-average flow rate. For arterial flow, both the cross-sectional area and the velocity change with time, so that ideally one would form the product of the instantaneous mean velocity and the cross-sectional area at the same time. In practice, such simultaneous measurement of velocity and diameter is not attainable, and most workers take the average of several diameter measurements on a real-time scan and multiply it by the time-averaged mean velocity.

Doppler Color Flow Mapping

The main application of duplex scanning is in the detailed study of well-defined anatomical regions. Such systems do not readily convey information about blood flow throughout the entire scan plane. Doppler color flow mappings are particularly helpful as they produce real-time two-dimensional images, color coded according to flow conditions, superimposed on real-time two-dimensional gray-scale pulse–echo images of anatomical structures. This facilitates evaluation of vessels within organs or those that are not readily delineated by conventional scanning. Color Doppler sonography is based on *Doppler autocorrelation flow detector*, which rapidly extracts Doppler signals line by line as the ultrasonic beam is scanned through the image plane. The resulting display image is a combination of Doppler and anatomical information. The output from the autocorrelation detector consists of directional real-time velocity (or Doppler frequency) signals. These are arranged to color code the real-time gray-scale image. Forward flow is usually presented in red color and reverse flow in blue color. The degree of turbulence is color coded in green. Best results are obtained by using electronically scanned linear or phased array.

THE TRANSVAGINAL IMAGE-DIRECTED DOPPLER SYSTEM

An image-directed Doppler system, or duplex system, is one that enables two-dimensional real-time scanning to guide the appropriate placement of an ultrasonic Doppler beam. In this way, the blood vessel from which the Doppler signals originate can be identified. The first part of the duplex scanning always begins with a real-time imaging so that the operator can get an anatomical image and identify the sites for Doppler studies. When applying the endovaginal ultrasonic probe, the full advantage of this imaging modality can be exploited. The physical principles upon which image formation is based were discussed before.

The transvaginal duplex system is benefited by the unique properties inherent in this system as previously described. The close proximity of the probe to the vessels of interest and the high resolution transducer makes it possible to identify and measure small vessels (10–15 mm). With this approach Doppler flow measurements of some pelvic vessels can be obtained at a smaller angle of insonation, thereby increasing the accuracy of the measurement (for optimal flow measurements the angle of insonation should not exceed 60°). With the probe situated close to the vessel, the limitation of the range velocity is largely overcome. This also makes it possible to use a higher frequency Doppler transducer and obtain a higher frequency shift at any given angle of insonation, thereby increasing the accuracy of measurement. The examination is performed with an empty bladder, which prevents distortion of the normal anatomy and vessel displacement. With the advent of color flow mapping it is possible to study the arrangement and flow patterns of complex vascular beds in the pelvis. All these properties turn the transvaginal duplex system into a versatile, accurate flow probe for measuring blood flow characteristics in the female pelvis.

SUMMARY

The properties of ultrasound in tissues and the factors governing image quality were discussed. Particular emphasis was placed on the vaginal probe, which forms the basis for a "new generation" of pelvic imaging and is the main theme of this book. Only by fully understanding the properties of ultrasound can the capabilities and limitations of this technique be appreciated. A good knowledge of the basic physical principles is mandatory for the clinician as well as the investigator in attaining the highest-quality results. Less emphasis was placed on the various technical aspects of operating ultrasound instruments, eg, machine controls, electronic image formation, scan converters, and techniques for preprocessing and postprocessing.

REFERENCES

Basic Principles of Ultrasound Imaging

1. Wells PNT: Biomedical Ultrasonics. New York, Academic Press, 1977.
2. McDicken WN: Diagnostic Ultrasonics: Principles and use of instruments. New York, John Wiley & Sons, 1981.
3. Nyborg WL: Biophysical Mechanisms of Ultrasound, in Repacholi MH, Benwell DA (eds): Essentials of Medical Ultrasound. Clifton, NJ, Humana Press, 1982.
4. Zagzebski J: Physics of Diagnostic Ultrasound, in Ansert SH (ed): Textbook of Ultrasonography, St. Louis, CV Mosby, 1983.
5. Zweibel WJ: Review of basic terms used in diagnostic ultrasound. Semin Ultrasound 1983;4:60.
6. Kremkau WF: Diagnostic Ultrasound: Principles, Instrumentation and Exercises. Orlando, Fla, Grune & Stratton, Inc., 1984.
7. Powis RL, Powis WJ: A Thinker's Guide to Ultrasonic Imaging. Baltimore, Urban & Schwarzenberg, 1984.
8. Maslak S: Computed Sonography, in Sanders R, Hil M (eds): Ultrasound Annual 1985. New York, Raven Press, 1985.
9. Hunter TB, Haber K: A comparison of real-time scanning with conventional static B-mode scanning. J Ultrasound Med 1983;2:363.
10. Carson PL, Fischella PR, Oughton TV: Ultrasonic power and intensities produced by diagnostic ultrasound equipment. Ultrasound Med Biol 1978;3:341.
11. Zagzebski J, Banjavic R, Madsen E, et al: Focused transducer beams in tissue-mimicking material. J Clin Ultrasound 1982;10:159.
12. Kossoff G: Analysis of focusing action of spherical curved transducers. Ultrasound Med Biol 1979;5:359.

13. Kossoff G, Garrett W, Carpenter D, et al: Principles and classification of soft tissues by grey scale echography. Ultrasound Med Biol 1976;2:89.
14. Gray J, Lisk K, Haddick D, et al: Test pattern for video displays and hard-copy cameras. Radiology 1985;154:519.
15. Thaler I, Manor D: Transvaginal imaging: applied physical principles and terms. J Clin Ultrasound 1990;18:235.
16. Schaaps JP, Soyeur D: Pulsed Doppler on a vaginal probe: necessity, convenience, or luxury? J Ultrasound Med 1989;8:315.

Doppler Physics and Methodology

1. Atkinson P, Woodcock JP: Doppler Ultrasound and Its Use in Clinical Measurement. London, Academic Press, 1982.
2. Wells PNT: Ultrasonic Doppler Equipment, in Fullerton GD, Zagzebski JA (eds): Medical Physics of CT and Ultrasound. New York, American Institute of Physics, 1980, pp 343–366.
3. Noordergraaf A: Circulatory System Dynamics. New York, Academic Press, 1978.
4. McDonald DA: Blood Flow in Arteries. London, Edward Arnold, 1974.
5. Eik-Nes SH, Marsal K, Kristoffersen K: Methodology and basic problems related to blood flow studies in the human fetus. Ultrasound Med Biol 1984;10:329.
6. Evans DH, Barrie WW, Asher MJ, et al: The relationship between ultrasonic pulsatility index and proximal arterial stenosis in canine model. Circ Res 1980;46:470.
7. Gill RW: Pulsed Doppler with B-mode imaging for quantitative blood flow measurement. Ultrasound Med Biol 1979;5:223.
8. Gill RW: Measurement of blood flow by ultrasound: Accuracy and sources of error. Ultrasound Med Biol 1985;4:625.
9. Namekawa K, Kasai C, Omoto R: Real-time two-dimensional blood flow imaging using ultrasound Doppler. J Ultrasound Med 1983;2:10.
10. Uematsu S: Determination of volume of arterial blood flow by an ultrasonic device. J Clin Ultrasound 1981;9:209.
11. Shung KK: Physics of blood echogenicity. J Cardiovasc Ultrasonogr 1983;2:401.
12. Wells PNT: Basic Principles and Doppler Physics, in Taylor KJW, Burns PN, Wells PNT (eds): Clinical Applications of Doppler Ultrasound. New York, Raven Press, 1988, pp 1–25.
13. Burns PN: Interpretation and Analysis of Doppler Signals, in Taylor KJW, Burns PN, Wells PNT (eds): Clinical Applications of Doppler Ultrasound. New York, Raven Press, 1988, pp 76–119.
14. Wells PNT: Instrumentation Including Color Flow Mapping, in Taylor KJW, Burns PN, Wells PNT (eds): Clinical Applications of Doppler Ultrasound. New York, Raven Press, 1988, pp 26–45.
15. Grant EG, Tessler FN, Perrella RR: Clinical Doppler imaging. AJR 1989;152:707.
16. Lewis BD, James EM, Charboneau JW, et al: Current applications of color Doppler imaging in the abdomen and extremities. Radiographics 1989;9:599.
17. Kurjak A, Jurkovitc D, Akfirevic Z, et al: Transvaginal color Doppler imaging. J Clin Ultrasound 1990;18:227.
18. Thaler I, Manor D, Brandes JM, et al: Basic principles and clinical applications of the transvaginal Doppler duplex system in reproductive medicine. J In Vitro Fertil Embryo Transfer 1990;7:74–85.

CHAPTER **2**

Transvaginal Sonography:
Equipment

David B. Peisner, MD

INTRODUCTION

The number of transvaginal ultrasound probes and machines has increased dramatically recently. A welcome side effect to this has been the development of new features for many of these machines. While the basic concepts of ultrasonography obviously do not change for the vaginal approach, there are a number of considerations, both practical and scientific, that affect the equipment for this diagnostic medium. The purpose of this chapter is to discuss equipment considerations and describe them for many machines. At the end of the chapter is a chart of features and specifications from many ultrasound machine manufacturers. This chart, similar to many domestic magazines, provides an efficient way for the potential buyer of these machines to compare the various models.

PHYSICAL CONSIDERATIONS

Physical considerations are important for a number of reasons. First, transvaginal sonography is often used for procedures or at the bedside. Therefore, the *dimensions* and *weight* of the machine may be a factor in choosing a machine. A smaller machine is obviously easier to manipulate in an operating room. In fact, the dimensions of some of the machines may be too large to fit through some doors. In that case, the machine may be inconvenient to use in some situations. While even the heaviest machines can be moved, some weigh several hundred pounds and this is a potential problem for a machine that might be moved frequently. Finally, a machine that is inconvenient to move may be more prone to damage.

Concerning the cables, their length and storage is an often overlooked consideration. The length of the power cord determines how mobile the machine can be and the length of the probe cables can be a limiting factor in a procedure. Some machines have a place to store cords and cables and some do not. For a machine with many probes, a camera, and a video recorder, the number of loose cables may become unwieldy.

Other characteristics such as *electrical power* become important for practical reasons. For example, voltage requirements are usually not a major problem since manufacturers are aware of differing specifications in various countries. However, the amount of power that a machine requires (measured in watts) may be important. In a room with many machines, one of the larger machines may overload the electrical system and cause a power outage. Careful planning prior to purchasing a machine can avoid this problem.

Along the same lines, the *environmental requirements* of the machine may be a consideration when a model is selected. While most machines operate in a variety of temperature and humidity conditions, some may not and this can be an important factor, especially in tropical areas. Since all electronic machines generate heat, the elimination of heat should be considered. A large machine may produce a significant amount of heat, which may raise the temperature of the examination room. Furthermore, some machines have fans and some do not. Those that do may produce more noise and in addition, may have filters that require frequent cleaning. Although filters may be inconvenient to use, they may prolong the life of the machine.

Other factors concern the *space on the cart/machine* for storing equipment and supplies. Some machines have space for gel bottles. Many clinics like to use a gel warmer and the ability to put it someplace on the machine may be a consideration. Most machines have a place for a camera and/or video recorder. However, additional space (shelves or other compartments) can be very useful for storing supplies, charts, probes, etc.

Physical considerations may affect the daily operation of the machine. For example, some machines have many *receptacles for probes* which usually allows them to be selected from the console. Those machines with a single receptacle force the user to plug and unplug the probes for their selection. Since some machines may be damaged if this is done with power turned on, this is potentially risky for machine longevity. The location of the probe receptacles is also a consideration. It can be very difficult to insert a big plug if the receptacle is near the floor at the rear of the machine. Therefore, a machine with probe selection controlled from a switch or keyboard is preferable.

Other connectors on the machine may be considered. A clinic often will have both a recorder and another camera or instant printer connected to the ultrasound machine. Some may wish to have an auxiliary monitor connected to allow the patient (or others) to observe the examination. All of these require connections to the machine which are not necessarily present on some scanners. In addition, some machines may provide connectors for other signals such as Doppler, ECG, and/or remote control of the auxiliary equipment.

The *location and size of the monitor* is a simple but important factor. While virtually all modern machines produce good ultrasound pictures, a picture on a small screen may be difficult to see if the operator is far away from the machine. Furthermore, some monitors are fixed in their cabinets and do not swivel. This can be a factor if the operator is moving around the patient.

TRANSDUCERS

The number and type of transducers vary widely among manufacturers. While the topic of this book is transvaginal sonography, the table of manufacturers at the end of this chapter includes all probes for completeness. Nevertheless, some characteristics will not apply to transvaginal probes. For example, linear transducers exist for abdominal sonography but not for transvaginal sonography where all probes produce sector images. The different types of sector probes are mechanical, phased array, and curvilinear.

The *mechanical sector transducer* consists of a rotating or oscillating crystal(s) in an oil bath. This method is the simplest way of scanning and allows the widest field of view. The field of view is dependent on the direction the crystal is pointing but is limited only by the mechanical characteristics of the transducer motor and the shape of the handle. In some machines, fields of view approaching 240° are possible. The field of view is one of the most important for the transvaginal probe. An exam may be severely limited if the field of view is less than 90°!

One disadvantage of the mechanical sector probe is inherent noise in the near field. For transvaginal sonography, this may seem to be a problem since pelvic structures may often lie within 1 cm of the transducer. However, the problem can be solved by slightly withdrawing the probe from the vagina to move the structure away from the near field. Another disadvantage of a mechanical transducer is the fact that it must be bathed in oil, and air bubbles will severely distort the image. Often the operator can refill the transducer through a valve on the probe but some manufacturers insist that their service technicians fill it and this can add to maintenance costs.

A *phased array sector transducer* consists of a fixed array of crystals that are sequentially triggered to aim the ultrasound beam in a sector. This methodology requires no moving parts, but electronically is more difficult to process. Therefore, these machines may be more expensive. Since there are no mechanical parts, these transducers are often smaller than their mechanical counterparts.

The *curvilinear sector transducer* consists of an array of crystals that are arranged along a tightly curved end of the probe. Since the beam from each crystal exits perpendicularly from the transducer surface, the curvature of the probe end yields a sector image from this array. Electronically, this arrangement is simpler than the phased array but has a similar image. However, the field of view of a curvilinear probe is fixed while a phased array may be variable. Both the curvilinear and phased array options have excellent near field noise characteristics.

When a probe is considered, the physical dimensions may be important. One of the most significant is the shape of the handle. Some transvaginal transducers have bent ("broken") handles (see the pictures at the end of this chapter) and some have straight handles. The probes with bent handles may be easier to manipulate if the patient is not on a gynecologic table. However, a transverse view of the lateral portions of the adnexa is difficult to examine with this type of probe unless the probe is rotated 180° for opposite sides of the pelvis. In addition, the operator must invert the image on the screen to maintain proper orientation when the probe is rotated. Those with straight handles are easier to aim and do not have to be rotated when the adnexa are examined. Finally, weight and dimensions of the transducer may make a difference for some operators. Mechanical probes are generally somewhat heavier and larger than the nonmechanical ones.

The number of *probe specifications* is considerable. For example, the *frequency* of transvaginal sonography is generally higher than transabdominal sonography. However, this may vary from 5 MHz to 7.5 MHz for various probes. Some probes may be capable of scanning at multiple frequencies, sometimes simultaneously in the same picture. This feature is a major advantage because there is no need to exchange the probe during an examination if the operator wants to improve the image by changing the frequency. As the frequency increases, the resolution of the image will increase but the depth of penetration will decrease (see Chapter 1).

Another consideration is the *focal zone* of the probe(s). Mechanical probes generally have fixed focal zones in the vicinity of 5 cm from the end of the probe. Nonmechanical transducers may also have fixed focal zones or may have multiple zones. Like the frequency specifications, some probes may be capable of multiple focal zones simultaneously in the same picture.

The *field of view* was previously mentioned and there are two characteristics that are important. First is the absolute width of the field, which is usually measured in degrees of a circle. Since there are 360° in a circle, a field of view of 120° is exactly one third of a circle (Fig 2.1). A probe with a larger field of view will be able to visualize more of a large organ such as a uterus with myomas. Some probes also have steerable fields of view. For example, a probe may have a field of view of 120°. If this is symmetric with respect to the end of the probe, the field of view will be 60° on either side of the imaginary line extending from the end of the transducer. However, for ovaries that are located laterally in the pelvis, examination may be difficult. For this reason, some probes can steer their field of view to one side of the midline. For the probe previously mentioned, the entire 120° field of view may be steered to one side of the midline or, in some cases, even farther. Finally, one recent development is the ability to scan in a plane perpendicular to the original scan plane, sometimes simultaneously with the primary array of crystals. In addition to steering the field of view, some transducers can also steer the scanning plane.

The *power output* of each probe may vary for each manufacturer and still be within the guidelines of AIUM standards. One exception where power outputs may be increased is Doppler flow applications. In this case, the operator should determine whether the power output of the probe is within the clinical guidelines for a particular application. More and more machines offer a switch for power selection.

Some probes may have machine controls mounted in the probe body. These may allow the operator to freeze the picture and/or do other operations. Most probes have biopsy or needle guides that attach to allow ultrasound-guided puncture procedures in the pelvis. These include follicle retrievals, drainage of cysts, and terminations of some pregnancies. If procedures are done with the probe, specially designed probe covers are available for some machines and not others. These are specified in the table at the end of the chapter. If a probe cover is not available, the author has had extensive experience with a surgical glove over the end of a variety of transvaginal transducers. This technique usually works quite well and is inexpensive.

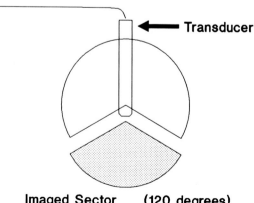

Figure 2.1 An imaged field of 120° corresponds to exactly one third of a circle.

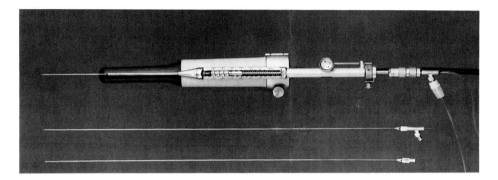

Figure 2.2 The Labotect puncture device.

For some puncture procedures, an interesting device is made by Labotect, GmbH (Fig 2.2), which is a *spring-loaded biopsy guide* that may be adapted to many transvaginal probes. This device literally "fires" a needle very rapidly to a preset depth along a needle path that is defined on the screen by software. While the principle of introducing a needle into a pelvic structure is not different than a free-hand approach, the rapidity of needle introduction by this device avoids much of the organ movement that may make the free-hand technique inaccurate. It also alleviates the need for analgesia.

For other procedures some companies now manufacture a *rotating transducer that fits in a narrow catheter*. An example of this is shown in Fig 2.3. While this is primarily used in blood vessels or the urethra/ureter, a catheter such as this may have some use to visualize endometrial lesions in the future.

There are a number of characteristics of the transducers that affect the *image* on the monitor. These comments will be directed toward transvaginal probes, but obviously apply to all probes. First, the power output of each probe will affect the image. As it is discussed in Chapter 1, increased power allows the ultrasound beam to penetrate deeper into tissue while increased frequency allows the beam to

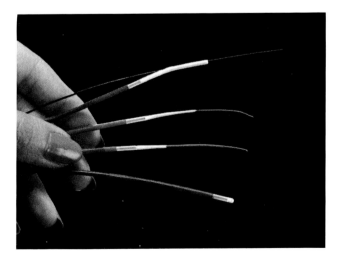

Figure 2.3 Picture of several catheter-type ultrasound transducers which can be inserted into blood vessels, ureter, etc.

penetrate less, but with a sharper image. While all machines transmit beams within AIUM guidelines, some machines may penetrate deeper than others with similar power and frequency specifications for their transvaginal probes.

As probes are being evaluated, the amount of power each produces may be a consideration as well as the claimed depth of penetration. The penetration depends not only on the power that the transducer produces but also the geometry of the crystals and the receiving electronics.

Another important factor is *resolution*. Since all transvaginal images are sectors, resolution is highly dependent on the depth of the image. Deeper structures are not as clear as more superficial structures. This depends on the number of crystals in the probe and also on the electronics, which may be able to electronically sharpen the image. Resolution may also increase with different focusing techniques. As resolution is being evaluated, note that horizontal and vertical resolution are specified separately because they depend on different factors in the probes. (See Chapter 1 for more information on this phenomenon.)

The appearance of the image may depend on *postprocessing*. This electronic technique allows the machine to manipulate the stored image electronically. The contrast spectrum is usually the primary application but edge enhancement, image enlargement, and other forms of image analysis are possible. Postprocessing may be more dependent on the machine than on the individual probes. However, a potential buyer of machines should investigate these specifications prior to the purchase of a machine.

Another factor is *contrast resolution*. This is a measure of how well the probe and machine can differentiate structures of similar echogenicity. If the contrast resolution is very high, then structures of similar echogenicity will be separate images on the screen. If contrast resolution is low, these images will appear to be a single item on the screen. While this is not a specification that is often quoted by manufacturers, an estimate can be obtained by looking at the number of gray levels that are displayed on the screen. If this number is high (128 or 256), then contrast resolution should be quite good. If this number is low (32 or 64), then the contrast resolution will be low and it may be difficult to distinguish a placenta from the uterine wall.

During the examination, the *frame rate* or number of images displayed per second on the monitor may be a factor. Most machines display an image 20 to 30 times per second, which is adequate. However, this may be different for various probes. If various zoom features and multiple focal zones are utilized, the frame rate may decrease dramatically. Consequently, a fetal heart that may be beating 150 times per minute or $2\frac{1}{2}$ times per second may be difficult to visualize with a frame rate of 5 per second.

Current *modalities* for ultrasound machines include B-mode (gray-scale image), M-mode (motion), Doppler (flow studies at a single point), and color Doppler (flow studies in an area of the image). While a full explanation of these modalities can be found elsewhere, color Doppler deserves one comment. Since the amount of processing required for this technique is immense, the frame rate of the image is usually much slower than gray-scale images. If the area of color display is large, the frame rate may be as slow as 2 frames per second. One consideration when evaluating a machine is whether or not a Doppler or M-mode image can be displayed simultaneously with a gray-scale image. When small structures are visualized, the author strongly recommends this simultaneous mode.

OPERATIONAL CONSIDERATIONS

The operation of the machine is often called the *user interface*. This consists of both the data input (transducers, keyboard, joystick, or trackball, and their physical characteristics) and the data processing (software for manipulating images and characters). This is an area that has a considerable amount of variability from machine to machine. However, due to operator preference, one type of interface may be wonderful for one physician and unacceptable for another. Therefore, these characteristics should be evaluated carefully, for they can affect the throughput of the clinic.

Most machines have *controls* only on the console. However, some have detachable control panels and/or keyboards. Some have auxiliary keyboards and a few have true remote controls to allow the machine to be some distance from the operator. This can be advantageous if one is doing a transvaginal examination on an obese patient. A handheld control may be much easier to manipulate in this situation. Some machines may even be operated primarily from a mouse, which may be quite convenient. Finally, some machines have limited remote control ability on the transducers themselves.

A *foot pedal* may be available for some machines. This may allow the operator to freeze the screen, take pictures, and/or operate a video recorder. When a transvaginal ultrasound examination is being performed, a foot pedal may be advantageous when the sonographer is holding the probe with one hand and manipulating the organs through the abdominal wall with the other hand.

The *keyboard* has many variations. There are true typewriter-style keys. There are membrane keyboards, such as those found on a calculator, and there are touch-sensitive pads, such as those found in elevators. All of these have advantages and disadvantages. The true typewriter keys are usually the easiest to use but may be the most prone to breaking due to mechanical failure and/or dust (flexible plastic keyboard covers may help the dust problem). The membrane keyboards are the cheapest to produce, are often found on inexpensive machines, and are impervious to dust. However, they may be difficult to operate due to the limited travel of the keys themselves. Finally, the touch-sensitive keys are the most rugged because they have no moving parts and are also impervious to dust. Again, they may be difficult to operate due to limited key travel. One other consideration for keyboards is their size. Smaller machines often have smaller keyboards and this may slow the operator's typing. The keyboard is not a major factor for a machine purchase but it should be considered.

When an ultrasound machine is turned on, it usually has the correct date and/or time on the screen. This *clock* is usually run by an internal battery. One minor consideration concerns whether or not this battery can be replaced by the operator. Battery life is another feature. Usually, the user-replaceable batteries will not last as long (a year or two) but are easy to replace. A nonuser-replaceable battery may last as long as ten years, but may cost several hundred dollars to replace if the machine is not covered by a service contract. Finally, some machines may contain an energy storage device which keeps the clock running without a battery. While these devices are very reliable, they may not work for more than a few days if the machine is left unplugged for an extended period of time.

In recent years, many machines have featured forms of *alternative data input*. These include a joystick, trackball, mouse, touch screen, barcode wand, and others. A *joystick* is usually an acceleration device. When the operator pushes the stick to one side, the cursor (spot on the screen) will move in that direction. When the stick is released, the cursor stops moving. Some joysticks may be position devices where the position of the cursor depends on the physical location of the stick. This type of operation may be more difficult to utilize due to inaccuracies in stick movement. The *trackball* and *mouse* are also position devices, but may be easier to use due to increased movement of the devices to produce a certain movement on the screen. Both are essentially similar in ease of use. The mouse requires a flat surface on the machine to operate, but is very easy to service if it stops working. The trackball takes less space on the console but is considerably more difficult to service if it fails. In the author's experience, trackballs rarely fail and consequently are a preferred device. The *touch screen* allows the operator to actually point at the screen to make a choice rather than using a trackball or joystick to electronically point at the screen. Finally, a *barcode wand* may be utilized in some situations to "read" patient information. While the author has not seen this feature in ultrasound machines, it is available in some laboratory equipment and is mentioned here for completeness.

The actual operation of the machine is usually controlled from a keyboard or from a separate set of keys/switches on the console. Some machines utilize *menus* or choices on the monitor screen. Other machines have dedicated keys or switches for major functions. These are noted in the table at the end of the chapter. If keys are used, these may be labeled with the function (such as "FREEZE") or may have an international symbol. The problem in ultrasound is that there is no international standard for *machine symbols* and, consequently, these can be very confusing in the author's experience. Other machines may use a combination of keys from the keyboard to control some functions. These work well but may not be readily obvious from either the keyboard or the monitor screen. The best systems in the author's opinion are either the dedicated keys with word labels or the screens with menus.

It is difficult to go into great detail about machine operation in a generic sense because the operation of the various features varies so much. *There are, however, a number of features that may be advantageous.* In the author's opinion, one of the most important features for transvaginal sonography is a *variable zoom* that allows a structure to be moved on the screen after the zoom is engaged. In other words, once the zoomed image is on the screen, the operator often will move the probe to get a slightly better view. When this happens, the structure of interest may move from the screen. If the zoomed area can also be moved without displaying the entire image again, the exam can be continued without waiting for the machine to reset itself. Some machines may allow the zoomed image to moved even after the image is "frozen." This feature really improves the efficiency of high-resolution transvaginal sonography.

Another aspect of the operation of the machine is the *speed of the software*. While this feature is not present in the table at the end of the chapter, a potential buyer of a machine should try the various features to see how long the machine takes to turn a feature on or off and how fast the cursor moves in response to a joystick or trackball. Since all of these machines are basically modified computers, some processors are faster than others and this can determine how fast the machine will react to a particular command from the operator.

FINANCIAL CONSIDERATIONS

The cost of a transvaginal ultrasound machine varies widely and depends on many factors including the features of the machine, the resolution of the transducer, and operational costs of the machine. This chapter does not cover this topic in great depth, but presents a limited view of each machine for comparison only. Since machines and prices may change rapidly, the figures in the chart should be considered approximations only.

The *basic cost* of the machine may be misleading because additional features such as M-mode, Doppler, and color Doppler can raise the price rapidly. Therefore, if many features are required, more expensive machines may be competitive with cheaper machines with the additional features. If a large institution is purchasing the machine, quantity discounts may be available.

Once a machine has been chosen, upgrade possibilities may be considered. As technology evolves, some machines may be upgraded. While these machines may be more expensive initially, the cost of upgrading may be less than purchasing a completely new machine. Thus, in the long run, the machine that can be upgraded may be cheaper than the machine that cannot.

Transducer probe cost should also be considered when a machine is purchased. If many are being obtained, their cost may equal or exceed the basic cost of the ultrasound machine. Furthermore, not all probes can be operated with some advanced features such as M-mode, Doppler, and color Doppler. If extra features do work with the probes, their purchase may not necessarily mean the extra features will work. Sometimes it is necessary to purchase additional electronic boards for these features.

Finally, maintenance costs should be considered. The warranty period may vary considerably among the manufacturers. Once the warranty has ended, the cost of maintenance (either fee for service or a contract) may be a large part of the machine cost. In this area, quantity discounts may also be available for service contracts on many machines at a single institution. Another consideration is the response time for service. A contract for rapid response can be expensive but this may be worthwhile to prevent costly "downtime."

CHART OF EQUIPMENT AND TRANSDUCERS

Undoubtedly, there will be more questions about machines than have been presented in this chapter. However, the chart that follows is designed to provide a working comparison among the various manufacturers. Since machines are continuously upgraded, this chart will not be entirely valid. However, it will help the sonographer by listing all of the various features that may be on various machines to allow one to look for an ultrasound machine that has the capability to match the clinical setting of the provider. Since the clinical setting is so variable, this chart includes many other machines and probes that are not transvaginal to provide a more complete picture of available ultrasound equipment for the obstetrician/ gynecologist.

While this chart was being prepared, an effort was made to contact all manufacturers. Unfortunately, some details were difficult to obtain and the chart is not complete. We apologize for any inconvenience due to missing information. If more than one model exists, these are listed separately. If an entry in the chart is blank, the information was not available.

Following the table are pictures of many of the vaginal transducers (Fig 2.4). Visualizing these probes may assist the reader to choose a system.

PHYSICAL CONSIDERATIONS

	Machine Weight (kilograms)	Machine dimensions (cm)	Voltage/Power (volts/watts)	Power cord length (cm)	Cable storage
Acoustic Imaging AI5200	204	129.5 x 69.8 x 104.1	120 (60 Hz) 800 watts (international version available)	366	Yes
Acuson	211	131.4 x 95.2 x 63.5	115, 220/240 1200 watts	457	Cable hanger
ADR/ATL Ultramark 4A	68-77	53.3 x 125 x 68.6	120 (60 Hz) 220/240 (50-60 Hz)	244	Bin
Ultramark 4 Plus	77-100	60 x 148 x 82	120 (60 Hz) 220/240 (50-60 Hz) 1000 watts	244	Bin
Ultramark 5	77-100	23.5 x 147.8 x 124	120 (60 Hz) 220/240 (50/60 Hz) 1000 watts	244	Bin
Ultramark 9	256	66 x 144.8 x 106.6	108-132 (60 Hz) 1380 watts	244	Cable management arm
Ausonics	14.4	45.8 x 15.6 x 39.6	110 or 220; 130 watts	200	None
Bruel & Kjaer 1849					
1846					
Corometrics 210	8	25 x 36.5 x 20	100/120 220/240 (50/60 Hz) 60 watts		None
Aloka 620	80	43 x 70 x 120	100/115 200/220 (50/60 Hz) 210 watts		None
633	85	45 x 88 x 121	115 (60 Hz); 280 watts		Cable hanger
650	180	54 x 134 x 85	115 (60 Hz); 480 watts		Cable hanger
680	155	54 x 91 x 148	100/115 220/240; 480 watts	305	Cable hanger
725	3 modules: 20 kg, 20 kg, 1.5 kg	35 x 46.5 x 28 35 x 20 x 55 25 x 15 x 6	100/115 200/240 (50/60 Hz)		None
870					None
Diasonics SPA1000	172	139.7 x 76.2 x 94	110 (60 Hz), 220 (50 Hz)		Bin on machine
DRF800	172	139.7 x 76.2 x 94	110 (60 Hz), 220 (50 Hz)		Bin on machine
Spectra	204	128.3 x 68.6 x 97.8	110 (60 Hz), 220 (50 Hz)		Bin on machine
Interventional	158.8	106.7 x 61 x 71.1	110 (60 Hz), 220 (50 Hz)		"Arm" on machine
Dynamic Imaging Concept 500/1000	12.5	33 x 23.5 x 50.6	100-250 (48-66 Hz)	450	None
Concept 2000	13.5	33 x 23.5 x 50.6	100-250 (48-66 Hz)	450	None
Elscint ESI1000	100	138 x 69 x 86	115 (60 Hz); 220 (50 Hz) 575 watts	200	None
ESI2000	100	138 x 69 x 86	115 (60 Hz); 220 (50 Hz) 575 watts	200	None
GE Medical Systems RT3200	80.3	53.3 x 78.7 x 119.4	115 (60 Hz); 220-240 (50 Hz); 250 watts		None
RT4000	136.1	57.2 x 59 x 141	115 (48-63 Hz)		None
Radius	210	65 x 136.7 x 104.3	110 (60 Hz); 220 (50 Hz)		None
Sonochrome					None
Hitachi EUB-200	9	25 x 40 x 25	120/220 (50/60 Hz) 90 watts	244	N/A
EUB-310	75	41 x 71 x 131	120/220 (50/60 Hz) 250 watts	244	Probe hanger
EUB-410	85	49 x 75 x 120	120/220 (50/60 Hz) 400 watts	366	Probe hanger
EUB-450	140	57 x 90 x 131	120/220 (50/60 Hz) 600 watts	366	Probe hanger
EUB-515	145	49 x 79 x 130	120/220 (50/60 Hz) 900 watts	366	Probe hanger
Kretz Combison 310	54.9	60 x 110 x 70	110-220 (50,60 Hz) 300 watts	213.4	Clips
Omron	150	54 x 92.5 x 132.2	100 (50/60 Hz) 1000 watts		
OTE Biomedica	14.4	21 x 38 x 40	100-115 (60 Hz); 220-240 (50 Hz) 70 watts		Slot on optional cart
Oxford Vasoflo 4 (Doppler only)	21.8	44.4 x 48.3 x 58.4	100,120,220,240 280 watts	300	None
Philips Orion					None
Platinum	204.1	134.6 x 61.0 x 96.5	110/220	457	Motorized reel
SDR1550			115/220		None
Pie Medical 150	12.7	38.1 x 55.9 x 43.2	100-240 (50/60 Hz) 120 watts	304.8	Hang from 'antenna'
1120B	44.4	55.9 x 63.5 x 119.4	100-240 (50/60 Hz) 300 watts	304.8	Hang from 'antenna'
1150	98.9	71.1 x 76.2 x 129.5	100-240 (50/60 Hz) 300 watts	304.8	Hang from 'antenna'
Quantum 2000	294.8	161.0 x 119.4 x 68.6	110, 220 (50/60 Hz) 1600 watts	256	"Bucket" which wraps around front and side
Siemens SL-1	68	61.5 x 120 x 80	100-120,220-240 (50-60 Hz) 210 watts		Hang from 'antenna'
CF	262	57.8 x 139 x 104	98-132,198-264 (47-63 Hz) 1700 watts		None

	Machine Weight (kilograms)	Machine dimensions (cm)	Voltage/Power (volts/watts)	Power cord length (cm)	Cable storage
Shimadzu SDL-32B	7.8	23 x 25 x 38	100-240 60 watts	245	Brackets
SDL-310	27	22 x 44 x 55	100-240 640 watts	245	Brackets
SDU-500	80	42 x 71 x 128	100-240 650 watts	204	Bracket
Teknar Proscan	19.5	23 x 43 x 46	100-120/200-240 (50-60 Hz)	295	None
Toshiba SSA-250A	121.6	50 x 85.1 x 133.1	120 1000 watts	182.9	Cable "arm"
SSA-270A	229.5	59.9 x 139.7 x 102.1	120 1500 watts	182.9	Cable "arm"

	Storage	Probe storage	# Probe connectors	Probe connector location	Other connectors
Acoustic Imaging	Gel bottles, charts, cameras	10	4	Front near floor	Video in/out, audio in/out, RGB, Y/C, camera control, parallel port
Acuson	Gel bottles, charts, cameras	11	2	Front (left and right)	Video in/out, RGB, Y/C
ADR/ATL Ultramark 4A	Gel bottles, charts, cameras	4	4	Front right near floor	Video in/out
Ultramark 4 Plus	Gel bottles, charts, cameras	4	4	Front right near floor	Video in/out, RS232
Ultramark 5	Gel bottles, charts, cameras	6	6	Front right near floor	Video in/out, RS232
Ultramark 9	Gel bottles, charts, cameras	6	6	Front right near floor	Video in/out, RS232, RGB
Ausonics	On optional cart	3	1	Front, right	Video in, video out, Doppler, ECG, Doppler control
Bruel & Kjaer 1849	Gel bottles, charts, cameras			Front	
1846	Gel bottles, charts, cameras			Front	
Corometrics 210	None	1	1	Right side	video in, video out
Aloka 620	Gel bottles, charts, cameras	2	2	Front, half way to floor	Video out
633	Gel bottles	3	3	Front, half way to floor	Video out
650	Gel bottles, charts, cameras	3	3		Video out
680	Gel bottles, charts, cameras	3	3	Right side	Video out (multiple), audio, VCR, color printer, RS232, SVHS
725	None on machine	None		Right side	Video out
870	Gel bottles, charts, cameras	5		Right side, part way to floor	
Diasonics SPA1000	Gel bottles, charts, cameras	5	2	Front under console	
DRF800	Gel bottles, charts, cameras	5	2	Front under console	
Spectra	Charts, cameras	5	2	Front near floor	
Interventional	Charts, cameras	5	2	Front under console	
Dynamic Imaging Concept 500/1000	On optional cart	2	1 (2 additional connectors optional)	Side	Video in/out
Concept 2000	On optional cart	2	2 (3 additional connectors optional)	Side and back	Video in/out, RS232
Elscint ESI1000	Gel bottles, charts, cameras	5	2 sector, 1 linear	Front under keyboard	Video in/out, RS232, VCR remote control
ESI2000	Gel bottles, charts, cameras	5	2 sector, 1 linear	Front under keyboard	Video in/out, RS232, VCR remote control, audio output
GE Medical Systems RT3200	Gel bottles, charts, cameras	4	2	Front	Video in/out
RT4000	Gel bottles, charts, cameras	4	2	Front	Video in/out, echo out
Radius		3	2	Front	Video in/out, audio in/out
Sonochrome		3	2	Front	Video in/out, audio in/out
Hitachi EUB-200	None	1	1	Rear	Video out
EUB-310	Gel bottles, charts, cameras	2	1	Right side	Video out
EUB-410	Gel bottles, charts, cameras	2	2	Right side	Video out
EUB-450	Gel bottles, charts, cameras	2	2	Front under keyboard	Video out
EUB-515	Gel bottles, charts, cameras	2	2	Front under keyboard	Video out
Kretz Combison 310	Gel bottles, charts, cameras	5	3	Right side	Video out (2)
Omron	Gel bottles, charts, cameras	4		Front, near floor	
OTE Biomedica	Gel bottles, charts, cameras on optional cart	1 on optional cart	1	Rear	

	Storage	Probe storage	# Probe connectors	Probe connector location	Other connectors
Oxford Vasoflo 4	On cart	2	2	Front	Video out, RS232, Centronics, analog inputs, footswitch, headphones, Doppler in/out
Philips Orion	Gel bottles, charts, cameras	4			
Platinum	Gel bottles (has warmer built in), charts, cameras	9	2	Front	NTSC/PAL/RGB video out, VCR in/out, Serial/parallel output, Digital image output, audio in/out, footswitch
SDR1550	None	None		Right side	Light pen
Pie Medical 150	Gel bottles, charts, cameras	2	2	Rear	VCR in/out, video out
1120B	Gel bottles, charts, cameras	5	3	Rear	VCR in/out, video out (2), RS232, keyboard control
1150	Gel bottles, charts, cameras	8	6	Rear	VCR in/out, video in, video out (2), RS232, keyboard control
Quantum 2000	Gel bottles, charts, cameras	6	1 (3 as of Nov, 1990)	Lower right on front of machine	RGB RS170A, NTSC RS170A, RS232, SVHS
Siemens SL-1	Gel bottles, charts, cameras	3	3	Front	
CF	Gel bottles, charts, cameras	2		Front near floor	Video in/out, RGB
Shimadzu SDL-32B	Gel bottle	1	1	Rear	Video in/out, footswitch
SDL-310	Optional	2	2	Right side	Video in/out, footswitch, camera
SDU-500	Gel bottle	3	3	Right side	Video in/out
Teknar Proscan	On cart	3	1	Front	Video in/out, footswitch
Toshiba SSA-250A	Gel, Cameras	6	6	Side	Video, RGB, S-VHS, RS232
SSA-270A	Gel, Cameras	4	4	Front	Video, RGB, S-VHS, RS232

	Monitor (size - cm)	Monitor location	Keyboard	Remote control	Other input
Acoustic Imaging	B/W 22.9 Color 30.5	Fixed in top of machine which swivels	Typewriter with extra keys and pushbuttons	Camera foot pedal	Trackball
Acuson	22.9 or 30.5, B/W or color	Fixed in machine	Typewriter with extra keys	None	Trackball
ADR/ATL Ultramark 4A	B/W 22.9 cm	Swivel	Typewriter, extra keys	M-line	Trackball
Ultramark 4 Plus	B/W 22.9 cm	Tilt, swivel, raise	Typewriter/ membrane keys	M-line, printer	Trackball
Ultramark 5	B/W 22.9 cm	Tilt, swivel	Typewriter/ membrane keys	M-line, Doppler sample, printer	Trackball
Ultramark 9	B/W 22.9 cm, Color 22.9 cm	Tilt, swivel	Typewriter and additional plasma keys	M-line, Doppler sample, printer, VCR	Trackball
Ausonics	B/W 12.7 cm	Fixed in machine	Membrane, hinge mounted with 8 dedicated keys	None	Trackball
Bruel & Kjaer 1849	B/W	Tilt/swivel	Elevator with extra keys, keyboard slides into machine		None
1846	B/W	Tilt/swivel	Elevator with extra keys, keyboard slides into machine		None
Corometrics 210	B/W 14 cm	Fixed in machine	Membrane, numbers only	None	None
Aloka 620	B/W 22.8 cm	Tilt/swivel	Membrane with extra keys	Foot pedal optional	Trackball
633	B/W 22.8 cm	Tilt/swivel	Membrane with extra keys	Foot pedal optional	Trackball
650	B/W 22.8 cm	Tilt/swivel	Membrane with extra keys	Foot pedal optional	Trackball
680	Color 30.5 cm	Tilt/swivel	Membrane with extra keys	None	Trackball
725	B/W 17.8 cm	Fixed in machine	Membrane with extra keys		Joystick
870	Color	Fixed in machine	Membrane with extra keys	Foot pedal optional	Trackball
Diasonics SPA1000	(2) B/W	One fixed in machine, other tilt/swivel	Membrane with extra keys		Trackball
DRF800	(2) B/W	One fixed in machine, other tilt/swivel	Membrane with extra keys		Trackball
Spectra	B/W and Color	Tilt/swivel	Membrane with extra keys		Trackball
Interventional	(2) B/W	Fixed in machine	Membrane with extra keys	Foot pedals	Trackball
Dynamic Imaging Concept 500/1000	B/W 17.8	Fixed in machine	Membrane with extra keys	Foot switch supplied	Trackball
Concept 2000	B/W 17.8	Fixed in machine	Membrane with extra keys	Foot switch supplied	Trackball

	Monitor (size - cm)	Monitor location	Keyboard	Remote control	Other input
Elscint	B/W 22.9	Tilt/swivel	Elevator with many extra keys	Foot pedal freeze optional	Joystick
	B/W 22.9 (image) B/W 22.9 (data)	Tilt/swivel	Elevator with many extra keys	Foot pedal freeze optional, Doppler remote	Joystick
GE Medical Systems　RT3200	B/W 30.5	Tilt/swivel	Membrane with extra keys	Footswitch	Trackball
RT4000	B/W 30.5	Tilt/swivel	Membrane with extra keys	Footswitch	Trackball
Radius	B/W 30.5 image; B/W data	Tilt/swivel	Typewriter with extra keys	Footswitch	Trackball
Sonochrome	Color 30.5 image; B/W data	Tilt/swivel	Typewriter with extra keys	Footswitch	Trackball
Hitachi　EUB-200	B/W 12.7	Fixed in machine	Membrane, numbers only	None	
EUB-310	B/W 22.9	Fixed on arm	Membrane with extra keys	None	Joystick
EUB-410	B/W 22.9	Tilt/swivel	Membrane with extra keys	None	Trackball
EUB-450	B/W 30.5	Tilt/swivel	Membrane with many extra keys	None	Trackball
EUB-515	Color 30.5	Tilt/swivel	Membrane with many extra keys	None	Trackball
Kretz Combison 310	B/W 22.9	Fixed in machine	Membrane	Footswitch	Trackball
Omron	B/W 30.5	Tilt/swivel	Membrane with many extra keys		Trackball
OTE Biomedica	B/W 20.3	Fixed in machine	Membrane, numbers only (alpha keyboard optional)		Joystick
Oxford　Vasoflo 4	Color 30.5	Fixed on top of machine	Membrane with extra keys	Footswitch, infrared keypad (12 keys)	
Philips　Orion	B/W	Tilt/swivel	Typewriter with extra keys		Joystick
Platinum	Color 35.6	Tilt/swivel	Typewriter with extra keys. Entire control console moves away from machine on "arm"	(Entire console moves away from machine), Mode control on probe	Mouse, 3 1/2" floppy disks
SDR1550	B/W	Fixed in machine	Membrane with extra keys labeled with symbols		None
Pie Medical　150	B/W (17.8 cm)	Fixed in machine	Membrane with dedicated keys; function keys next to screen	None	Joystick
1120B	B/W (22.9 cm)	Tilt/swivel	Membrane with dedicated keys; function keys for menus	None	Joystick
1150	B/W (22.9 cm)	Tilt/swivel	Membrane with dedicated keys; function keys for menus	Mouse	Trackball/Mouse External keyboard
Quantum　2000	Color (image) 33 B/W (menus/data)	Swivel	Typewriter with many extra dedicated keys	Wired remote with all controls used during scanning	Trackball
Siemens　SL-1	B/W 20.3 B/W 22.9	Fixed in machine Tilt/swivel	Membrane with extra keys labeled with symbols	Freeze control on some probes; infrared remote	Trackball
CF	(2) Color 22.9	Tilt/swivel	Typewriter	Footswitch	Trackball
Shimadzu　SDL-32B	B/W 14	Fixed in machine	Membrane (numbers) with extra keys	Footswitch (freeze)	N/A
SDL-310	B/W 22.9	Fixed in machine, optional second monitor	Membrane with extra keys	Footswitch (freeze)	Trackball
SDU-500	B/W 30.5	Tilt/swivel	Membrane with extra keys	N/A	Trackball
Teknar　Proscan	B/W 22.9	Fixed in machine	Typewriter ("XT" type custom keyboard)	Separate trackball with 3 keys	Trackball, foot pedal
Toshiba　SSA-250A	B/W 30.5	Tilt/swivel	Membrane with many extra keys	Pedal (expose, freeze)	Touch sensitive screen, trackball
SSA-270A	Color 30.5	Tilt/swivel	Membrane with many extra keys	Pedal (expose, freeze)	Touch sensitive screen, trackball

	Temperature (°C) Humidity (%)	Fan & Filters	Battery	VCR/Camera control from machine
Acoustic Imaging	16-35°, 15-95%	Fan, user serviceable filter	Lithium battery, lasts 5 years, not user replaceable	Camera
Acuson	15-32°, <90%	6 fans, 3 user serviceable filters	Yes - lasts 3 years, not user replaceable	Camera, VCR

	Temperature (°C) Humidity (%)	Fan & Filters	Battery	VCR/Camera control from machine
ADR/ATL Ultramark 4A	10-40°, 15-95%	Fan	Yes	Printer
Ultramark 4 Plus	10-40°, 15-95%	Fan	Yes	Camera, VCR, printer
Ultramark 5	10-40°, 15-95%	Fan	Yes	Camera, VCR, printer
Ultramark 9	10-40°, 15-95%	Fans, filters	Yes	Camera, VCR
Ausonics	-10 to +40; <90%	Fan	10 year lithium, not user replaceable	None
Bruel & Kjaer 1849 1846				
Corometrics 210 Aloka	10-40°, 30-75%		NiCad battery continuously charged, not user replaceable	None
620		Fan		Camera
633		Fan		Camera
650		Fan		Camera
680		Fan, user serviceable filter		Variety possible
725				
870				Camera
Diasonics SPA1000	10-40°, 10-90%			
DRF800	10-40°, 10-90%			
Spectra	10-40°, 10-90%			
Interventional	10-40°, 10-90%			
Dynamic Imaging Concept 500/1000	10-40°, 10-90%	Fan	NiCad holds charge 3 months, lasts 5-7 years	N/A
Concept 2000	10-40°, 10-90%	Fan	NiCad holds charge 3 months, lasts 5-7 years	N/A
Elscint ESI1000	10-40°, 10-90%	Fan, user can clean 1 filter	AA, user replaceable	VCR (Panasonic only)
ESI2000	10-40°, 10-90%	Fan, user can clean 1 filter	AA, user replaceable	VCR (Panasonic only)
GE Medical Systems RT3200	10-40°, 5-85%	Fan	Yes	Camera, VCR
RT4000	15-40°, 5-85%	Fan	Yes	Camera, VCR
Radius	10-40°, <90%	Fan, filters	Yes, AA	Camera, VCR
Sonochrome	10-40°, 30-75%	Fan, filters	Yes, AA	Camera, VCR
Hitachi EUB-200	5-35°, 30-85%	Fan	Battery optional	No
EUB-310	5-35°, 30-85%	Fan	Yes	No
EUB-410	5-35°, 30-85%	Fan	Yes	No
EUB-450	5-35°, 30-85%	Fan	Yes	Camera/VCR control optional
EUB-515	5-35°, 30-85%	Fan	Yes	Camera/VCR control optional
Kretz Combison 310	10-40°, <90%	Fan, user can change filter	NiCad continuously recharged, not user replaceable	None
Omron				Camera
OTE Biomedica				None
Oxford Vasoflo 4	10-35°, <90%	Fan, user can change filter	Lithium lasts 10 yrs, not user replaceable	None
Philips Orion				
Platinum		Fan, airflow from top to bottom of machines, no filters	Continuously recharged power cell, not user replaceable	Camera, VCR
SDR1550				
Pie Medical 150	8-40°	Fan, user can change filters	NiCad, holds charge 3 months; lasts 5-7 years	None
1120B	8-40°	Fan, user can change filters	NiCad, holds charge 3 months; lasts 5-7 years	None
1150	8-40°	Fan, user can change filters	Lithium, lasts 10 years, not user replaceable	Camera
Quantum 2000	0-40°, 15-95%	Fan, user can clean filters	Lithium, lasts 10 years, not user replaceable	VCR
Siemens SL-1	10-40°			
CF	10-40°			Camera, VCR

		Temperature (°C) Humidity (%)	Fan & Filters	Battery	VCR/Camera control from machine
Shimadzu	SDL-32B	10-35°	Fan	N/A	N/A
	SDL-310	0-40°, 35-85%	2 Fans	Yes	Camera, VCR
	SDU-500	10-35°, 35-85%	2 Fans	NiCad rechargeable	Camera, VCR
Teknar	Proscan	15-40°, 0-90%	Fans	Lithium, lasts 10 years, not user replaceable	None
Toshiba	SSA-250A	3-35°, 35-85%	Fans, filters	Yes, rechargeable	None
	SSA-270A	5-35°, 35-85%	Fans, filters	Yes, rechargeable	VCR

OPERATIONS

	Image modes (all have gray scale except as noted)	Inversion	Reverse Video	Zoom	Frame averaging
Acoustic Imaging	M-mode, Doppler, Color Doppler	Right-left, up-down	Yes	Yes, size and location cannot be changed after selection, not movable in freeze	Up to 6 frames
Acuson	M-mode, Doppler, Color Doppler	Right-left, up-down	Yes	Continuous adjustment, cannot be moved with image frozen	Up to 6 frames
ADR/ATL Ultramark 4A	M-mode, Doppler	Right-left, up-down	Yes	Adjustable up to 5X, movable in live and freeze, digital	2 algorithms, up to 4 frames, variable persistence
Ultramark 4 Plus	M-mode, Doppler	Right-left, up-down	Yes	Adjustable up to 5X, movable in live and freeze, digital	
Ultramark 5	M-mode, Doppler	Right-left, up-down	Yes	Adjustable up to 5X, movable in live and freeze, digital	
Ultramark 9	M-mode, Doppler, Color Doppler	Right-left, up-down	Yes	Adjustable up to 8X, movable in live and freeze, digital	
Ausonics	M-mode, Doppler, ECG, VCR playback	Right-Left, up-down	Yes	Yes all modes, not movable after image is frozen, not variable size	Yes, adjustable except < 150 mm scales
Bruel & Kjaer 1849					
1846				Yes	
Corometrics 210 Aloka					
620	M-mode	Right-left	Yes		
633	M-mode, Doppler	Right-left	Yes	4 sizes	
650	M-mode, Doppler	Right-left, up-down	Yes	Yes, variable size, not movable after freeze	Adjustable, all modes and probes
680	M-mode, Doppler, Color Doppler	Right-left, up-down	Yes	Yes, variable size, not movable after freeze	Adjustable, all modes and probes
725	M-mode, Doppler	Right-left, up-down	Yes		
870	M-mode, Doppler, Color Doppler, Color M-mode				
Diasonics SPA1000	M-mode, spectrum analysis				
DRF800	M-mode, spectrum analysis				
Spectra	M-mode, Doppler, Color Doppler, spectrum analysis			Yes	
Interventional					
Dynamic Imaging Concept 500/1000	M-mode (Note: Concept 500 uses linear probes only)	Right-left	Yes	Yes 1.0, 1.5, 2.0 magnifications	Yes
Concept 2000	M-mode	Right-left, up-down	Yes	Yes, 1.0, 1.5, 2.0, 3.0 magnifications	Yes
Elscint ESI1000	A-mode, M-mode	Right-left, up-down	Yes	2X zoom, also M-mode, movable at all times	All modes, all probes
ESI2000	A-mode, M-mode, Doppler	Right-left, up-down	Yes	2X zoom, also M-mode, movable at all times	All modes, all probes
GE Medical Systems RT3200	M-mode	Right-left, up-down	Yes		Yes
RT4000	M-mode, Doppler	Right-left, up down	Yes		Yes
Radius	M-mode, Doppler	Right-left, up-down	Yes	Yes	Adjustable
Sonochrome	M-mode, Doppler, Color Doppler	Right-left, up-down	Yes	Yes	Adjustable
Hitachi EUB-200	M-mode	Right-left	Yes	Yes 1.5, 2.0 magnification	Yes
EUB-310	M-mode	Right-left	Yes	Yes 1.2, 1.5, 2.0 magnification	Yes

	Image modes (all have gray scale except as noted)	Inversion	Reverse Video	Zoom	Frame averaging
Hitachi EUB-410	M-mode	Right-left, up-down	Yes	Yes 0.8, 1.2, 1.5, 2.0 magnification	Yes
EUB-450	M-mode, Doppler	Right-left, up-down	Yes	Yes 0.8, 1.2, 1.5 magnification	Yes
EUB-515	M-mode, Doppler, Color Doppler	Right-left, Up-down	Yes	Yes 5 steps	Yes
Kretz Combison 310	M-mode	Right-left, up-down	Yes	Variable zoom all modes, not moveable in freeze	Yes, all modes and probes
Omron	M-mode			X3, X6, X12	
OTE Biomedica	M-mode				
Oxford Vasoflo 4	Doppler Spectrum (CW, PW) ONLY	N/A	N/A	N/A	N/A
Philips Orion		Up-down			
Platinum	M-mode, Doppler, Color Doppler	Right-left, up-down	Yes	Yes, all modes, moveable	Yes, all modes, programmable persistence
SDR1550	M-mode	Right-left	Yes	Yes	
Pie Medical 150	M-mode	Left-right, up-down	Yes	None	One selection
1120B	M-mode, Doppler CW & PW	Left-right, up-down	Yes	Yes, movable and adjustable at all times in all modes	One selection
1150	M-mode, Doppler, Color Doppler	Left-right, up-down	Yes	Yes, movable and adjustable at all times in all modes	One selection
Quantum 2000	Doppler, Color Doppler (M-mode and CW Doppler available Fall, 1990)	Left-right, up-down	Not available	Yes, variable, works in freeze mode, all probes	Adjustable in all modes for all probes
Siemens SL-1	M-mode	Left-right, up-down	Yes	Yes, (limited)	
CF	M-mode, Doppler (PW & CW), Color Doppler	Left-right, up-down	Yes	Yes	
Shimadzu SDL-32B		Left-right	Yes	Yes	N/A
SDL-310	M-mode	Left-right, up-down	Yes	Yes	Yes
SDU-500	M-mode, Doppler, ECG	Left-right, up-down	Yes	Yes	Yes
Teknar Proscan		Up-down	Yes	Yes, (limited)	N/A
Toshiba SSA-250A	M-mode, Doppler	Left-right, Up-down	Yes	Yes, moveable	8 choices
SSA-270A	M-mode, Doppler, color Doppler	Left-right, Up-down	Yes	Yes, moveable	8 choices

	Image depth (cm)	Multiple images	Pre/Post Process	Calipers	Calculations
Acoustic Imaging	21.5	2, side by side for linear probes	8 sliding TGC; 4 levels persistence, 3 levels edge enhance, 8 levels compression; 5 post processing curves	2 linear, 1 ellipse/area	Obstetrics, vascular
Acuson	24	Two, side by side for linear probes	Many software controlled options and user definable curves	2 pairs/ellipses, automatic circle/ellipse	Obstetrics, cardiology, vascular
ADR/ATL Ultramark 4A	26.5	Dual in sector and linear	Edge enhancement, gray scale, dynamic range, 8 sliding TGC	2 distance and 2 planimeter per image	Obstetrics, cardiology, vascular
Ultramark 4 Plus	26.5	Dual in sector and linear	Edge enhancement, gray scale, dynamic range, 8 sliding TGC	2 distance and 2 planimeter per image	Obstetrics, cardiology, vascular
Ultramark 5	26.5	Dual in sector and linear	Edge enhancement, gray scale, dynamic range	2 distance and 2 planimeter per image	Obstetrics, cardiology, vascular
Ultramark 9	38	Dual cineloop	Multiple curves and filters under user control	Multiple calipers, ellipse	Obstetrics, cardiology, vascular
Ausonics	7.5-27.5	No	TGC manual adjust software controlled; edge enhance & dynamic range soft. cont.; Post processing key selected soft. cont.	4 distances/image all probes & modes; one area/circum per image	Obstetrics, abdominal, cardiac tables; can be upgraded
Bruel & Kjaer 1849					
1846			Yes	Yes	

	Image depth (cm)	Multiple images	Pre/Post Process	Calipers	Calculations
Corometrics Aloka 210	28.2		Near field and far field only	One set	
620		2, side by side	Two rotary controls, 8 slide TGC controls	Two sets, one circle	Obstetrics
633	24	2, side by side	Two rotary controls, 8 slide TGC controls	Two sets, one circle	Obstetrics
650	25.5	4, two by two	2 rotary, 11 slide TGC controls, 4 mode gray scale enhancement	Two sets, one circle	Obstetrics, cardiology
680	25.5	4, two by two	3 Steps preprocessing, 10 step AGC, multiple post processing curves	4 sets, all probes and modes	Obstetrics, cardiology, vascular
725			AGC, FTC	Two sets	Cardiology, vascular
870				Two sets	
Diasonics SPA1000	5-23			Yes	Obstetrics, cardiology, vascular
DRF800	5-23			Yes	Obstetrics, cardiology, vascular
Spectra	3-23		Multiple software controlled options	Yes	Obstetrics, cardiology, vascular
Interventional			Multiple curve and options selections	Yes	
Dynamic Imaging Concept 500/1000	22	2, side by side	N/A	Yes, 3 sets	Obstetrics, neonatal
Concept 2000	22	2 screens	4 curve selections	Yes, 3 sets	Obstetrics, cardiology, neonatal
Elscint ESI1000	4-24, 7 steps	2, side by side 4, two by two	Automatic TGC, 8 manual TGC controls, 3 preset & 2 user gray curves	3 pairs of calipers, 3 regions of interest	Obstetrics, cardiology
ESI2000	4-24, 7 steps	2, side by side 4, two by two	Automatic TGC, 8 manual TGC controls, 3 preset & 2 user gray curves	2 pairs of calipers, 3 regions of interest	Obstetrics, cardiology, Doppler ratios
GE Medical Systems RT3200	7.5-20	3, side by side		Yes	Obstetrics, vascular
RT4000	7.5-20	2, side by side	Slide TGC controls	Yes	Obstetrics, vascular
Radius	22	Yes	Slide TGC controls, many software controlled options	Yes	Obstetrics, cardiology, vascular
Sonochrome	22	Yes	Slide TGC controls, many software controlled options	Yes	Obstetrics, cardiology, vascular
Hitachi EUB-200	18	Yes, linear mode	Pre processing only	Yes	N/A
EUB-310	21	Yes, linear mode	Pre processing only	Yes	
EUB-410	21	Yes, linear mode	Multiple controls	Yes	
EUB-450	21	Yes, linear mode, Up to 8 images	Slide TGC plus multiple sofware controls	Yes	Obstetrics, cardiology, vascular
EUB-515	24	Yes, linear mode	Slide TGC with multiple software controls	Yes	Obstetrics, cardiology, vascular
Kretz Combison 310	6-21	Two, side by side	Threshhold, dynamic range, grayscale options	6 sets/image, all modes, automatic circle/ellipse	Obstetrics
Omron	0-4		Slide TGC	Yes	
OTE Biomedica	6-24 (7 settings)		Slide TGC with selectable pre/post processing options	Yes	Obstetrics
Oxford Vasoflo 4	0-14	Up to 16 side by side	Automatic and manual, selection of threshold	Yes	Obstetrics, Vascular, Transcranial
Philips Orion				2 sets	
Platinum	5-24	Dual or quad image, all modes	Dynamic range, edge enhancement, persistence, 48 gray scale curves	8 measurements per screen, all modes, circumferences and areas measured multiple ways	Obstetrics, cardiology, radiology, vascular
SDR1550	4.5-20		4 selectable input curves	Yes	
Pie Medical 150	5-20 cm in 4 steps	2, side by side	4 TGC slide controls	16 measurements per image; area; circle	Software on SmartCards; 6 OB tables, 2 user tables
1120B	5-20 cm in 5 steps	2, side by side 4, two by two	6 TGC slide controls 4 Pre & 4 Post processing curves	16 measurements per image; area; circle; draw; ellipse	6 OB tables, 2 user tables
1150	5-20 cm in 6 steps	2, side by side 4, two by two	8 TGC slide controls 4 Pre & 4 Post processing curves	16 measurements per image; area; circle; draw; ellipse	Software on SmartCards; 6 OB tables, 2 user tables
Quantum 2000	4-20 cm	2, side by side available Fall, 1990	Multiple pre and post processing options including slide TGC controls and rotary controls	At least 4 measurements per image, more if just distance, circle & ellipse available, draw, multiple image measurements	Obstetrics, vascular, cardiology

	Image depth (cm)	Multiple images	Pre/Post Process	Calipers	Calculations
Siemens SL-1	6-20 cm		5 slide TGC controls, dynamic range, edge enhance, 5 gray scale curves	Yes	Obstetrics, cardiology
CF	4-24	Yes	10 slide TGC controls, many software controlled pre/post processing options	Yes	
Shimadzu SDL-32B	20	Dual	Near & far fields	Yes	
SDL-310	22	Dual	4 preset TGC, 4 enhancements, 4 dynamic ranges, 4 reject, 4 gamma	2 sets	Obstetrics, cardiology
SDU-500	22	3 images	8 steps STC, 4 enhancements, 4 dynamic ranges, 4 reject, 4 gamma	4 distance, 2 areas, circles, angles, volume	Obstetrics, cardiology, vascular, pediatric
Teknar Proscan	1.5-25	Two, side by side	Software controlled	3 sets	Volume, planemetric, ellipsoidal, 2 plane
Toshiba SSA-250A	24	Dual/quad screen, cine	Many choices dynamic range, edge enhance, persistance, multiple curves	4 sets of calipers, all modes	
SSA-270A	24	Dual/quad screen, cine	same as above	4 sets of calipers, all modes	

	Power adjust	Probe Selection	Frame rate per second
Acoustic Imaging	Ten settings	Keyboard	4-42
Acuson	Three settings	Key on console	5-56
ADR/ATL Ultramark 4A	Adjustable	Console control	6-65
Ultramark 4 Plus	Adjustable	Console control	6-65
Ultramark 5	Adjustable	Console control	6-65
Ultramark 9	Adjustable	Console control	Up to 156
Ausonics	40 increments, software controlled	(Only one plugged in)	13, 19, 27; key selected
Bruel & Kjaer 1849			
1846			
Corometrics 210 Aloka		Only one plugged in	Adjustable, maximum 30
620	Yes	Single key	Adjustable, maximum 30
633	Yes	Console control	Adjustable, maximum 30
650	Yes	Console control	Adjustable, maximum 30
680	Adjustable in 10 steps	Console control	Adjustable, maximum 30
725	Yes		Adjustable, maximum 30
870	Yes	Console control	
Diasonics SPA1000		Keyboard	4-30
DRF800		Keyboard	4-30
Spectra		Keyboard	4-42
Interventional		Keyboard	
Dynamic Imaging Concept 500/1000	No	Keyboard	16
Concept 2000	No	Keyboard	16-24
Elscint ESI1000	4 settings	Switch	8-60, depends on image size, user adjustable
ESI2000	6 settings	Switch	8-60, depends on image size, user adjustable
GE Medical Systems RT3200	Switch selectable	Key on console	up to 30
RT4000	Switch selectable	Key on console	up to 30
Radius		Key on console	
Sonochrome		Key on console	
Hitachi EUB-200	No	Only 1 plugged in	
EUB-310	No	Only 1 plugged in	
EUB-410	Yes	Keyboard	
EUB-450	Keyboard, 3 choices	Keyboard	Variable
EUB-515	Keyboard, 3 choices	Keyboard	Variable
Kretz Combison 310	15 choices	Keyboard (2 strokes)	(6.7-20) not adjustable
Omron			

	Power adjust	Probe Selection	Frame rate per second
OTE Biomedica	Adjustable	Only 1 plugged in	25 (not adjustable)
Oxford Vasoflo 4	5 settings	Keyboard	N/A
Philips Orion			
Platinum	4 steps, set by mouse	Probe is selected by removing it from holder	2-52
SDR1550			
Pie Medical 150	No	Keyboard 1-2 keys	11 or 22; keyboard selected
1120B	No	Keyboard 1-2 keys	Sector 6-18; Linear/curved 2-60; keyboard selected
1150	No	Keyboard 1-2 keys	Sector 6-18; Linear/curved 2-60; keyboard selected
Quantum 2000	Variable in 1 dB steps, 0-20 dB	Dedicated key	Maximum 30
Siemens SL-1		Dedicated keys	Sector 5-30; Linear 6-31
CF	7 adjusments	Keyboard	Up to 60
Shimadzu SDL-32B		Only 1 plugged in	Depth dependent
SDL-310		Keyboard	8-28
SDU-500	Yes	Console control	8-30
Teknar Proscan	Adjustable	Only 1 plugged in	Depends on probe
Toshiba SSA-250A	Adjustable 16 steps	Console button	Depends on probe and mode
SSA-270A	Adjustable 16 steps	Console button	Depends on probe and mode

TRANSDUCER PROBES

Types: M--mechanical sector C--curvilinear P--phased array sector L--linear A--annular crystals
B--biplane S--steerable plane of scan TV--transvaginal TR--transrectal SH--straight handle BH--bent ("broken") handle
Note: Not all probes can be used on all machines.

	Type	Weight (grams)	Dimensions (mm, diam x length)	Freq. (MHz)	Cable length (cm)	Cost (x $1000)	Field of view (cm or degrees)
Acoustic Imaging	C (13 probes)	800	60 x 120	3.5,5,7.5	187	8.5	48-114°
	L (3 probes)		70 x 120	3.5,5,7.5			8 to 12 cm
	C,TV			7.5		12.5	
	C,TR			5		12.5	
Acuson	L (5 probes)	675-1100 includes cable & plug		3.5,5,7	213	(other probes	3.8, 5.8, 8.2, 12 cm
	P (7 probes)			2.5,3.5,5,7		9.5-27.5)	90°
	P,TV,SH (2 probes)			5,7	254	12	90°
	P,TR,SH (2 probes)			5,7			90°
	L,TR,SH			7			5.0 cm
ADR/ATL	L (4 probes)			3.5,5,7.5	206		11.9,8.3,3.8 cm
	M (15 probes)	454		2.25,3.5,5.0, 7.5, 10	206		90°
	C (5 probes)			3.5,5	206		60°, 90°
	P (3 probes)			2.25,3.5,5			
	CW (4 probes)			2.25,3,5,10			
	M,TV,SH (3 probes)			3,5,7.5	206		90°
	C,TV,SH			5	206		150°, (3 90° steps)
Ausonics	M	480	28 x 155	2.5	200	4-6	90°
	M	480	23 x 152	3.5	200	4-6	90°
	M	480	28 x 155	3.5	200	4-6	90°
	M	480	23 x 152	5	200	4-6	90°
	M	480	23 x 152	7.5	200	4-6	90°
	M	600	64 x 190	7.5	200	5-7	50°
	M,TV,SH	580	28 x 320	7.5	200	7-10	90°
	M,TR,SH,B	660	21 x 327	7.5	200	12-15	90°
Bruel & Kjaer	M (4 probes)			4,6,7,3-5			
	M,TV,SH			7			
	M,TR,SH (2 probes)			4-7			
Corometrics Aloka	L (7 probes)			3.5,5.7.5		6.5-14	3.8-12.5 cm
	C (7 probes)			3.5,5			34-90°
	M (10 probes)			2,3,3.5,5,7.5			
	P,TV,BH			5			60
	P,TV,BH			5			88
	P,TV,BH			5			90
	L-P,TR,SH (2 probes)			5,7.5			2 cm, 90°
Diasonics	L (2 probes)			3.5,5			6,8 cm
	P (2 probes)			3.5,5			90°
	C (2 probes)			3.5,7.5			48-53°
	M,TV,SH (2 probes)		15 x 322	7,7.5			30-110°
	M,TR,SH			7			30-110°
	Interventional catheter			20			360°
Dynamic Imaging	L (5 probes)			3.5,5,7.5			6,8,12 cm
	C (5 probes)			3.5,5,7, 7.5			50°
	A (2 probes)			3.5,5			90°
	M (5 probes)			2.5,3.5,5,7.5, 10			90°
	M,TV,SH			7.5			90°
	M,TR,SH			7.5			90°

	Type	Weight (grams)	Dimensions (mm, diam x length)	Freq. (MHz)	Cable length (cm)	Cost (x $1000)	Field of view (cm or degrees)
Elscint	L	400		3.5	200	7	12 cm
	M (4 probes)	250	42 x 125	3.5,5,6.5,10	200	5-6	30-105°
	M Duplex Doppler	300		10	200	8	30-70°
	M,TV,SH	270	27.5 x 266	6.5	200	7	30-105°
	M,TR,SH	700	19 mm diam	7.5	200	14	30-110°
GE Medical Systems	L (5 probes)			3.5,5,7.5			6-13 cm
	P (3 probes)			2.5,3.5,5			90°
	C (3 probes)			3.5,5			60°
	P,TV,BH (2 probes)			5,7			90°
Hitachi	L (7 probes)			3.5,5,7.5		4-13	
(Not all probes work on all machines)	C (6 probes)			3.5,5			60-100°
	L-C,TR,SH			5			
	C,TV,BH		22 x 140	6.5			120°
	C,TV,B		23 x 150	5,6.5			100° sagital 120° axial
	C,TV, held on finger			5,7.5			60°
Kretz	M (3 probes)	392	40 x 140	3.5,5,7	200	7-13	60°, 90°
	M,TV,SH (2 probes)	420	21 x 150 26 x 150	5,7.5			90,240°
	M,TR,SH	896	20 x 200	7.5			Transverse: 360° Longitundinal: 90°
Omron	L (2 probes)			15,30			1.3, 2.7 cm
OTE Biomedica	M,A (4 probes)			3.5,5,7.5			
Oxford Vasoflo 4	Pencil CW (2 probes)			4,8			N/A
	Pencil pulsed			2			N/A
	Flat			8			N/A
	TV,SH (2 probes)			4,8			N/A
Philips	L (4 probes)			3.5,5,7.5		8.5-12	3.8-9.7 cm
	C (9 probes)			3.5,5,7.5			25-90°
	P,TV,SH (2 probes)			7			
	P,TR			7.5			
Pie Medical 150	M			3.5		8-12	60-150°, 4 steps
150	M			5			60-150°, 4 steps
150	M,TV,SH			5			60-150°, 4 steps
1120B	L			3.5			12 cm
1120B	L			5			6.7 cm
1120B	L			7.5			3.4 cm
1120B, 1150	P,A			3.5			90°
1120B, 1150	P,A			5			73°, 90°
1120B, 1150	P,A,TV,SH			5			73°, 90°, 150°
1150	L			3.5			10.5 cm
1150	L			5			5.25 cm
1150	L			7.5			3.5 cm
1150	C			3.5			100°
1150	C			5			100°
Quantum	L (2 probes)			5,7.5		10-15	3.0, 4.5 cm
	C (3 probes)			3,5			
	C,TV			7.5			
Siemens	L (6 probes)	450		3.5,5,7.5			6.4,8.4,11.3 cm
	M (5 probes)	250		3.5,5,7.5			60-100°
	P (7 probes)			2.25,3.5,5,7			30-90°
	CW Pencil (2 probes			2,4			N/A
	M,TV,SH			5,7			100°
Shimadzu SDL-32B	L (8 probes)			3.5,5,7.5	183		4 - 10 cm
SDL-310	L (7 probes) 3 intraop.			3.5,5,7.5	183		2.9 - 10 cm
SDL-310	C (4 probes)			3.5,5	183		60 - 109°
SDL-310	C,TV			5	183		115°

	Type	Weight (grams)	Dimensions (mm, diam x length)	Freq. (MHz)	Cable length (cm)	Cost (x $1000)	Field of view (cm or degrees)
Shimadzu SDL-310	L,TR			5	183		6.1 cm
SDU-500	L (10 probes) 3 intraop.			3.5,5,7.5	183		2.9 - 10 cm
SDU-500	C (3 probes)			3.5,5			60 - 109°
SDU-500	P (3 probes)			2.5,3.75,5			90°
SDU-500	C,TV (avail. 11-90)			5	183		115°
Teknar Proscan	M	142	13.1 x 33.4	5		7.5	90°
	M,TR,SH,B	595	2.8 x 14.3	7.5		9.5	Longitudinal-150° Transverse-360°
Toshiba	M					4-18	
	L						
	C						
	A						
	P,TV,BH						

	Type	Focal Area (mm²)	Focal Length (cm)	Steer?	Biopsy guide?	Probe covers?	User service?
Acoustic Imaging	C (13 probes)			Yes	Yes	Yes	N/A
	L (3 probes)			Yes	Yes	Yes	N/A
	C,TV			Yes	Yes	Yes	N/A
	C,TR			Yes	Yes	Yes	N/A
Acuson	L (5 probes)		Electronically variable including multiple zones		No	Yes	N/A
	P (7 probes)				Some probes	Yes	N/A
	P,TV,SH				Yes	Yes	N/A
	P,TR,SH (2 probes)				Yes	Yes	N/A
	L,TR,SH				Yes	Yes	N/A
ADR/ATL	L (4 probes)		0-5.5, 0-16, 0-20		Yes	Yes	N/A
	M (15 probes)		Many choices 1.5-13	No	Yes	Yes	Some types
	C (5 probes)			No	No	Yes	N/A
	P (3 probes)				Yes	Yes	N/A
	CW (4 probes)						N/A
	M,TV,SH (3 probes)		4.5 (3-6) 3.6 (2.6-5.4) 2.6 (0.75-4)	No	Yes	Yes	N/A
	P,TV,SH			Yes	Yes	Yes	N/A
Ausonics	M		6.2 (4.5-11)		Yes	Yes	No
	M		5.8 (4.1-12.7)		Yes	Yes	No
	M		6.6 (5.1-15)		Yes	Yes	No
	M		5.6 (4.2-10.5)		Yes	Yes	No
	M		3.6 (2-7.9)		Yes	Yes	No
	M		6.5 (4-10)		Yes	Yes	No
	M,TV,SH		3.6 (2-7.9)		Yes	Yes	No
	M,TR,SH,B		2.7 (1.7-4.5)	plus or minus 45°	Yes	Yes	No
Bruel & Kjaer	M (4 probes)				Yes		
	M,TV,SH				Yes		
	M,TR,SH				Yes		
Corometrics Aloka	L (7 probes)						
	C (7 probes)						
	M (10 probes)						
	P,TV,BH		Electronic focus		Yes		
	P,TV,BH				Yes		
	P,TV,BH				Yes		
	P-L,TR,SH (2 probes)				Yes		

	Type	Focal Area (mm²)	Focal Length (cm)	Steer?	Biopsy guide?	Probe covers?	User service?
Diasonics	L (2 probes)		Multiple focal zones		Yes		
	P (2 probes)				Yes		
	C (2 probes)				Yes		
	M,TV,SH (2 probes)		1-5	+ or - 110°	Yes		
	M,TR,SH		1-5		Yes		
	Interventional catheter				Yes		
Dynamic Imaging	L (5 probes)		Dynamic		Yes		
	C (5 probes)		Dynamic				
	A (2 probes)		Dynamic	Yes			
	M (5 probes)		4,8	Yes			
	M,TV,SH		4	Yes through 180°			
	M,TR,SH		4	Yes			
Elscint	L		Electronic variable				
	M (4 probes)		3-8	Yes	Yes	Yes	Yes
	M Duplex Doppler		3		No	No	
	M,TV,SH		3	Yes	Yes	Yes	Yes
	M,TR,SH		2.5	Yes, also steerable plane of scan	Yes, 2 types	Yes	Yes
GE Medical Systems	L (5 probes)						
	P (3 probes)						
	C (3 probes)						
	P,TV,BH (2 probes)				Yes		
Hitachi	L (7 probes)		4 focal zones, electronically adjustable		Yes	Yes	N/A
	C (6 probes)				Yes	Yes	N/A
	L-C,TR,SH				Yes	Yes	N/A
	C,TV,BH				Yes	Yes	N/A
	C,TV,B				Yes	Yes	N/A
	C,TV,held on finger						N/A
Kretz	M (3 probes)		2.4,6.5	No	Yes	Yes	No
	M,TV,SH (2 probes)		2,3	No	Yes	Yes	No
	M,TR,SH		2,3	No	Yes	Yes	No
Omron	L (2 probes)						
OTE Biomedica	M,A (4 probes)						
Oxford Vasoflo 4	Pencil CW (2 probes)		2.5-2.8,0.8-1.2	N/A	N/A		
	Pencil pulsed			N/A	N/A		
	Flat		0.6-1.0	N/A	N/A		
	TV,SH		2.5-3.0	N/A	N/A		
Philips	L (4 probes)		Variable, up to 12 zones under software control	N/A	Yes	Yes	No
	C (9 probes)			No	Yes	Yes	No
	P,TV,SH (2 probes)			No	Yes	Yes	No
	P,TR			No	Yes	Yes	No
Pie Medical 150	M	5.1	3.2	Yes, 75°	Yes	Yes	Yes
150	M	2.7	2.5	Yes, 75°	Yes	Yes	Yes
150	M,TV,SH	1.4	2.5	Yes, 75°	Yes	Yes	Yes
1120B	L	4.3	5.1	No	Yes	Yes	Yes
1120B	L	3.0	3.6	No	Yes	Yes	Yes
1120B	L	1.4	2.7	No	Yes	Yes	Yes

	Type	Focal Area (mm²)	Focal Length (cm)	Steer?	Biopsy guide?	Probe covers?	User service?
Pie Medical 1120B, 1150	P,A	1.8	2.7	No	Yes	Yes	Yes
1120B,1150	P,A	1.5	2.6	No	Yes	Yes	Yes
1120B,1150	P,A,TV,SH	2.7	2.4	No	Yes	Yes	Yes
1150	L	4.8	5.8	No	Yes	Yes	Yes
1150	L	2.4	3.5	No	Yes	Yes	Yes
1150	L	1.1	2.0	No	Yes	Yes	Yes
1150	C	6.7	5.4	No	Yes	Yes	Yes
1150	C	2.8	3.3	No	Yes	Yes	Yes
Quantum	L (2 probes)		All dynamically focused	No	No	Yes (CIVCO Medical Inst.)	No
	C (2 probes)			No	Yes (Fall, 1990)		No
	C,TV			No	No		No
Siemens	L (6 probes)		4.2-11.9				
	M (5 probes)		1.6-6.0				
	P (7 probes)						
	CW pencil						
	M,TV,SH			Yes through 220°	Yes	Yes	
Shimadzu SDL-32B	L (8 probes)		1-20 cm	N/A	Some types		N/A
SDL-310	L (7 probes)		1-22 cm	N/A	Some types	Yes	N/A
SDL-310	C (4 probes)		1-22 cm	N/A	N/A	Yes	N/A
SDL-310	C,TV		1-17 cm	Yes	Yes	Yes	N/A
SDL-310	L,TR		1-17 cm	N/A	Yes	Yes	N/A
SDU-500	L (10 probes)		1-22 cm	N/A	Some types	Some types	N/A
SDU-500	C (3 probes)		1-22 cm	Yes	Some types	Some types	N/A
SDU-500	P (3 probes)		1-22 cm	Yes	Yes	Yes	N/A
SDU-500	C,TV (avail. 11-90)		1-17 cm	Yes	Yes	Yes	N/A
Teknar Proscan	M		6-12	No	Yes	Yes	No
	M,TR,SH,B		1.6-4.1	No	Yes	Yes	No
Toshiba	M			No	No	Yes	No
	L			No	No	Yes	
	C			No	No	Yes	
	A			No	No	Yes	
	TV			No	Yes	Yes	No

	Type	Power (SPTA mW/cm²)	Modes	Resolution mm A-axial L-lateral	Contrast resolution	Penetration depth (cm)
Acoustic Imaging	C (13 probes)	1.7 to 58.5	All modes, all probes, simultaneous images available		128 gray levels	3.5 MHz: 17 5.0 MHz: 14 7.5 MHz: 8
	L (3 probes)					
	C,TV					
	C,TR					
Acuson	L (5 probes)	B:2-15 M:21-67 Doppler:32-718	All modes, all probes, simultaneous images available		128 gray levels	24
	P (7 probes)	B:2-29 M:6-66 Doppler:13-713				24
	P,TV,SH	B:5 M:13-39 Doppler:50-140				14 cm
	P,TR,SH (2 probes)	B:9-14 M:12-37 Doppler:36-424				10
	L,TR,SH	B:6 Doppler:29-402				10

54   D. PEISNER

	Type	Power (SPTA mW/cm²)	Modes	Resolution mm A-axial L-lateral	Contrast resolution	Penetration depth (cm)
ADR/ATL	L (4 probes)	Varies (listed in manual)	M-mode	Varies	Models 4&5:	Differs with probes and systems
	M (15 probes)		M-mode, Doppler	Varies	64 gray levels	
	C (5 probes)		M-mode, Doppler, Color	Varies		
	P (3 probes)					
	CW (4 probes)					
	M,TV,SH (3 probes)	Varies (listed in manual)		A-0.5 to 1.2 L- <2 to 3	Model 9: 256 gray levels	
	P,TV,SH		M-mode, Doppler, Color	A-0.5 L-1.5		
Ausonics	M	B:59 M:135	All modes	A-1.05 L-2.24		15
	M	B:66 M:144	All modes	A-1.0 L-2.2		13
	M	B:112 M:197	All modes	A-0.75 L-1.92		13.5
	M	B:37 M:85	All modes	A-0.7 L-1.6		11
	M	B:19 M:48	All modes	A-0.45 L-1.4		6
	M	B:17 M:48	All modes	A-0.45 L-1.3		6
	M,TV,SH	B:19 M:48	All modes	A-0.45 L-1.4		6
	M,TR,SH,B	Long B:44 M:33 Transv B:22 M:51	All modes	A-0.3 L-0.85		6
Bruel & Kjaer	M (4 probes)					
	M,TV,SH					
	M,TR,SH					
Corometrics Aloka	L (7 probes)	B: 1.2-7 M: 34-57 Doppler: 210-280			Models 620, 633: 64 gray levels	
	C (7 probes)	B: 1.2-17 M: 43-91 Doppler: 25-290			Models 650, 680: 256 gray levels	
	M (10 probes)	B: 1.2-4.6 M: 43-91 Doppler: 37-490				
	P,TV,BH			A-0.5, L-1.7		
	P,TV,BH					
	P,TV,BH					
	P-L,TR,SH (2 probes)					
Diasonics	L (2 probes)			A-0.6,0.9 L-1.4,1.5		14,20 cm
	P (2 probes)			A-0.6,0.9 L-1.1,1.4		18,23 cm
	C (2 probes)			A-0.45,0.9 L-0.4,1.5		8,20 cm
	M,TV,SH (2 probes)			A-0.4,0.45 L-0.7,1.0		10,11 cm
	M,TR,SH			A-0.45 L-1.0		11 cm
	Interventional catheter					
Dynamic Imaging	L (5 probes)					13.2, 22
	C (5 probes)					11.8,12.6,20.9
	A (2 probes)					
	M (5 probes)					
	M,TV,SH					
	M,TR,SH					
Elscint	L				64 gray levels	18
	M (4 probes)		All modes, simultaneous images available	6.5: A-0.8 L-3.0 10: A-0.5 L-2.0	64 gray levels	4-18
	M Duplex Doppler			A-0.5 L-2.0	64 gray levels	4
	M,TV,SH			A-0.8 L-3	64 gray levels	8
	M,TR,SH		All modes	A-0.3 L-1.0	64 gray levels	7
GE Medical Systems	L (5 probes)		All modes	A-0.3 L-1.0	64 gray levels	12
	P (3 probes)					
	C (3 probes)					
	P,TV,BH (2 probes)					
Hitachi	L (7 probes)	All within FDA limits	All modes, all probes (not all machines accept all probes, not all machines have all features)	N/A	N/A	3.5 MHz: 20.8 5.0 MHz: 13.8 7.5 MHz: 11.1
	C (6 probes)			N/A	N/A	

	Type	Power (SPTA mW/cm²)	Modes	Resolution mm A-axial L-lateral	Contrast resolution	Penetration depth (cm)
Hitachi	L-C,TR,SH			N/A	N/A	
	C,TV,BH			N/A	N/A	
	C,TV,B			N/A	N/A	
	C,TV,held on finger			N/A	N/A	
Kretz	M (3 probes)	18.7	All modes		64 gray levels	
	M,TV,SH (2 probes)	0.46, 63.8	All modes	A- <1 L- <1		
	M,TR,SH	0.46	All modes	A-0.5 L- <0.8		
Omron	L (2 probes)		All modes			
OTE Biomedica	M,A (4 probes)					
Oxford Vasoflo 4	Pencil CW (2 probes)	40-260	N/A	N/A	N/A	Depends on tissue, signal, etc
	Pencil pulsed	25-1400	N/A	N/A	N/A	
	Flat		N/A	N/A	N/A	
	TV,SH		N/A	N/A	N/A	
Philips	L (4 probes)	"Within FDA guidelines for all probes, modes, and applications"	All modes, all probes with many simultaneous options	Not specified by company		3.5 MHz: 24 5.0 MHz: 18 7.5 MHz: 14
	C (9 probes)					
	P,TV,SH (2 probes)					
	P,TR					
Pie Medical 150	M	B:<27 M:146	M-mode	A-1.2; L-1.5	64 gray levels	20
150	M	B:<7.7 M:54	M-mode	A-0.9; L-1.0	64 gray levels	16
150	M,TV,SH	B:<14 M:180	M-mode	A-0.9; L-0.8	64 gray levels	12
1120B	L	B:<0.28 M:2.6	M-mode, Doppler	A-1.2; L-1.5	256 gray levels	20
1120B	L	B:<1.17 M:5.1	M-mode, Doppler		256 gray levels	16
1120B	L	B:<0.91 M:4.5	M-mode, Doppler		256 gray levels	7
1120B, 1150	P,A	B:<11 M:101	M-mode, Doppler	A-1.2; L-1.0	256 gray levels	20
1120B, 1150	P,A	B:<5.8 M:84	M-mode, Doppler		256 gray levels	16
1120B, 1150	P,A,TV,SH	B:<6.5 M:37	M-mode, Doppler		256 gray levels	12
1150	L	B:3.5 M:74	M-mode, Color Doppler		256 gray levels	20
1150	L	B:8.4 M:153	M-mode, Color Doppler		256 gray levels	16
1150	L	B:2.4 M:48.2	M-mode, Color Doppler		256 gray levels	7
1150	C	B:2.1 M:50	M-mode, Color Doppler		256 gray levels	20
1150	C	B:4.2 M:101	M-mode, Color Doppler		256 gray levels	16
Quantum	L (2 probes)	All preset values below 100 mW/sq cm SPTA value written on screen	All modes, all probes, simultaneous images available	Proprietary	120 gray levels	8,10
	C (3 probes)					14,15,20
	C,TV					9
Siemens	L (6 probes)				256 gray levels	
	M (5 probes)					
	P (7 probes)					
	CW pencil					
	M,TV,SH					
Shimadzu SDL-32B	L (8 probes)		All modes	A-1, L-2	32 gray levels	20
SDL-310	L (7 probes)	0.4 - 15.7	All modes	A-1, L-2	32 gray levels	22
SDL-310	C (4 probes)	0.3 - 4.7	All modes	A-1, L-2		22
SDL-310	C,TV	0.8 - 3.5	All modes	A-1, L-2		17
SDL-310	L,TR	0.7 - 3.0	All modes	A-1, L-2		17
SDU-500	L (10 probes)	2.2 - 318	All modes	A-1, L-2	64 gray levels	22
SDU-500	C (3 probes)	0.5 - 108.6	All modes	A-1, L-2		22
SDU-500	P (3 probes)	2.8 - 671	All modes	A-1, L-2		22
SDU-500	C,TV (avail. 11-90)		All modes	A-1, L-2		17
Teknar Proscan	M			A-1.2 L-2.0	128 gray levels	
	M,TR,SH,B	B:18 M:296		A-1.0 L-1.0		
Toshiba	M					
	L					
	C					
	A					
	TV					

FINANCIAL CONSIDERATIONS

	Machine cost (x $1000)	Quantity discount?	Warranty	Upgrade possibilities	Maintenance
Acoustic Imaging	100-150	Yes	1 year (extended 1 year if machine is down at any time during first year)	Yes	5-10%
Acuson	100-350	No	1 year	Fully upgradeable	5.5-10%, many plans, 99% uptime guarantee
ADR/ATL Ultramark 4A	20-30	Yes	1 year	Many possibilities, all machines	Variable, all machines
Ultramark 4 Plus	35-50	Yes	1 year		
Ultramark 5	45-90	Yes	1 year		
Ultramark 9	150-225	Yes	1 year		
Ausonics	15-25	Yes	1 year	Hardware modules; software	About 10% of machine cost; separate probe plans
Bruel & Kjaer 1849					
1846					
Corometrics 210 Aloka	8-15	Yes			
620	30-45	Yes	99% uptime guaranteed		Available
633	40-65	Yes			Available
650	80-120	Yes			Available
680	150-170	Yes		Available	Available
725		Yes		Available	Available
870		Yes		Available	Available
Diasonics SPA1000					
DRF800					
Spectra				Software upgrades on floppy disks	
Interventional					
Dynamic Imaging Concept 500/1000	10-12	Yes	1 year	C500 to C1000	
Concept 2000	15-30	Yes	1 year	Yes	
Elscint ESI1000	30-50	Yes	1 year	Software and most hardware	10% of system cost, separate probe plan
ESI2000	45-60	Yes	1 year	Software and most hardware	
GE Medical Systems RT3200			1 year		Available
RT4000			1 year		Available
Radius			1 year		Available
Sonochrome			1 year		Available
Hitachi EUB-200	11-24	Yes	1 year	No	Available
EUB-310	18-30	Yes	1 year	Software	Available
EUB-410	35-50	Yes	1 year	Software	Available
EUB-450	65-120	Yes	1 year	Doppler, ECG, etc	Available
EUB-515	110-150	Yes	1 year	Doppler, color, etc	Available
Kretz Combison 310	30	Yes	1 year	Software	Available for machine and/or probes
Omron					
OTE Biomedica					
Oxford Vasoflo 4	13.7	Negotiable	1 year	Pulsed Doppler, software upgrades	10% of purchase price
Philips Orion					
Platinum	Not specified by company	Not specified by company	1 year, 99% uptime guaranteed	Hardware and software	Handled by local offices
SDR 1550					
Pie Medical 150		Yes	1 year	SmartCard exchange	About 8% of machine; 5% of probes
1120B		Yes	1 year		About 8% of machine; 5% of probes
1150		Yes	1 year	SmartCard exchange	About 8% of machine; 5% of probes
Quantum 2000	175-225	Yes	1 year	Yes	About 8%

	Machine cost (x $1000)	Quantity discount?	Warranty	Upgrade possibilities	Maintenance
Siemens SL-1				Upgradeable software	
CF					
Shimadzu SDL-32B			1 year	Yes	N/A
SDL-310			1 year	Yes	Available
SDU-500			1 year	Yes	Available
Teknar Proscan	40-50	Yes	1 year	Hardware, Software	Various plans - 5-10% of machine cost
Toshiba SSA-250A	110-150	Yes		Software only	6-7%
SSA-270A	115-200	Yes		Software only	6-7%

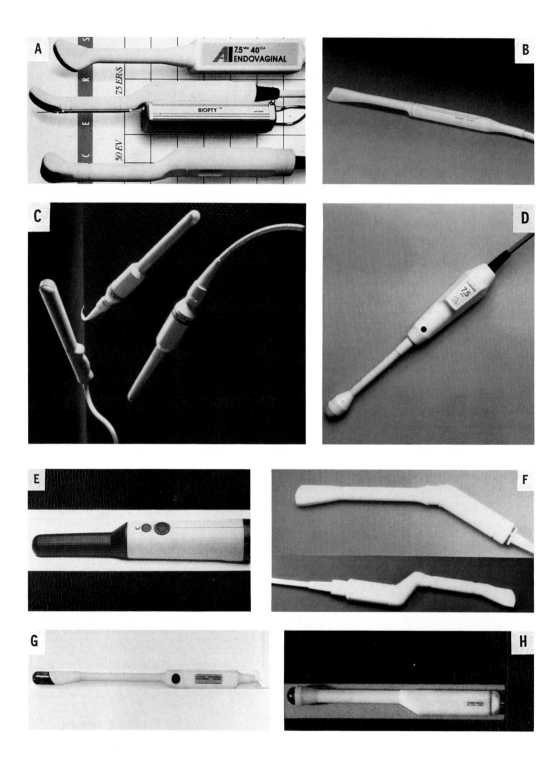

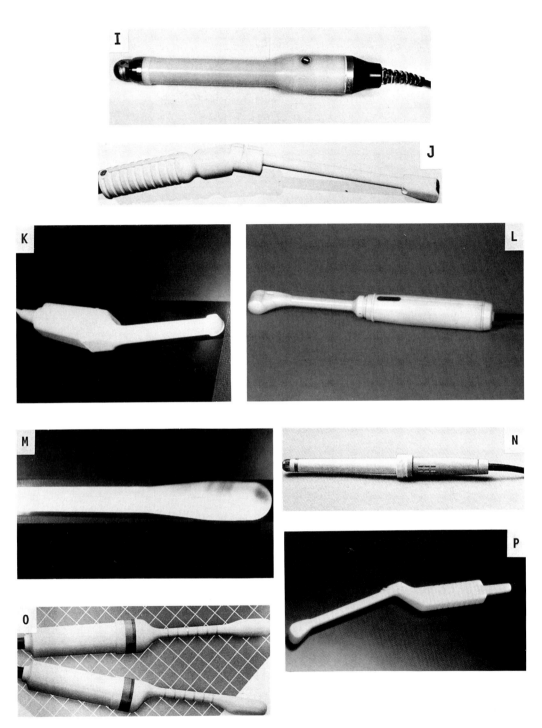

Figure 2.4 Photographs of the transvaginal transducer probes are listed in alphabetical order: A—Acoustic Imaging, B—Acuson, C—ATL/ADR, D—Ausonics, E—Bruel & Kjaer, F—Corometrics (Aloka), G—Diasonics, H—Dynamic Imaging, I—Elscint, J—General Electric, K—Hitachi, L—Kretz, M—Phillips, N—Pie Medical, O—Siemens, P—Toshiba.

CHAPTER **3**

The Technique of Transvaginal Sonography

Etan Z. Zimmer, MD
Ilan E. Timor-Tritsch, MD
Shraga Rottem, MD

INTRODUCTION

The introduction of the transvaginal scanning technique resulted in some confusion, since the relationship between the observer, the beam path, and the anatomy are altered when compared with the traditional transabdominal scanning technique. However, the technique will appear natural to those who are accustomed to a bimanual gynecologic examination. As a systematic approach to the scanning technique develops, the examination becomes much easier to perform. The user can achieve a confident level of skill within a short period of time, and as the results are so rewarding, even the novice will maintain interest and continue its use.

The aim of this chapter is to equip the transvaginal sonographer with the necessary information for obtaining the best results when using this technique.

THE EXAMINATION TABLE

For most of the scanning procedures, utilizing an ''in-line'' transducer probe (a probe that has an end-firing scanhead with its shaft and handle on the same axis), a flat ultrasound examining table is appropriate. If a probe with an angle between the shaft and the handle is used, a gynecological examination table is required. The elevated thighs enable free movement of the probe in the horizontal plane by the operator. All surgical procedures performed by vaginal approach require a gynecological examination table with popliteal support. If a regular flat examination table is used, a special 15–20 cm thick foam cushion should be inserted below the pelvis after the head and upper body of the patient are elevated. This cushion allows free movement of the examiner's hand in tilting the transducer probe in the vertical plane to achieve maximum angling.

It is important to avoid placing the patient in the Trendelenburg position (pelvis elevated and upper body too low) since the minimal amount of pelvic fluid that is often present in the normal exam can help in outlining pelvic organs and, most importantly, the tubes. For this reason, we encourage the use of a slightly reversed Trendelenburg position during examination.

61

PREPARATION OF THE PATIENT FOR THE EXAMINATION

Empty or Full Bladder?

The first and perhaps most important *prerequisite* for transvaginal sonographic examination should be a thorough and *complete emptying of the urinary bladder*, for three reasons: (1) a full bladder may "occupy" most of the pelvis and also the screen, displacing important "target organs" to be scanned; (2) sound waves passing through a bladder filled with a low-impedance fluid creates the well-known effect of enhancement (this high-echo area below the bladder interferes with a proper gain setting); (3) a full bladder distorts pelvic anatomy by compressing pelvic organs in addition to displacing possible ovarian or tubal pathology beyond the reach of the transducer.

In many laboratories, if the patient is seen for the first time, transabdominal scanning is first performed; requiring a full bladder. This prevents the need of filling the bladder at a later stage in those cases where an unsatisfactory transvaginal image is obtained, and a transabdominal scan is considered necessary.

However, an experienced observer who knows how to handle the vaginal transducer probe, and to use his other hand to manipulate the position of the pelvic organs, will find the vaginal technique sufficient in most cases.

In a patient presenting with a full bladder and scanned for a suspected ectopic gestation, transabdominal should precede transvaginal scanning and the patient should not be allowed to drink at all.

Minimal distension of the bladder might be useful on two occasions: (1) patients with a severely anteflexed uterus—in order to "straighten them out" relative to the imaging plane; (2) imaging of a low-lying placenta or placenta previa. In this case, the bladder will help in outlining the anterior lip of the cervix and the internal os.

Pelvic Examination

A thorough bimanual pelvic examination provides the gynecologist with additional valuable information. This examination should, therefore, precede the transvaginal ultrasound examination. A pelvic examination may be performed any time the sonographer has trouble understanding the ultrasonographic image or if a discrepancy exists between the obtained image and the expected diagnosis.

Patient Information

A short explanation of the procedure will prevent patient anxiety. Most patients do not associate ultrasound scanning with a vaginal examination; therefore, it is necessary to inform the patient about this relatively "new way" of performing the sonographic examination. One should mention the similarity between the vaginal transducer and the familiar vaginal speculum or a Pap test the patient has experienced before.

The patient should be reassured that the probe is smaller than most specula and is only inserted a short distance. Thus, it should cause less discomfort than an internal examination. Some laboratories permit the patient to place the tip of the probe in the vagina themselves.

THE EQUIPMENT AND THE TRANSDUCER

The ultrasound equipment should be programmed before the transducer probe is introduced into the vagina.

The patient's identification data, last menstrual period, and other important observations should be typed in through the keyboard. Permanent recording devices, such as multiformat cameras, VCRs, and printers should be switched to "standby" position. A foot-pedal switch for freezing the screen and taking hard copies of the image should be available since in most patients, the operator will use both hands for manipulation of the probe and scanned organ. These preparations will reduce the actual examination time.

The transducer tip is then *covered* with ultrasound coupling gel and introduced into a protective rubber sheet. Care should be taken to avoid trapping any air bubbles, which create unwanted artifacts on the screen. The probe should be covered with either a commercially available probe cover, or with a plain surgical rubber glove using one of the digits. A condom can also be employed, but there are two possible disadvantages: first, condoms may break because they are too thin; second, some condoms contain a spermicidal or embryocidal material and are not to be used in exams of infertility patients.[1] A small amount of *coupling gel* or any lubricating gel can be applied to the outside of the probe before insertion into the vagina.

However, Schwimmer et al[2] have recommended caution in employing the commonly used ultrasound coupling gels for vaginal transducer lubrication in patients who will undergo insemination immediately after transvaginal examination. Some of the most commonly used coupling gels were found to adversely affect sperm motility.

At or close to midcycle, when this may become relevant, the cervix ordinarily produces enough mucus to enable a good sound coupling between the transducer probe and the vaginal vault. It is, therefore, technically feasible to perform a vaginal scan at midcycle without artificially lubricating the tip of the probe.

The microorganisms that cause sexually transmittable diseases may be transferred with medical instruments. Therefore, the possibility of *cross infection* should be a major concern since the transducer is used within the vagina. In addition to the use of probe covers, the probe should be disinfected after each examination.[1] While a *disinfectant* may be safe for some transducers, it may be destructive to others, and probe manufacturers should provide information about safe and effective cleaning and disinfecting. Some disinfectant solutions have the ability to disinfect within 10 min, thus enabling more frequent use of the transducers. If at the end of an examination the probe is immersed in a disinfectant solution, by the time the report is written and the next patient has been prepared, the probe will be disinfected. A variety of disinfectants are available, and their bactericidal and virucidal effects have been discussed by Odwin et al[1] and are presented in Table 3.1. If the patient is known to have an infectious disease, double protective sheets may be used. The examiner should always wear gloves during the examination.

TABLE 3.1 High-Level Disinfectant Products

Manufacturer	Brand Name	Effect on Microorganisms
Sporicidin International	Sporicidin disinfectant spray* Sporicidin disinfectant solution* Sporidicin towelettes*	Herpes 1 and 2, polio 1 and 2, Coxsackie virus B-1, Cytomegalovirus, Rotavirus, HIV-1, Influenza A2 parovirus, vaccinia, Bacillus subtilis, Clostridum sporogenes
Central Solutions Inc.	Pheno-Cen disinfectant spray*	Salmonella choleraesuis. Trichophytom mentagrophytes, Staphylococcus aureus, Pseudomonas aeruginosa, HIV-1.
Surgikos, Inc.	Cidex Plus disinfectant solution* Cidex disinfectant solution*	Herpes 1 and 2, HIV-1, Cytomegalovirus, adenovirus type 2, poliovirus type 1, rhinovirus, Coxsackievirus B1, B subtilis, C sporogenes.
Metrex Research Corporation	MetriCide 29 disinfectant solution* MetriCide disinfectant solution*	Herpes 1 and 2, HIV-1, Cytomegalovirus, rhinovirus vaccinia, adenovirus, T mentagrophytes, Mycobacterium bovis, S aureus, S choleraesuis.

* Registered with the EPA as an inactivator of HIV-1 (AIDS virus).

After: Odwin CS et al. Probe covers and disinfectants for transvaginal transducers. J Diagn Med Sonograph 1990;6:130–135.

SCANNING TECHNIQUE

To obtain images in varying directions, planes, and depths, the following maneuvers can be employed:

1. *tilting* or angling the shaft by its handle so as to point the tip of the probe to any direction in the pelvis;
2. *pushing-pulling* the whole probe to bring a deeper or closer organ into the focal region or actually into the focal length;
3. *rotating* the handle slowly along the longitudinal axis of the probe to change the scanning plane along a 360° range.

Figures 3.1**A**–3.1**C** illustrate the above-discussed scanning planes and directions achieved by the examiner.

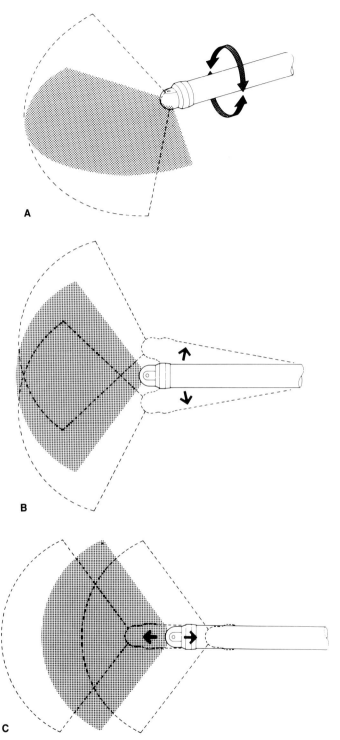

Figure 3.1 Basic scanning directions, planes, and depths achieved by moving the probe. Any combination of the following may be used to obtain the best possible image: (**A**) rotating the probe along its longitudinal axis; (**B**) angling the shaft, pointing it in any desired direction; (**C**) pushing or pulling the probe, ''positioning'' deeper or closer structures within the focal range of the transducer.

"Combined" Manual Help and TVS:

1. The examiner should place the other hand on the lower abdomen to bring pelvic structures closer to the tip of the probe, as in a regular bimanual pelvic–abdominal scan.

2. In the case of *pelvic pain*, localization of the point of maximal intensity under direct vision and gentle pressure with the tip of the transducer probe may be attempted.

3. *Diagnosis of pelvic adhesions* or adherence of different organs becomes possible by the *sliding organs sign*: The transducer tip is pointed at the uterus, ovaries, or any pelvic finding (eg, ovarian mass, tubo-ovarian complex) and a gentle push-pull movement of several centimeters is begun. If no adhesions are present, the organs will move freely in the pelvis. This displacement of organs is perceived on the screen as a sliding movement. One may, for instance, observe the free sliding of an ovarian mass over the lateral wall of the pelvis which, of course, is static. In the case of a tubo-ovarian complex, the relative locations of the uterus, tube, and ovary will not change under the pushing motion of the probe, because of extensive adhesions preventing normal and physiological sliding of these organs. If the patient is being scanned to help diagnose pelvic pain it is possible to probe each of the pelvic organs if they are painful. If, during bimanual pelvic–abdominal examination, a palpable finding is obvious, one may perform a one-finger vaginal examination and introduce the probe along this finger, directing it to the finding in question. This makes palpable findings instantly "visible." Some probes are sufficiently thin to enable this combined mode of examination.

Sometimes the region of interest is very close to the transducer; thus, "noise-ridden," and unclear pictures appear on the screen. This is more prevalent with mechanical sector scanners which are known to produce "noise" in the near field. Probes using electronic scanning create a better near field image. In a case of "noise," the transducer should be pulled outward 1 or 2 cm until the picture clears. This procedure may help when the cervix is examined. If the far end of the picture is blurred, the transducer is pushed gently into the vagina until a "sharper" picture is obtained. Both maneuvers are based on bringing the region of interest into the focal area of the transducer.

In addition to these manual manipulations of the probe, the symmetrical end-firing "fan" of the beam in some ultrasound machines can be steered in an off-axis scanning direction by the appropriate electronic controls. Thus, scanning of the whole pelvis is possible. In other machines the scanning plane can be changed without angling the probe. Most transvaginal transducer probes utilize a symmetrical end-firing probe with various scanning angles from 90° to 240°. Other probes use a built-in, fixed upward tilt of the scanning plane in addition to a second angle between the handle and the shaft carrying the transducer itself. Probes with electronically or mechanically steered scanning directions or planes have a distinct advantage over the fixed off-axis firing or "broken-handle" probes. The latter usually requires switching the picture orientation on the screen since angling these probes may require a 180° rotation to enable their pointing in the required direction. (The properties, specification, and possibilities of the different transducers should always be examined in advance by the potential buyer.)

To end the scanning, the probe should be pulled out slowly from the vagina while constantly observing the screen. New and heretofore undetected findings may be revealed.

Reminder

The effective focal zone of the 6.5 MHz transducer ends at 7–8 cm. Structures deeper than 8 cm may be diagnosed, but they appear "blurred" and are irregularly outlined. A fairly large mass may be missed by vaginal scanning if, because of its size, it does not extend deep enough into the pelvis. If a pelvic mass has to be ruled out or is suspected, a 5.0 MHz vaginal probe should be used or an additional transabdominal scan should be performed.

The Scanning Routine

It is suggested that a relatively strict scanning routine should be followed. The "natural" plan of scanning we found useful is:

1. In the beginning, as the probe advances, scan the *cervix*, at least passingly.
2. The *uterus* should be found and evaluated. At this point the *cervix* should be included.
3. If the patient is pregnant, study the *gestation*.
4. Go to the *adnexa*, study the ovaries and tubes (if feasible), and look for possible masses.
5. One of the most important places to scrutinize is the *cul-de-sac*.
6. Other places, structures, and additional pathologies can now be addressed.

It is still important to use the largest possible magnification that still enables orientation as well as recognition of the organs or the pathology. Magnification does not alter the resolution using high-frequency probes.

Orientation

Orientation of transvaginal images is different from conventional transabdominal images as the vaginal scanning angle is initially perpendicular compared with the abdominal approach (Fig 3.2**A,B**).

In the United States, it is customary to standardize the image orientation for pelvic scans.

1. On a sagittal longitudinal plane, the filling bladder should appear on the upper left side of the screen with the cervix to the right side of the picture. If an anteverted uterus is scanned, the fundus of the uterus will appear on the lower left side of the screen.
2. On the cross-sectional (horizontal or coronal) plane, the patient's right side, ie, the right ovary, will appear on the left side of the screen, as if reading a coronal x-ray image.

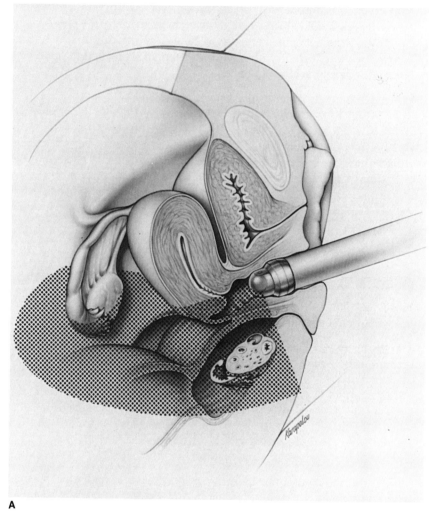

A

Figure 3.2 The anatomical relation to the transvaginally inserted probe and the pelvic organs demonstrates (**A**) the horizontal plane, and (**B**) the vertical, or sagittal, scanning plane.

Almost all machines offer left-right as well as upside-down "image-invert" switches. Some European countries, as well as individuals, feel that displaying the cervix on the lower part of the image, and the fundus on its upper part, seems more reasonable. The "apex-invert" switch can be activated, if desired.

It is of *utmost importance* to label each and every image taken or taped for easy evaluation.

Images obtained by transvaginal sonography do not generally correspond to the normal anatomical planes, since the vagina runs superiorly and posteriorly and the pelvis itself is tilted at an angle of 30° to the long axis of the body. Dodson and Deter[3] suggested that instead of referring to coronal, sagittal, or longitudinal images a terminology of TRANS pelvic plane and AP-plane should be used. A TRANS pelvic plane refers to a plane imaged when the sound beam is directed across or from side to side in the pelvis. An AP-plane refers to an image obtained when the sound beam is directed anteriorly and posteriorly.

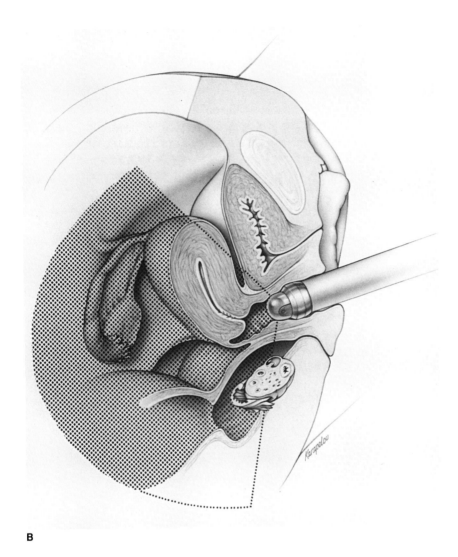

B

A different approach to orientation is to focus on target organs rather than anatomic pelvic planes.[4] This is called ''organ-oriented'' scanning. The main reasons for this new concept are as follows:

1. There is a very short distance between the high-frequency vaginal probe and the scanned area. A close-up image is generated, encompassing a single organ or only part of it.
2. The angle between the probe and the pelvic organs is being continually changed during the examination at the operator's convenience.
3. A 360° rotation is applicable in using the transvaginal probe.

The organ-oriented transvaginal scanning can be considered as a modified bimanual examination providing a detailed image of the organ on the screen. Using this technique the sonographer will search for every specific organ as the main target. Therefore it is practical to address the longitudinal axis of the uterus (or any other organ) specifically, instead of the orientation of the scanning plane to the pelvic coordinates.

THE EXAMINATION

Cervix

The cervix is the first structure on the path of the vaginal probe to its final place of scanning, the pelvis. If the cervix has to be scanned, it may be done as the probe penetrates 2.5–3 cm into the vagina, 2–3 cm before the tip of the probe reaches the cervix itself. This prevents the picture from being obscured by air that may be trapped in the fornices at the end of a prolonged or repeated examination. The cervix may also be examined after locating the uterus and then pulling the probe slowly outward. A horizontal and vertical plane in which the central structure to be imaged is the cervical canal should always be obtained.

The mucus within the endocervical canal usually appears as an echogenic interface. This may become hypoechoic during the periovulatory period as the cervical mucus has a higher fluid content.[5] The uterine vessels can be seen as punctate anechoic structures at the level of the internal cervical os. Cystic structures adjacent to the cervical canal and external os are frequently seen. They represent endocervical cysts and Nabothian cysts.

Nomograms of cervical length throughout pregnancy have been established.[6] An accurate measurement of cervical length may be important as it could improve the risk assessment for preterm labor and delivery.

Cervical pregnancy should always be kept in mind and sought if ectopic pregnancy is suggested. Scanning of the cervix during pregnancy is primarily for ruling out cervical incompetence and placenta previa. Experience reveals that transvaginal sonography might be useful in early recognition and staging of cervical malignancy.

Uterus

The most prominent landmark in the pelvis is usually the uterus. If the uterus is detected on the screen the routine examination should start systematic scanning. The scanning should go from the back to the front using the horizontal plane first. If the uterus is anteverted and anteflexed, the first cross section to be seen is the cervix. A slow upward scan will reveal the body and, finally, the fundus of the uterus. With the same sequence (scanning from the back to the front) in a retroverted uterus, the fundus is imaged first and the cervix last. The transverse or horizontal scan should be followed by the vertical scanning plane, which will reveal the entire uterus with its endometrial lining. The endometrium has a variety of appearances depending on its stage of development.[5] In the proliferative phase the endometrium tends to measure 4–8 mm in AP dimension. This measurement includes both endometrial layers combined. In the periovulatory phase the endometrium is multilayered, measuring 6–10 mm. The secretory phase has the thickest endometrium, usually measuring 7–14 mm.

In postmenopause, the uterus becomes gradually smaller and usually loses its anteversion and anteflexion. It has a uniform echogenicity with an extremely thin endometrial lining, which is hard to differentiate from the myometrium. In some patients a sonolucent area can be seen in the uterine cavity. It is possible that in these cases uterine secretions have accumulated as a result of variable degrees of cervical stenosis.

Scanning of the lateral uterine margin on either side may reveal the ingoing, outgoing, and pulsating vascular packets at the level of the junction between the cervix and the body of the uterus. Blood flow is readily seen in these vessels with the high-frequency transducer. Blood flow measurements of the uterine artery and vein may be done using this site.

A high proportion of women who have an intrauterine device have various symptoms attributed to the device. With transvaginal sonography it is possible to locate the device and indicate whether it is in the uterine cavity, it has moved into the region of the lower uterus and upper cervix or it is embedded in the myometrium.

In cases where it is technically difficult to depict an enlarged uterus, the widest possible angle should be used. Another possibility is to use the "split-screen" technique, which consists of subsequent imaging of the sagittal sections of the uterine corpus on split screens. The total size of the uterus is obtained by adding up the measurements on the two screens. However, if the uterus seems to be excessively enlarged a transabdominal scanning should be added to enable a better examination.

Ovaries

In the premenopausal woman, the ovaries are usually imaged along the side of the uterus between the fundus uteri and iliac vessels. They are found in close proximity, lying in the area called "Waldeyer's Fossa." More rarely the ovary is found in the cul-de-sac or behind the uterus. If the ovary is not depicted in these places, the probe should be angled anteriorly while pushing the ipsilateral anterior abdominal wall with the free hand. This may bring down the ovary that is located higher than usual toward the focal zone of the transducer. The ovaries have a distinct appearance because of their relatively lower echogenic texture as well as the different-sized Graafian follicles. The follicles appear as echo-free, translucent, round structures from several millimeters to 2 cm in diameter. During the reproductive years, these follicles serve as sonographic "markers" of the ovaries. The uterine and iliac vessels should not be confused with follicles in the ovary. If there is any uncertainty as to the origin of a round cystic structure, a longitudinal plane should be imaged.

After menopause it is hard to find the ovaries because the above-described "markers" (ie, the follicles) are not present, the ovaries themselves atrophy and there is less pelvic fluid to provide an acoustic interface. With the recent introduction of color coded Doppler flow imaging, by finding the color coded flow of the ovarian artery or vein one can better detect the otherwise sonographically "nondetectable" ovaries.

As the ovaries are imaged the use of the abdominal hand, mentioned earlier, becomes even more important for manipulating the ovaries into the "scanning-sight" of the probe.

If the ovaries are imaged in the postmenopausal patient, this should be clearly mentioned in the sonographic report, and a workup of the case is advisable.

Fallopian Tubes

The normal fallopian tube is difficult to image because of its small size and serpiginous course. If found, they are usually lateral to the uterus behind the ovaries or in the cul-de-sac. They appear as 1 cm wide echogenic tortuous structures. Sonographic delineation of the tube is facilitated by intraperitoneal fluid present in the cul-de-sac. It is possible to enhance detection of the tube by selecting a midcycle day for the scan, because a large number of patients have increased pelvic fluid at that time. Placing the patient in a reverse-Trendelenburg position may be helpful as fluid can be collected in this region. When a large amount of fluid is present the tube may often be located in a higher position. In such a case the same maneuver as described for the high-positioned ovary should be used.

In some patients the flaring of the fimbriated end of the tube can be seen as it approximates its nearby ovary.

The pathologic tube is more easily recognized because the fluid, pus, or blood in the lumen or in the surrounding area facilitates the demonstration of typical lesions. If the tube is detected longitudinal and serial, cross sections should be made by rotating the probe around its longitudinal axis. The wall, luminal content, and possible adherence to the surroundings should be examined.

Cul-de-sac

The cul-de-sac, or pouch of Douglas, may be found by directing the probe posteriorly. In many cases a small amount of fluid may be present in this space under normal conditions. Free fluid outlines the posterior wall of the uterus and sometimes even the ovaries. As mentioned before, it is disadvantageous to place the patient in the Trendelenburg position since some of the fluid will spill from the pouch of Douglas to other lower-lying spaces. Because of the high resolution of the pictures, even a small amount of fluid in the cul-de-sac may impress the novice sonographer, leading to a false interpretation, namely ''a large fluid collection'' (Fig 3.3).

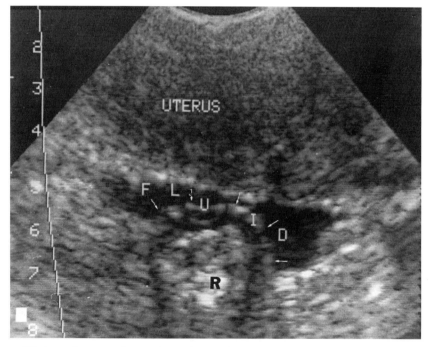

Figure 3.3 A small amount (approximately 5–8 mL) of pelvic fluid is present in the cul-de-sac, behind the uterus. A cross section of the rectum (R) and its peritoneal cover (arrows) is visible.

When a large amount of fluid is present, such as in ascites, the near field findings are clearly displayed. But the uterus and ovaries may be pushed beyond the focal length of the probe. Evaluation of the cul-de-sac for presence or absence of fluid, with or without blood clots, is important in the differential diagnosis of unruptured or ruptured ectopic pregnancy.

Pregnancy

One of the most valuable applications of transvaginal sonography is the early identification of a normal or abnormal pregnancy. On the average this technique can detect embryonic or fetal structures one to two weeks earlier than transabdominal sonography. Warren et al[7] documented the early stages of embryonic development starting at 4 wk of gestation.

The diagnosis of very early abnormal pregnancy is at times difficult. Keeping in mind the temporal appearance of embryonic and extraembryonic structures, one could evaluate the presence or absence of an abnormal pregnancy if the correct dating of pregnancy itself is known. When any doubt concerning the dating exists, serial ultrasound scans are appropriate for clinical follow-up.

Other Pelvic Structures

Iliac Vessels

The vein and artery are easily located by pointing the transducer tip to the side of the pelvis and searching for them in the transverse as well as the vertical plane. Blood flow is seen in the vein; the vein appears medially and closer to the pelvic organs than the common iliac artery, which lies in a lateral position, and pulsates passively, moving the adjacent vein. The internal iliac artery has a width of 5–7 mm and the vein is approximately 10 mm. These two large vessels are of great importance as the lateral landmarks of the pelvis during the sonographically guided removal of oocytes, since the ovaries are sometimes in very close proximity (even adherent) to the covering peritoneum. Color coded Doppler flow images of the pelvic vessels are expected to generate more information, which in turn may help in the accurate diagnosis of certain pathologies.

Bowel

At present no detailed studies have been published on the bowel examination with transvaginal ultrasound. However, the rectum, sigmoid colon, and terminal coils of the ileum can be seen. They usually demonstrate a sonolucent ring like muscularis and a fluid-filled or gas-containing central core. If there is peristalsis, the detection becomes an easy task. This is a usual occurrence in the small bowel. The large bowel moves more slowly; therefore, more time should be spent to observe its peristalsis. It is important to note that if static films are read they may confuse the reader.

Lower Urinary Tract

Scanning of the lower urinary tract (the bladder and the urethra) is a relatively new use of the vaginal probe. Thin probes have advantage over thicker ones by virtue of their not distorting the anatomy. The probe should only be partially introduced into the vagina. "Tilted" angle probes create a better field of view and are able to penetrate below the symphysis. Patients are usually scanned with a full as well as empty bladder and in a sitting position using a specially designed chair. More information can be found in Chapter 8.

Limitations of the Technique

Findings larger than 7 cm to 10 cm or those outside the pelvis are difficult to scan with the vaginal probe because of its limited focal length. Using the manual manipulation previously described may help in localizing these structures, which are "missed" by vaginal scanning. However, in patients with a large myomatous uterus, part of the finding may still be outside the focal zone of the transducer. Furthermore, the rigid bulky myomas may limit the operator's ability to maneuver the probe.

The patient with an intact hymen might present a problem. Detailed explanation, patience in manner, and gentle technique will be helpful in these patients. In elderly patients the vagina has less elasticity, and this limits the maneuverability of the probe. The novice operator may experience difficulties and feel the need to complete the evaluation with transabdominal sonography in some of these patients.

COLOR CODED DOPPLER FLOW STUDIES

This is a new technique to interrogate certain areas or pathological structures for the presence and/or the absence of blood flow. It seems to have become an increasingly used technique which is still under careful evaluation. Its use is described in Chapter 17.

PERINEAL SCANNING

Perineal scanning is a technique of ultrasonic imaging of the pelvis with a transducer placed on the perineum. The patient is examined in the same position employed in transvaginal scanning. Ultrasonic gel is applied on the perineum and the covered transducer is placed on it. Examination can be done with a minimally filled bladder. To enhance tissue differentiation the patient is asked to perform a Valsalva maneuver. This produces relative motion of different tissue layers and pelvic structures and facilitates their identification.[8] A linear array or sector scanner transducer can be used. At present, there are only a few studies reporting on this technique. Because of the limitation of the transducer's focal range it seems that an accurate image can be obtained only from the cervix, lower uterine segment, bladder, and urethra.

Perineal scanning can be of value in patients with imperforated hymen or agenesis of the vagina. It is also important in the study of stress incontinence.[9] This technique should also be used in cases of cervical incompetence, suspected cord presentation or placenta previa, where the transabdominal image previously obtained was inadequate, and where the patient refused vaginal scanning.

Documentation

All important and necessary findings should be documented by means of a video recorder, video printer, multiformat files camera, etc. The scanning plane, localization of the structure, and marking of the left and right side are crucial for later evaluation and reference.

REFERENCES

1. Odwin CS, Fleischer AC, Kepple DM, Chiang DT: Probe covers and disinfectants for transvaginal transducers. J Diagn Med Sonograph 1990;6:130–135.
2. Schwimmer SR, Rothman CM, Lebovic J, Oye DM: The effect of ultrasound coupling gels on sperm motility in vitro. Fertil Steril 1984;42:946–947.
3. Dodson MG, Deter RL: Definition of anatomical planes for use in transvaginal sonography. J Clin Ultrasound 1990;18:239–242.
4. Rottem S, Thaler I, Goldstein SR, Timor-Tritsch IE, Brandes JM: Transvaginal sonographic technique: targeted organ scanning without resorting to "planes." J Clin Ultrasound 1990;18:243–247.
5. Fleischer AC, Gordon AN, Entman SS, Kepple DM: Transvaginal sonography (TVS) of the endometrium: current and potential clinical applications. Crit Rev Diagn Imaging 1990;30:85–110.
6. Kushnir O, Viggil DA, Izquierdo L, Schiff M, Curet LB: Vaginal ultrasonographic assessment of cervical length changes during normal pregnancy. Am J Obstet Gynecol 1990;162:991–993.
7. Warren WB, Timor-Tritsch IE, Peisner D, Raju S, Rosen MG: Dating the early pregnancy by sequential appearance of embryonic structures. Am J Obstet Gynecol 1989;161:747–753.
8. Jeanty P, d'Alton M, Romero R, Hobbins JC: Perineal scanning. Am J Perinat 1986;3:289–295.
9. Kölbl H, Bernaschek G, Wolf G: A comparative study of perineal ultrasound scanning and urethrocystography in patients with genuine stress incontinence. Arch Gynecol Obstet 1988;244:39–45.

CHAPTER 4

Transvaginal versus Transabdominal Ultrasound

Marcia J. Lavery, RDMS
Carol B. Benson, MD

INTRODUCTION

With the development of high frequency transvaginal probes, high resolution images of organs in the pelvis can now be obtained. The transducer can be placed closer to the structures to be evaluated and, therefore, less penetration is required. Transducers with frequencies of up to 7.5 MHz are best for this sonographic examination. Transabdominal scanning (TAS) requires deeper penetration and, therefore, a lower frequency transducer, usually 3–5 MHz, must be used. This limits resolution.

For TAS a full urinary bladder is required to provide a window for imaging pelvic organs and to displace bowel gas. Transvaginal scans (TVS) should be performed with an empty urinary bladder, thus eliminating patient discomfort. The empty bladder is required to keep the organs within the focal zone of the transducer. Even a partially distended bladder can distort the pelvic anatomy or push the organs out of the field of view. Because TVS is performed with an empty urinary bladder, pelvic ultrasounds can be performed immediately, without the delay required by TAS studies for filling of the bladder.[1,2]

The TVS approach is advantageous in patients with large or unusual body habituses. In particular, obese patients, previously subject to limited evaluation transabdominally, can be examined with the same high resolution probes as non-obese women (Fig 4.1). Significant anterior abdominal wall scarring need not restrict evaluation of the pelvis, as the TVS probe may be used as an alternative approach. Distended air-filled loops of bowel can be bypassed by TVS scanning.[1]

As opposed to passive scanning transabdominally, the TVS probe can be used actively to enhance evaluation of a patient with pelvic symptoms. The tip of the probe can be used to locate sites of maximum tenderness. The diagnosis of pelvic adhesions can be suggested based on movement of pelvic structures in response to the pressure of the probe. Procedures can be facilitated by guidance with the TVS probe.[1] Overall, patient acceptance of TVS has been excellent.[1,3]

Studies comparing TVS to TAS show that the TVS provided as much diagnostic information or more diagnostic information than TAS in 96–99% of cases.[2,4,5] Imaging transvaginally was as good as or better than imaging transabdominally in 82–90% of cases.[5] The sonographic appearance of the pelvic organs and early intrauterine pregnancy by both approaches, TAS and TVS, will be discussed and compared below.

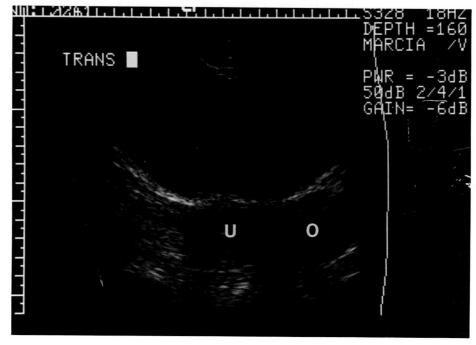

A

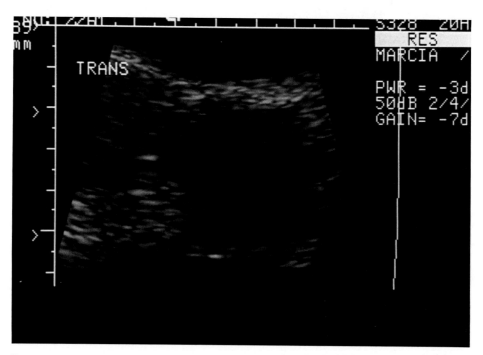

B

Figure 4.1 TAS versus TVS scan in obese women. (**A**) Transverse TAS image of pelvis showing indistinct uterus and left ovary. (**B**) On magnified view of left ovary, no individual follicles are identified. (**C**) TVS view of ovary demonstrating multiple small follicles and (**D**) one large, dominant follicle.

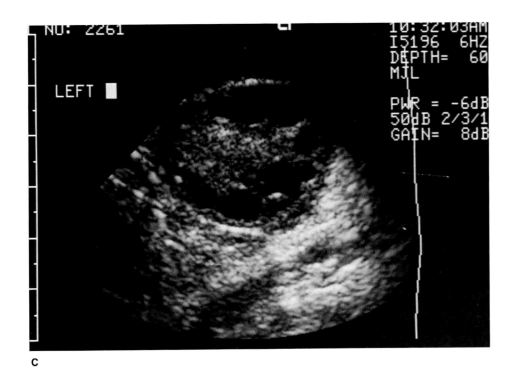

C

D

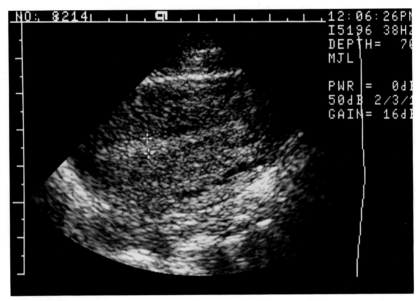

NO: 8214 ⊓ 12:06:26PM
I5196 38H2
DEPTH= 7
MJL

PWR = 0d
50dB 2/3/
GAIN= 16d

A

Figure 4.2 Endometrium by TVS scan. (**A**) Proliferative endometrium (between calipers) on sagittal image. (**B**) Periovulatory endometrium (between calipers), thicker than proliferative endometrium. (**C**) Thick secretory endometrium (between calipers).

UTERUS

TAS ultrasound of the uterus requires a full bladder in order to displace bowel gas and provide an acoustic window. The degree of bladder filling is important, and is thus a limiting factor to this type of examination. The bladder must be full enough to extend over the fundus of the uterus, but not so full that it compresses the uterus and its contents. The endometrial canal cannot always be seen, especially with retroflexed or retroverted uteri, or those containing fibroids.

Transvaginally the endometrial cavity can be imaged almost all the time (Fig 4.2). Endometrial thickness and echogenicity, as a function of the menstrual cycle, can easily be determined by TVS. Intrauterine contraceptive devices and retained products of conception in the uterine cavity (Figs 4.3 and 4.4) can be seen. In one study, the endometrial cavity was better evaluated by TVS in 40% of cases, and added diagnostic information in 23% of the cases after TAS had been performed. Equivalent evaluation was possible by the two modalities in the remaining cases.[6,7]

The size, position, and shape of the uterus can be evaluated by both modalities. Retroverted and retroflexed uteri, however, are better imaged transvaginally (Fig 4.5). Transvaginal probes can be rotated and angled to scan 360° around the pelvis, increasing the areas visible to the probe (Fig 4.6).

Uterine myomata alter the uterine contour. They may be exophytic or intramural. When the uterus is very large with multiple fibroids, the TAS may be limited by its narrow field of view and because the high-frequency beam may not be able to penetrate the enlarged uterus (Fig 4.7). In these cases, TVS sonography is required. TVS scanning can contribute to the evaluation of a patient with fibroids. In some cases the endometrial canal can only be seen transvaginally (Fig 4.8). Improved imaging of the adnexa in these cases may be possible, as well.

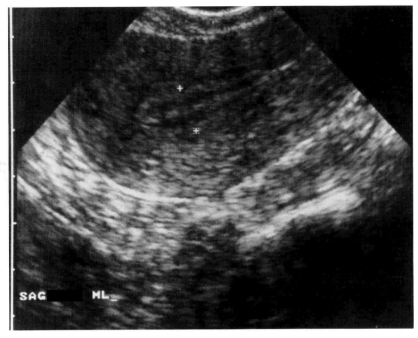

B

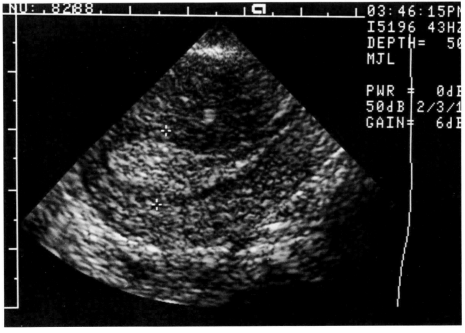

C

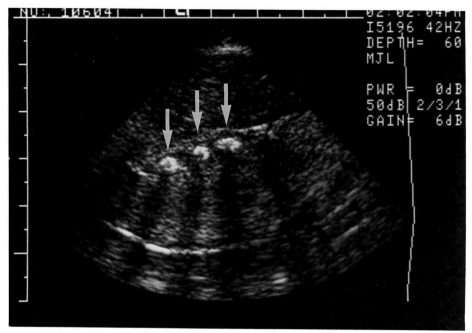

Figure 4.3 IUD in uterine cavity. Sagittal TVS image showing bright echoes of Lippes' Loop (arrows) contained within uterine cavity.

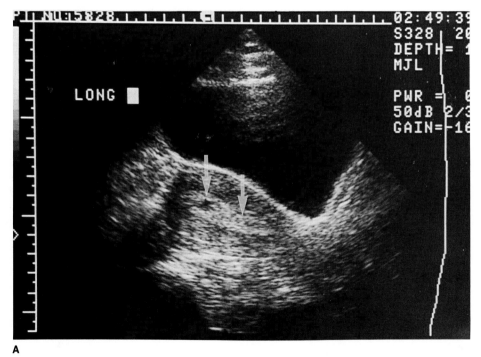

A

Figure 4.4 Blood and clot in uterine cavity. (**A**) Sagittal TVS scan shows anechoic and echogenic material (arrows) within uterine cavity. (**B**) Coronal image of complex material (arrows) within the uterus.

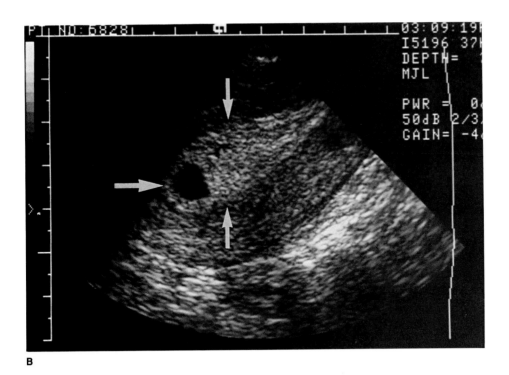

B

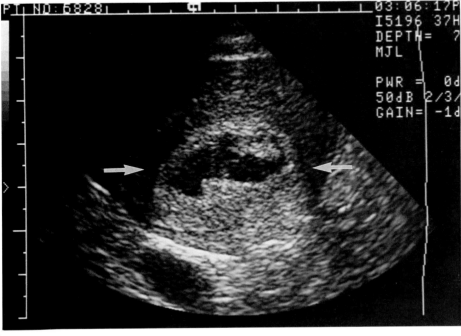

C

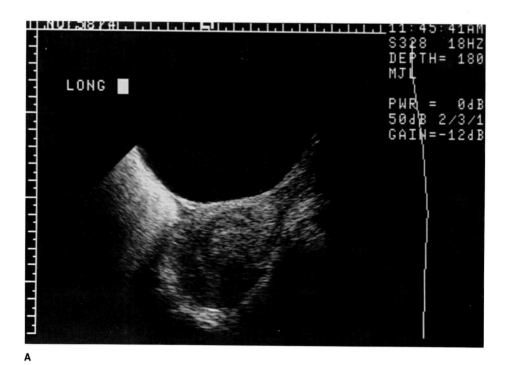

A

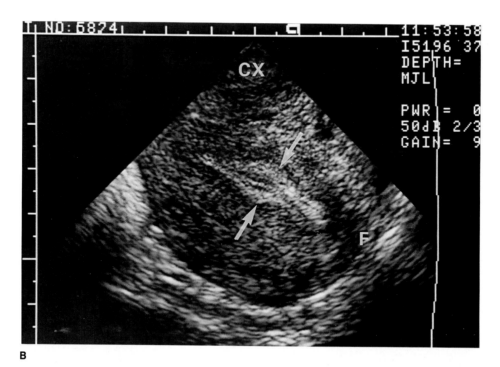

B

Figure 4.5 Retroverted retroflexed uterus. (**A**) TAS sagittal image through full urinary bladder showing retroverted uterus. Uterine cavity is not well seen. (**B**) TVS sagittal image of uterus with fundus (F) caudal and posterior to cervix (CX). Endometrium is clearly seen (arrows).

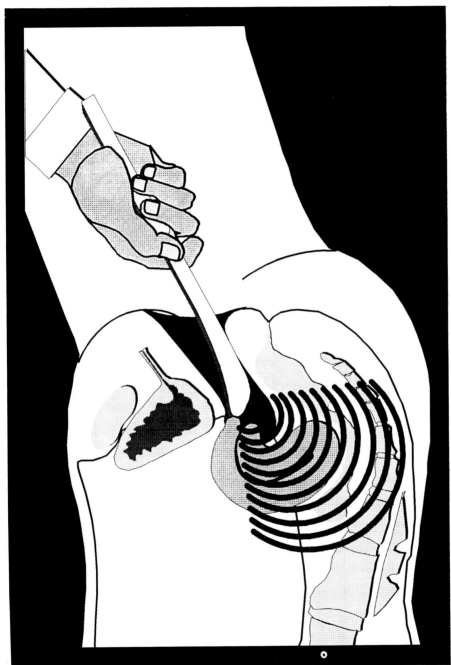

Figure 4.6 Posterior orientation of vaginal probe. Diagram of vaginal probe with beam directed posteriorly to scan retroverted retroflexed uterus. The probe can be rotated 360° to scan all possible angles.

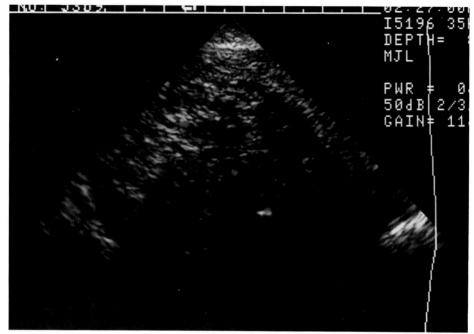

A

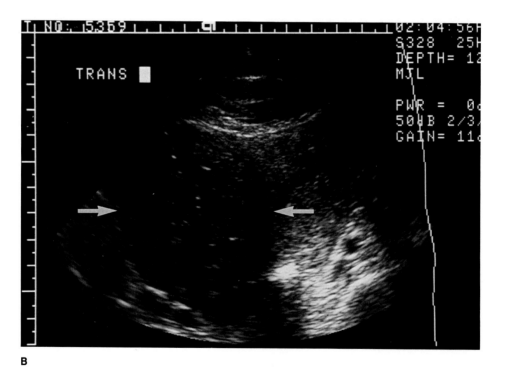

B

Figure 4.7 Fibroid uterus. (**A**) TVS coronal image showing poor penetration of beam and inability to visualize uterine contour or extent of fibroid. (**B**) TAS transverse view showing large fibroid (arrows) arising from uterus.

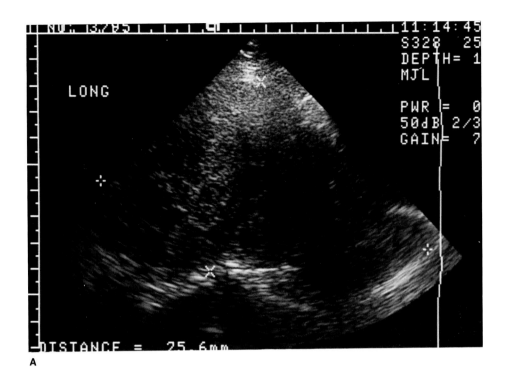

A

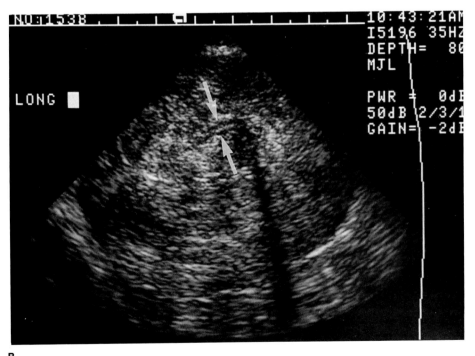

B

Figure 4.8 Endometrium in fibroid uterus. (**A**) TAS image of large fibroid uterus (calipers) (7.6 × 13.3 cm). Endometrial cavity cannot be identified. (**B**) TVS view of uterus showing endometrial cavity (arrows) in fibroid uterus. Beam penetration is poor with this higher frequency transducer, so that the uterine contour is poorly defined.

FALLOPIAN TUBES

The fallopian tubes are rarely visible by TAS except in cases with fluid within the tube. In such cases, the fluid-filled tube may be seen in the adnexa, but it may be impossible to distinguish the hydrosalpinx from the ovary or other pelvic collections. By TVS the normal tube is occasionally visible (Fig 4.9). Usually the proximal end of the tube may be visible at its junction with the cornua of the uterine fundus (Fig 4.9**A**). Fluid-filled salpinges can be distinguished from the ovaries because of the better resolution provided by the vaginal probes (Fig 4.10).[8,9]

OVARIES

As for imaging of the uterus, TAS of the ovaries requires a distended bladder. Maternal body habitus may limit resolution of the ovaries and its morphology. By transvaginal approach, the ovaries are usually easily located with their small developing follicles serving as sonographic markers (Fig 4.11). Enlarged ovaries may be imaged by either modality, but internal architecture is better defined on TVS (Fig 4.12). Studies report that TVS provided more information about ovarian anatomy and pathology than TAS in 76–85% of cases, and equivalent information in most other cases.[10,11]

The composition of ovarian masses is usually better defined by TVS. Apparently simple cysts on TAS may prove to be complex on higher resolution TVS (Figs 4.13 and 4.14). The contents of solid or complex masses may be better defined transvaginally for improved diagnosis (Fig 4.15), but if the mass is very large, TAS may provide more diagnostic information than the TVS because of its wider field of view (Fig 4.16).[10,11]

In the postmenopausal patient, the ovaries are often difficult to identify, especially by TAS. By transvaginal approach, 82% of ovaries were identified in postmenopausal women in one study.[12] This imaging modality may prove valuable for screening women for early diagnosis of ovarian malignancy.[12,13]

Adnexal masses may be separate from both the fallopian tube and ovary. By TVS, accurate distinction among the adnexal structures can often be made, so that the tube and ovary can be distinguished from the adnexal mass, and the differential diagnosis can be narrowed (Fig 4.17).

Ovarian follicular growth must be closely monitored in patients on ovulation induction drugs for infertility. Transvaginal measurement of follicular size and number yields findings similar to TAS measurement in most cases (Fig 4.18), but better resolution is achieved transvaginally.[14–17] In a few cases TVS will identify more follicles than can be seen transabdominally.[17] Only rarely, when the ovary is positioned unusually high, will the TAS approach yield more information than can be gained transvaginally. Infertility patients require multiple examinations. Because the discomfort and inconvenience of repeatedly filling the bladder is avoided if transvaginal monitoring is routine, TVS has recently become the primary imaging modality for the initial workup and subsequent monitoring of follicular growth.[14–17]

Most TVS probes are equipped with biopsy guides which can be used to direct needles for follicular aspiration and cyst and abscess drainage with real-time sonographic imaging.[18–20]

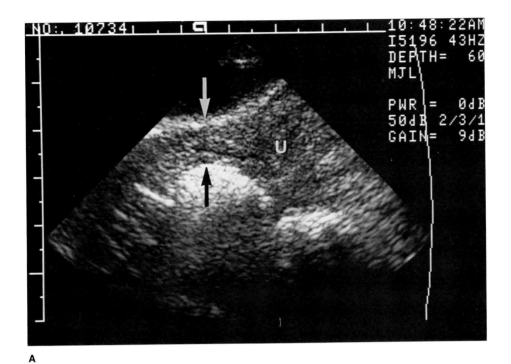

A

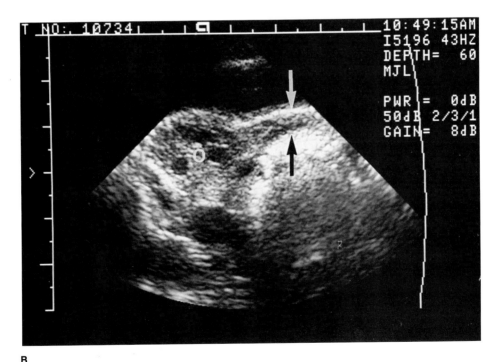

B

Figure 4.9 Fallopian tube seen transvaginally. (**A**) Transverse image showing right fallopian tube (arrows) entering the uterus (U). (**B**) Transverse image to the right of **A** showing proximal tube (arrows) adjacent to right ovary (O).

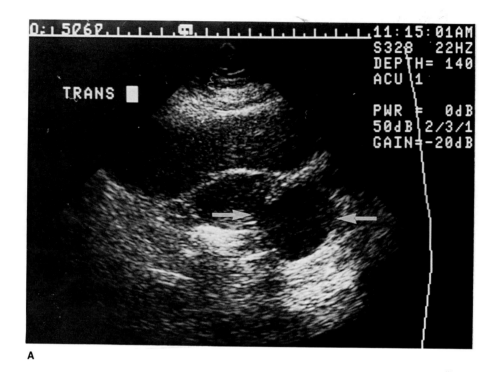

A

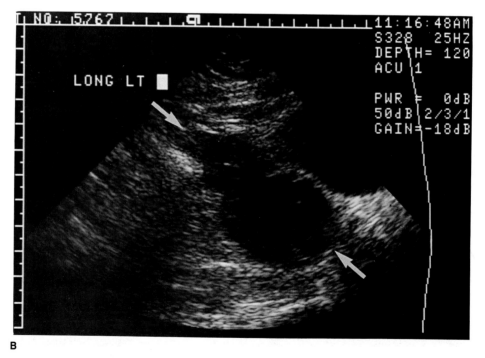

B

Figure 4.10 Hydrosalpinx and ovarian cyst. Transverse (**A**) and longitudinal (**B**) TAS images showing indistinct complex cystic left adnexal mass. (**C**) and (**D**) Coronal TVS images show the complex adnexal mass has two components, a hydrosalpinx (H) and a simple left ovarian cyst (C).

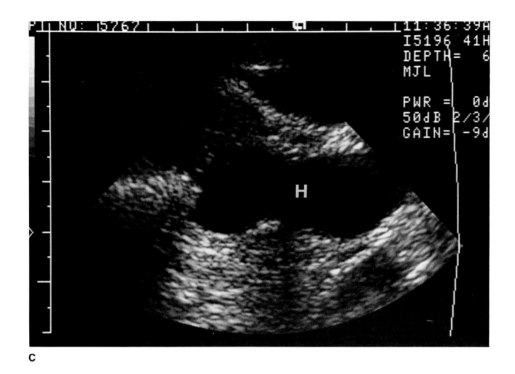

C

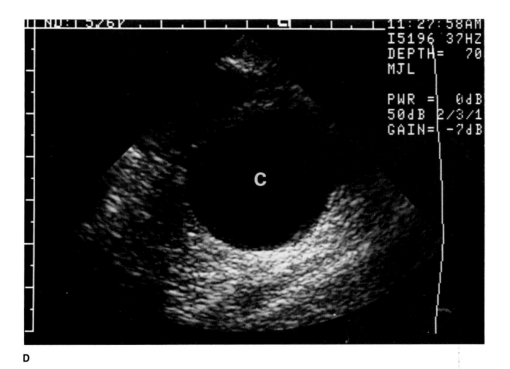

D

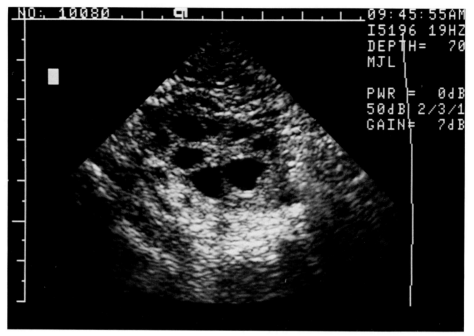

Figure 4.11 Normal ovary. TVS view showing multiple small follicles within ovary.

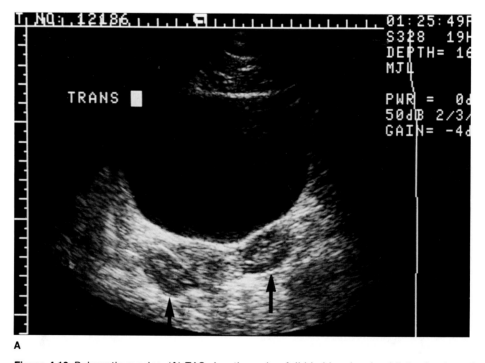

A

Figure 4.12 Polycystic ovaries. (**A**) TAS view through a full bladder showing bilateral enlarged ovaries (arrows). (**B**) By TVS scan multiple follicles are identified in the enlarged ovary.

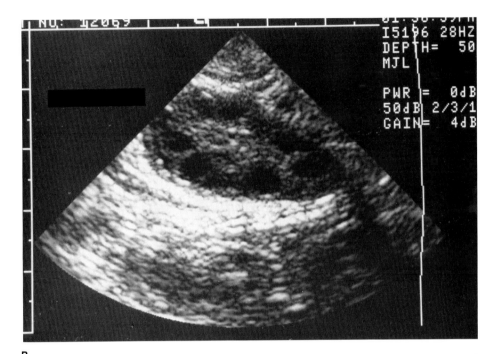

B

Figure 4.12 (continued)

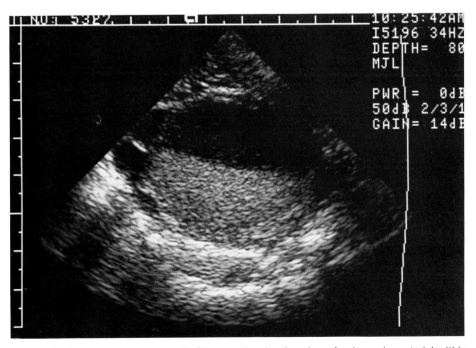

Figure 4.13 Complex ovarian cyst. TVS image showing layering of echogenic material within complex cyst.

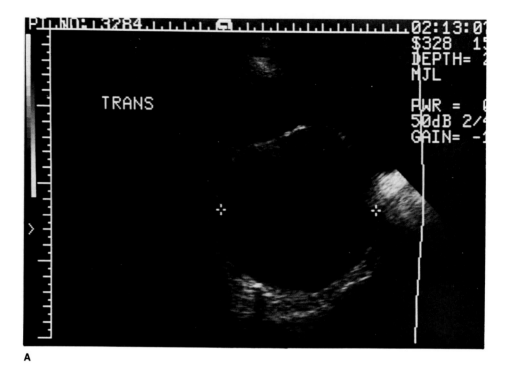

A

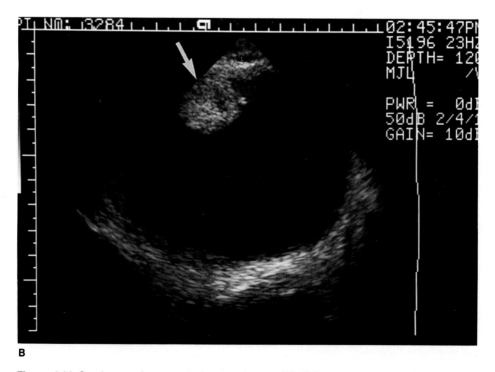

B

Figure 4.14 Ovarian mucinous cystadenocarcinoma. (**A**) TAS transverse scan showing large adnexal cyst (calipers) extending behind uterus. (**B**) By TVS scan, a tumor nodule (arrow) is identified in wall of cyst and low-level echoes in cyst fluid.

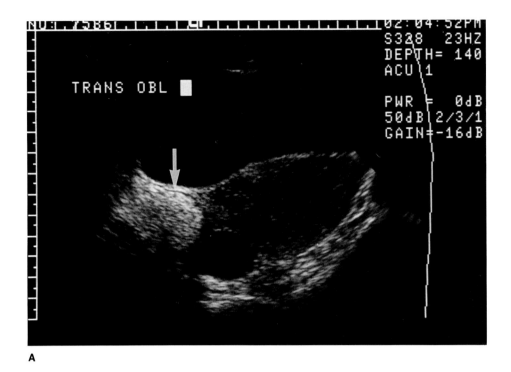

A

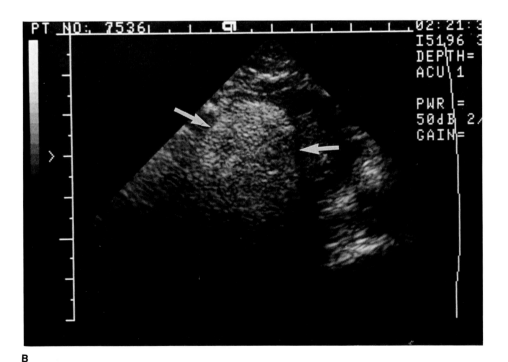

B

Figure 4.15 Ovarian dermoid tumor seen better transvaginally. (**A**) TAS transverse image show-ing poorly defined echogenic material in right adnexa (arrows) representing either bowel gas or ovarian pathology. (**B**) TVS image of echogenic dermoid tumor arising from ovary (arrows).

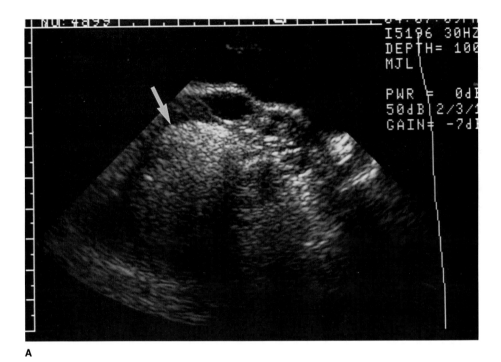

A

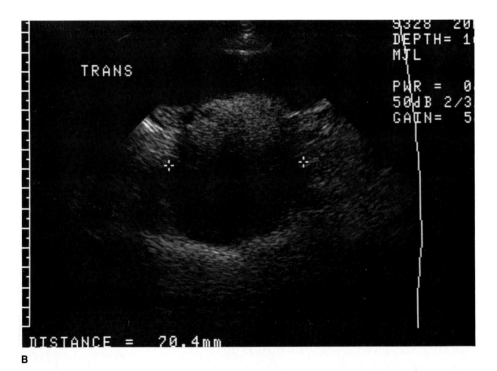

B

Figure 4.16 Ovarian dermoid tumor seen better transabdominally. (**A**) TVS sonogram showing poorly defined echogenic area or mass (arrow). TAS transverse (**B**) and longitudinal (**C**) images of large adnexal mass (**B**, calipers; **C**, arrows) containing echogenic material due to fat in dermoid tumor.

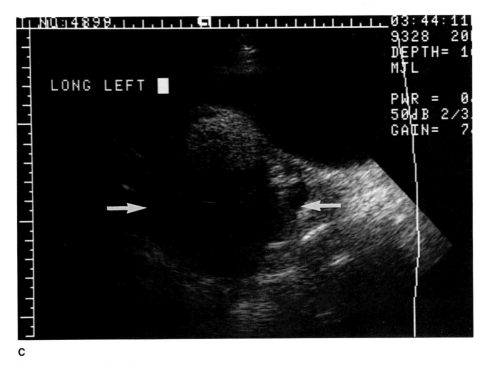

C

Figure 14.16 (*continued*)

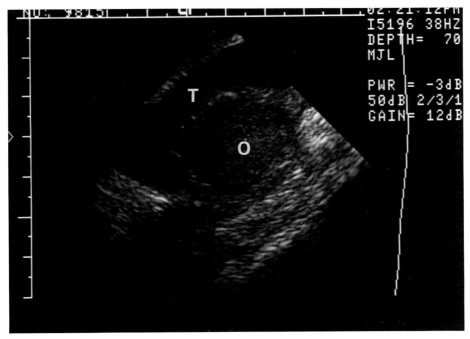

Figure 4.17 Tubo-ovarian abscess. TVS scan of complex adnexal mass showing fluid-filled fallopian tube (T) draped over edematous ovary.

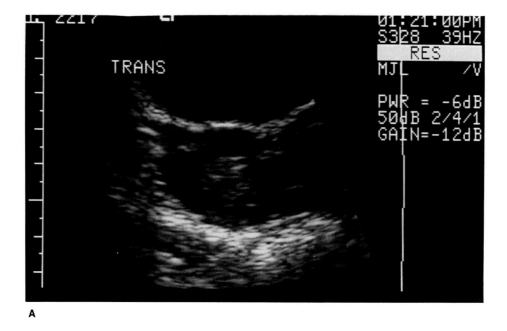

A

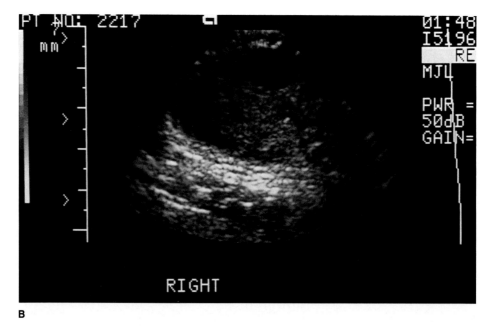

B

Figure 4.18 Ovarian follicles. (**A**) TAS, and (**B**) TVS images demonstrate similar number, sizes, and shapes of developing follicles.

EARLY PREGNANCY

The sonographic milestones of early intrauterine pregnancy prior to identification of the embryo include the detection of the "double-sac sign,"[21] a yolk sac within the gestational sac, and the "flicker" of the embryonic heart. These findings can be seen transvaginally several days before they can be seen transabdominally.[22] If the uterine cavity is empty and the adnexae are normal by TAS in a patient with a positive pregnancy test, TVS should be performed in search of an intrauterine or ectopic gestation (Fig 4.19). Similarly, if a gestational sac containing no yolk sac or embryonic pole is identified in the uterine cavity by TAS, a TVS should be performed in an attempt to identify a yolk sac or embryonic pole to prove the intrauterine collection is, in fact, a pregnancy (Fig 4.20). The embryonic heartbeat may be seen next to the yolk sac by high-resolution TVS earlier than by TAS, thus confirmation of embryonic viability is possible sooner in pregnancy (Fig 4.21).

As a result of increased spatial resolution provided by the transvaginal probe, the definitive diagnosis of an ectopic pregnancy with imaging of a live fetal pole is often possible after a negative or equivocal TAS (Fig 4.22).[23] TVS is reported to identify an adnexal mass in 88–92% of patients with ectopic pregnancies. Only 35–50% of these patients had adnexal masses by TAS.[24]

TVS, in addition to offering more information and better resolution in patients with suspected ectopic pregnancies, has the added advantage that the patient can be scanned immediately without delay for filling of the urinary bladder.[25]

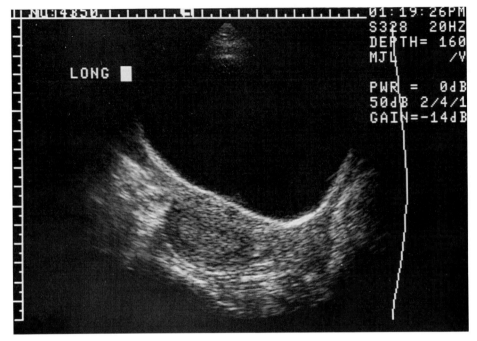

A

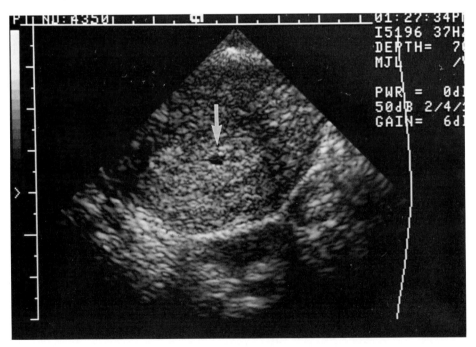

B

Figure 4.19 Very early intrauterine gestation seen only transvaginally. (**A**) TAS sagittal image of uterus containing no gestational sac. (**B**) Small gestational sac (arrow) identified in uterine cavity by TVS approach.

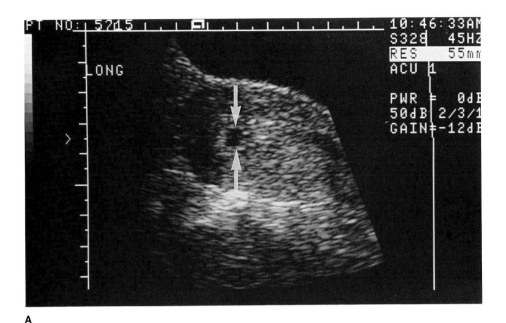

A

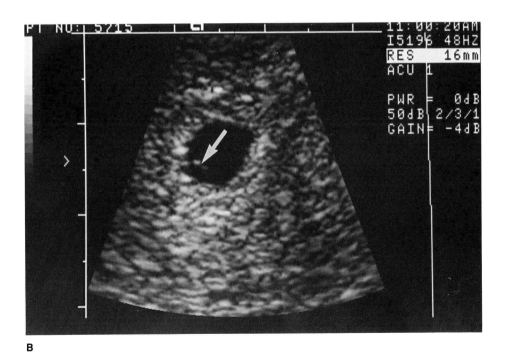

B

Figure 4.20 Early intrauterine pregnancy. (**A**) TAS scan showing intrauterine gestational sac (arrows). (**B**) By TVS ultrasound a yolk sac (arrow) is identified within the gestational sac.

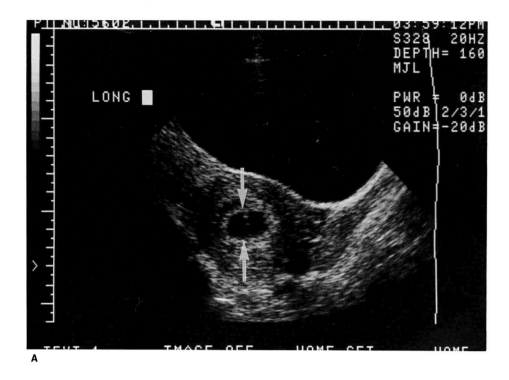

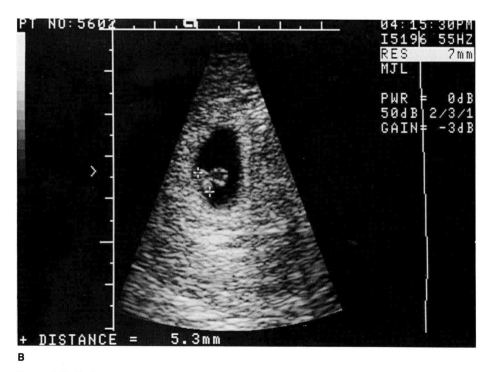

Figure 4.21 Early embryonic pole. (**A**) TAS image of gestational sac (arrows) containing a yolk sac. (**B**) Embryonic pole (calipers) identified transvaginally. (**C**) TVS M-mode documenting embryonic cardiac activity.

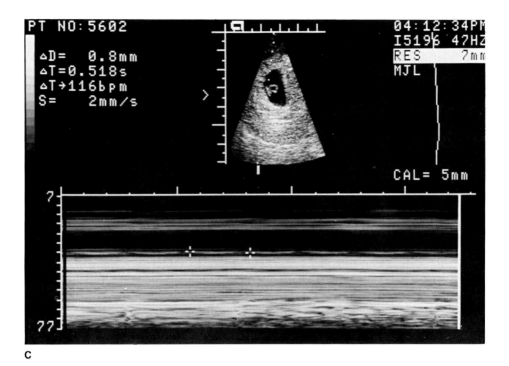

c

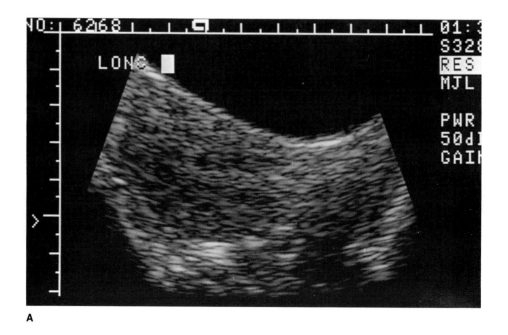

A

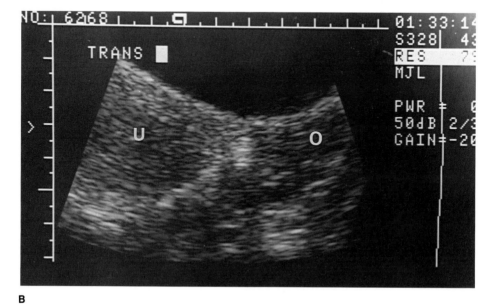

B

Figure 4.22 Ectopic pregnancy. (**A**) Sagittal TAS image in a pregnant patient showing no gestational sac in the uterus. (**B**) Transverse image transabdominally showing adnexal fullness between uterus (U) and left ovary (O). (**C**) Ectopic gestational sac and embryonic pole identified transvaginally. (**D**) TVS M-mode of live ectopic gestation.

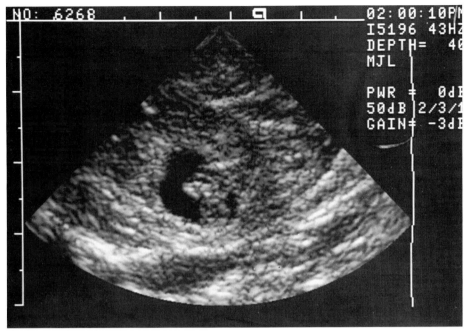

C

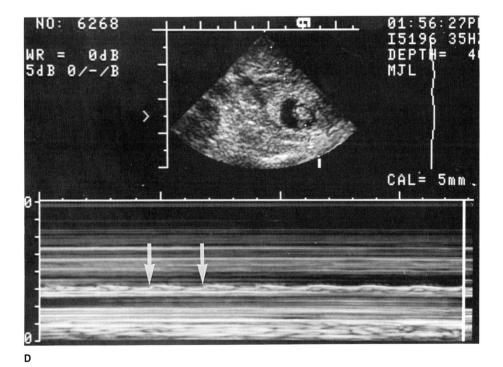

D

PLACENTA PREVIA

The exact relationship between the *internal os* and the *placenta* can be seen better by TVS. This issue will be discussed in Chapter 10.

SUMMARY

In summary, TVS permits high-resolution imaging of the pelvis in patients regardless of body habitus, abdominal wall scarring, or bowel gas. The exam is accepted well by most patients, and avoids the delay and discomfort of filling the urinary bladder required for TAS evaluation. TVS has the added advantage over TAS that the probe can be used actively to locate sites of pelvic tenderness and evaluate for pelvic adhesions. In cases where there is a large pelvic mass, such as large uterine fibroids or an ovarian neoplasm, TAS is necessary for complete evaluation because of its larger field of view. TVS probes do have limited penetration.

TVS and TAS are complementary imaging modalities for evaluation of the pelvic organs. In the majority of cases, the uterus and its contents, fallopian tubes, and ovaries are better evaluated by TVS, but TAS plays an important role as well.

REFERENCES

1. Timor-Tritsch IE, Rottem S, Thaler I: Review of TVS ultrasonography: a description with clinical application. Ultrasound Quarterly 1988;6:1–34.
2. Tessler FN, Schiller VL, Perrella RR, et al: TAS versus endovaginal pelvic sonography: prospective study. Radiology 1989;170:553–556.
3. Timor-Tritsch IE, Bar-Yam Y, Elgali S, Rottem S: The technique of TVS sonography with the use of a 6.5 MHz probe. Am J Obstet Gynecol 1988;158:1019–1024.
4. Coleman BG, Arger PH, Grumbach K, et al: TVS and TAS sonography: prospective comparison. Radiology 1988;168:639–643.
5. Mendelson EB, Bohm-Velez M, Joseph N, Neiman HL: Gynecologic imaging: comparison of TAS and TVS sonography. Radiology 1988;166:321–324.
6. Mendelson EB, Bohm-Velez M, Joseph N, Neiman HL: Endometrial abnormalities: evaluation with TVS sonography. AJR 1988;150:139–142.
7. Welker BG, Gembruch U, Diedrich K, et al: TVS sonography of the endometrium during ovum pickup in stimulated cycles for in vitro fertilization. J Ultrasound Med 1989;8:549–553.
8. Timor-Tritsch IE, Rottem S: TVS ultrasonographic study of the fallopian tube. Obstet Gynecol 1987;70:424–428.
9. Tessler FN, Perrella RR, Fleischer AC, Grant EG: Endovaginal sonographic diagnosis of dilated fallopian tubes. AJR 1989;153:523–525.
10. Leibman AJ, Kruse B, McSweeney MB: TVS sonography: comparison with TAS sonography in the diagnosis of pelvis masses. AJR 1988;151:89–92.
11. Lande IM, Hill MC, Cosco FE, Kator NN: Adnexal and cul-de-sac abnormalities: TVS sonography. Radiology 1988;166:325–332.
12. Rodriguez MH, Platt LD, Medearis AL, et al: The use of TVS sonography for evaluation of postmenopausal ovarian size and morphology. Am J Obstet Gynecol 1988;159:810–814.
13. Higgins RV, van Nagell JR, Donaldson ES, et al: TVS sonography as a screening method for ovarian cancer. Gynecol Oncol 1989;34:402–406.
14. Yee B, Barnes RB, Vargyas JM, Marrs RP: Correlation of TAS and TVS ultrasound measurements of follicle size and number with laparoscopic findings for in vitro fertilization. Fertil Steril 1987;47:828–832.
15. O'Shea RT, Forbes KL, Scopacasa L, Jones WR: Comparison of TAS and TVS pelvic ultrasonography for ovarian follicle assessment in in vitro fertilization. Gynecol Obstet Invest 1988;26: 52–55.
16. Schwimer SR, Lebovic J: TVS pelvic ultrasonography: accuracy in follicle and cyst size determination. J Ultrasound Med 1985;4:61–63.

17. Andreotti RF, Thompson GH, Janowitz W, et al: Endovaginal and TAS sonography of ovarian follicles. J Ultrasound Med 1989;8:555–560.
18. Feichtinger W, Kemeter P: TVS sector scan sonography for needle guided TVS follicle aspiration and other applications in gynecologic routine and research. Fertil Steril 1986;45:722–725.
19. Schwimer SR, Mark J, Lebovic J: Percutaneous ovarian cyst aspiration using continuous TVS ultrasonographic monitoring. J Ultrasound Med 1985;4:259–260.
20. Nosher JL, Winchman HK, Needell GS: TVS pelvic abscess drainage with US guidance. Radiology 1987;165:872–873.
21. Bradley WG, Fiske CE, Filly RA: The double sac sign in early intrauterine pregnancy: use in exclusion of ectopic pregnancy. Radiology 1982;148:223–226.
22. Jain KA, Hamper UM, Sanders RC: Comparison of TVS and TAS sonography in the detection of early pregnancy and its complication. AJR 1988;151:1139–1143.
23. De Crespigny LC: Demonstration of ectopic pregnancy by TVS ultrasound. Br J Obstet Gynecol 1988;95:1253–1256.
24. Shapiro BS, Cullen M, Taylor KJW, DeCherney AH: TVS ultrasonography for the diagnosis of ectopic pregnancy. Fertil Steril 1988;50:425–429.
25. Urquhart DR, Fisk NM: TVS ultrasound in suspected ectopic pregnancy. Br Med J 1988;296:465–466.

CHAPTER **5**

Transvaginal Sonography of Uterine Disorders

Arthur C. Fleischer, MD
Donna M. Kepple, RT, RDMS
Stephen S. Entman, MD

INTRODUCTION

Transvaginal sonography (TVS) affords detailed delineation of the uterus and its myometrium, endometrium, and vessels.[1] Because of this, several uterine disorders may be evaluated by TVS. After discussion of normal anatomy and scanning technique, this chapter will discuss the use of TVS in the evaluation of a variety of both benign and malignant uterine disorders.

NORMAL ANATOMY AND SCANNING TECHNIQUE

The uterus can be imaged in three major scanning planes with TVS. These include views in its long axis, an oblique semicoronal or semiaxial plane, and a short axis view (Fig 5.1**A**,**B**,**C**). The long axis image is obtained when the transducer/probe is introduced into the vagina and the uterus is imaged in greatest long axis. The semicoronal depiction of the uterus is obtained when the transducer is turned 90° to long axis and imaged in its greatest longitudinal plane. For anteflexed uteri, the probe handle is held posteriorly with the beam directed anteriorly; the opposite maneuver is used for retroflexed uteri. In the semicoronal scanning plane, the uterus is imaged in its width. The short axis view is obtained by retracting the transducer/probe into the midvagina and directing it anteriorly through the fornix.

The uterus varies in its size and shape, depending on the patient's parity and whether or not the patient is pre- or postmenopausal (Table 5.1). TVS should not be attempted until the late teens; therefore, the discussion of uterine anatomy will begin in patients that are nulliparous and postpubertal. The size of the uterus in these patients is approximately 6 cm in length, 3–4 cm in both anteroposterior (AP) and transverse dimension. In the parous patient, the uterine long axis can be up to 8 cm in length, whereas in the postmenopausal woman, the uterus decreases in size to approximately 4–6 cm in long axis. (Fig 5.1**D**,**E**).

If the uterus is anteflexed and the scanning is done in the semicoronal plane, the first structure to appear on the screen is the cervix. If a retroflexed uterus is present, the transducer will first reveal the fundus of the uterus, which in this case is close to the sacrum. Scanning in the longitudinal plane will reveal the exact position of the cervix in the pelvis.

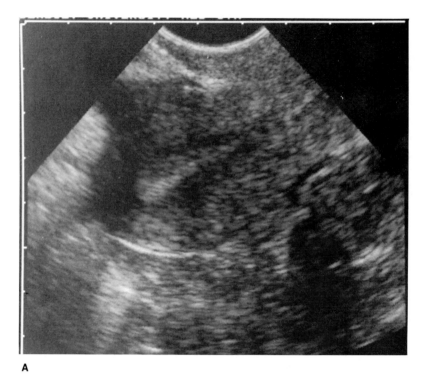

A

B

Figure 5.1 Normal uterus. (**A**) In long axis. (**B**) In semicoronal. (**C**) In short axis. (**D**) The atrophic uterus (4.2 × 2.2 × 2.5 cm) of a postmenopausal patient is outlined by the anteriorly situated bladder (B) and the small arrows. The cavity is filled with a small amount of fluid. No vaginal bleeding was evident in this patient.

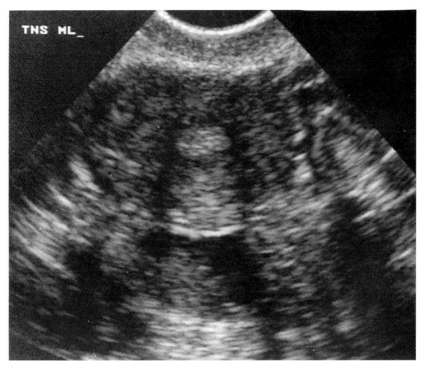

C

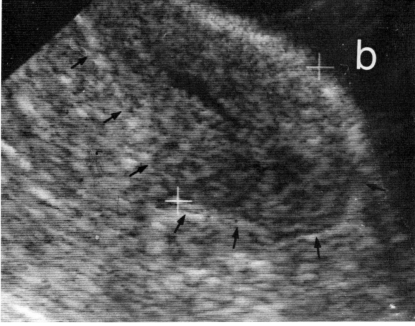

D

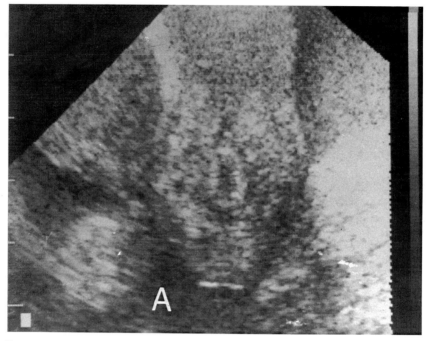

E

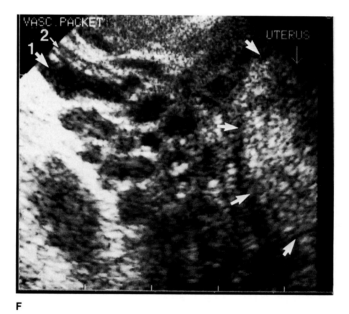

F

Figure 5.1 (*continued*) (**E**) The atrophic retroverted uterus (5.0 × 2.5 × 2.5 cm) is surrounded by ascitic fluid (A) and several pelvic masses. On the basis of TVS, an endometrial origin of the malignancy was excluded by the sonographer. The report of the pathologist was adenocarcinoma of the ovary. (**F**) Transverse section of the right parametrium at the level of the internal cervical os. The vascular packet consists of the uterine vein (1) and artery (2), as well as the rich vascular web approaching the uterus (outlined by small arrows), of which only a portion is included in this scan.

TABLE 5.1 Uterine Size (cm)*

	Length	Width	AP	Volume (cc)	Cx: Corpus/ Fundus
Adult (nulliparous)	6–8	3–5	3–5	30–40	1 : 2
Adult (parous)	8–10	5–6	5–6	60–80	1 : 2
Pubertal and postmenopausal	3–5	2–3	2–3	14–17	4 : 1/1 : 1

* Gray's Anatomy, p. 1356.

The vaginal portion of the cervix with the external os may be examined. Nabothian cysts of different sizes may appear as anechoic, extremely thin-walled round structures (Fig 5.2**D,E**). The cervix should be examined using the vertical plane, by turning the transducer plane 90°. This will cause the endocervical canal to become the most prominent structure on the screen. Sometimes, cystic formations of various sizes (0.5–3 cm) may appear along the endocervical canal. These probably represent dilated (obstructed) endocervical glands. The most important differential diagnosis of this finding may be the extremely remote possibility of a very early cervical pregnancy.

At the level of the internal os, close to the lateral aspect of the cervix, a paired group of blood vessels may be recognized (Fig 5.1**F**). Blood flow within the vessels is occasionally seen on real-time scanning as low-level echoes coursing within the lumen of the vessels. The two major vessels, the uterine artery and vein, are usually quite easily recognized. Doppler flow (pulsed and color) measurements can be obtained from these vessels as a means of assessing overall uterine perfusion. The resistive (RI) or pulsatility index (PI) can be used as a means to quantitate relative blood flow (RI = peak systolic velocity − end diastolic/mean velocity). Alternatively, the relative shape of the diastolic portion of the waveform can be used to roughly assess perfusion.

The uterus is supplied by the uterine artery, which is a branch of the hypogastric. After the uterine artery courses toward the cervix, it parts into an ascending branch, which runs along the corpus, and a descending branch, which courses toward the upper vagina. After coursing through the outer myometrium, the uterine artery gives rise to the arcuate arteries, which course in a concentric pattern within the outer third of the myometrium. Studies performed with duplex transvaginal Doppler show a steady rise in the PI in the follicular phase followed by a drop in the secretory.[2] The venous structures are more prominent than the arterial (Fig 5.2**B,C**). One can obtain triplex color Doppler of these vessels and assess the relative uterine perfusion (Fig 5.3**A,B**).

Variations in the normal anatomy of the central endometrial interfaces can be detected in patients who have fusion abnormalities of the uterus. Specifically, the bicornuate uterus can be readily identified due to the two echogenic endometrial lumina. Other anatomic variations (Fig 5.2**A,B,C**) include prominence of myometrial arcuate vessels and calcification of these vessels in the elderly patient as well as cervical inclusion cysts usually due to obstructed glands (Fig 5.2**D,E**).

The myometrial fibers are arranged in a specific pattern. These provide effective contraction of the uterus in the normal cycle.[3] Occasionally, a sustained contraction can appear as a hypoechoic rounded area. These contractions can be detected on TVS if the study is recorded and played in a fast-forward mode on a videocassette recorder. In this way, one can appreciate the direction and intensity of the uterine contractions. During menses, these contractions begin at the fundus

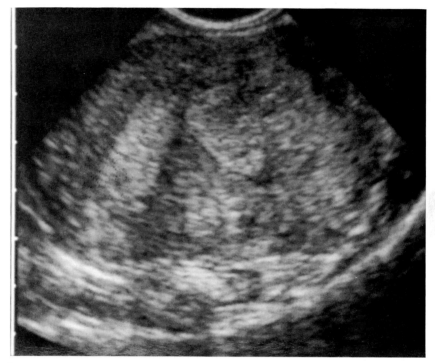

A

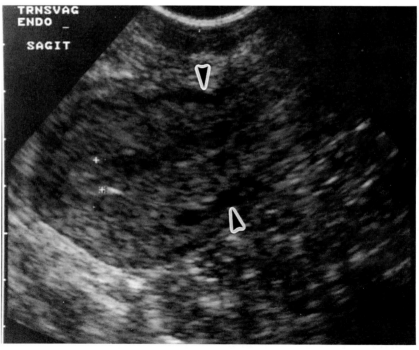

B

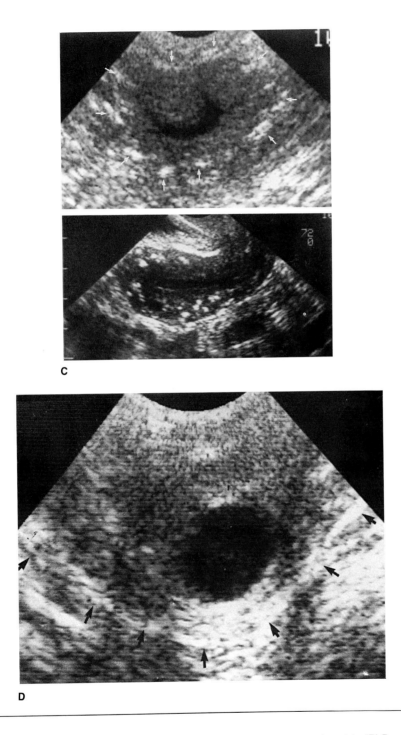

C

D

Figure 5.2 Normal variants. (**A**) Bicornuate uterus demonstrating two endometria. (**B**) Prominent arcuate vessels (arrowheads). (**C**) Extensive calcification within arcuate vessels. (**D**) Cross section of the cervix close to the external os. The 9 × 11 mm Nabothian cyst (confirmed by speculum examination) is situated in the posterior lip, which is delineated by small arrows. (*continued*)

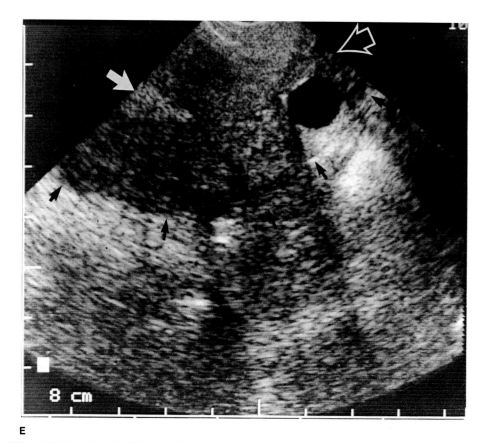

E

Figure 5.2 *(continued)* **(E)** Longitudinal section of the same Nabothian cyst in Fig. 5.2**D** shown at a smaller scale. Note endometrium on the left side (thick arrow). The external os is on the right side, approximately near the open arrow. The posterior aspect of the uterus is outlined by small black arrows.

and extend to the cervix. In midcycle, they are propagated in the opposite direction. Perhaps these contractions have a role in affecting efficacy of sperm transport, thereby optimizing the chances of implantation; this is tempting to speculate.

Transvaginal sonography clearly depicts changes in the endometrial texture and thickness during the menstrual cycle (Fig 5.4**A**–**D**). In the menstrual phase, the endometrium appears as an interrupted interface that is thin and has some hypoechoic areas related to extravasated blood and sloughing tissue (Fig 5.4**A**). In the proliferative phase, the endometrium appears as isoechoic to the myometrium (Fig 5.4**B**). During the preovulatory phase, the endometrium may have a multilayered appearance with an inner hypoechoic layer and an echogenic outer layer (Fig 5.4**C**). The inner hypoechoic layer probably represents the inner myometrium, which is relatively edematous. In the secretory phase, the thickness measures between 8 and 14 mm, and the endometrium is echogenic (Fig 5.4**D**). This is probably related to mucous and glycogen stored in the endometrial glands and the echogenic interfaces provided by the tortuous glands. Table 5.2 includes the relative thicknesses of the endometrium throughout the cycle. The thickness myometrium numbers are specified and include both layers as measured in the greatest AP dimension.

The endometrium of a postmenopausal woman is typically thin and atrophic (less than 10 mm in total anteroposterior width). Occasionally, a small amount

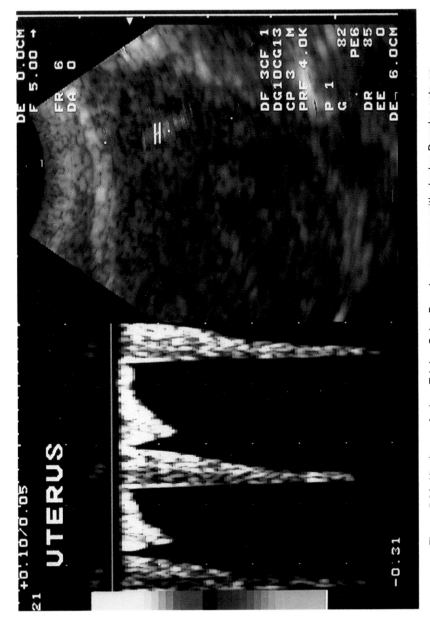

Figure 5.3A Uterine perfusion. Triplex Color Doppler sonogram with duplex Doppler gate on main uterine artery (in blue).

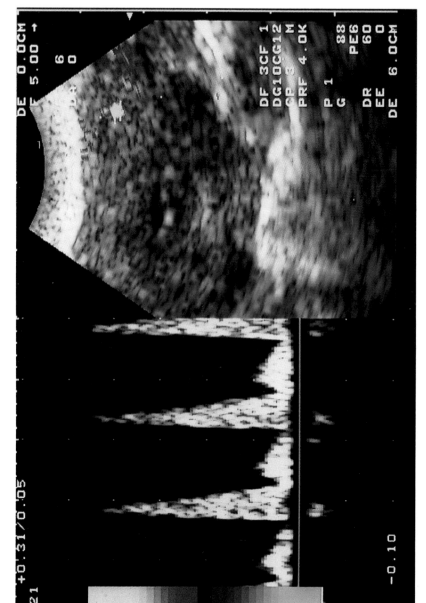

Figure 5.3B Same patient as in Figure 5.3A showing arcuate vessels within the myometrium of the fundus.

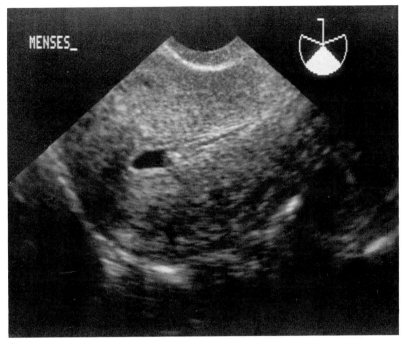

A

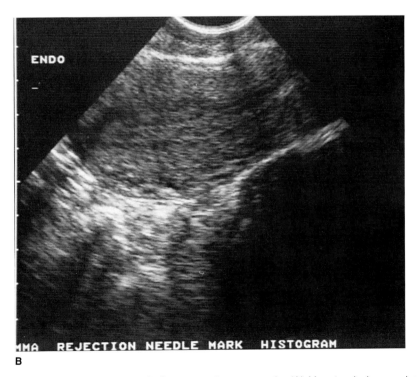

B

Figure 5.4 Endometrial changes during a spontaneous cycle. (**A**) Menstrual phase—showing sloughing of the endometrium. (**B**) Proliferative phase—isoechoic to myometrium. (*continued*)

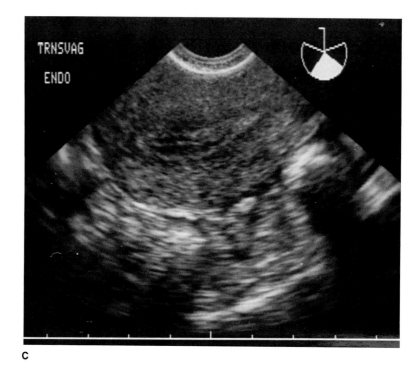

C

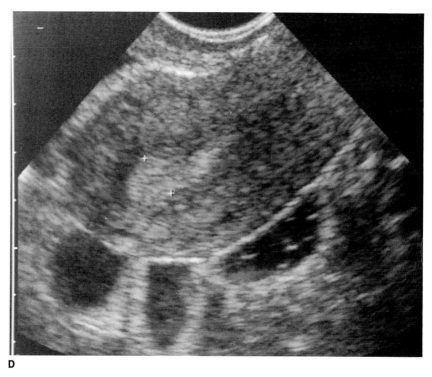

D

Figure 5.4 (*continued*) (**C**) Periovulatory period—multiple layers due to edema of the compactum layer. (**D**) Secretory phase—echogenic and thick due to mucus and glycogen stored within glands (between +s).

TABLE 5.2 Endometrial Thickness

	Range (mm)
Proliferative phase	4–8
Secretory phase	7–14
Postmenopausal (no HRT)	4–8
Postmenopausal (HRT)	6–10

HRT = hormone replacement therapy

(2–3 cc) of intraluminal fluid may be present particularly in women with ascites. If present on repeat scans, this finding should be considered suspicious for an endometrial disorder. Polypoid growths are particularly well seen when surrounded by intraluminal fluid (Fig 5.6**F**).

Leiomyoma

Leiomyomas are common tumors consisting of smooth muscle and connective tissue. They arise from the soft tissue and smooth muscle covering the intramyometrial arcuate vessels. They can remain intramural or, if they extend into the uterine lumen, submucosal, or outward become pedunculated and subserosal. Leiomyomas have a variety of sonographic textures ranging from hypoechoic to echogenic with a calcified border (Fig 5.5**A,B,C**). This is to be expected since these tumors have a varying amount of smooth muscle and connective tissue.

One can utilize TVS as a means of monitoring the size of leiomyomas. Color Doppler sonography may be helpful to identify those leiomyomas that are vascular and may be responsive to GnRH analog (Lupron[R]) treatment.[4] TVS is particularly helpful in identifying intraligamentous fibroids and the pedicle of pedunculated subserosal fibroids as well as differentiating these from intramural ones (Fig 5.5**C**).

Endometrial Hyperplasia

Dysfunctional bleeding in the postmenopausal woman is a fairly common disorder. This condition may be related to the atrophic endometrium, which is prone to hemorrhagic ulceration. A more common condition occurs when there is an excess of circulating estrogen promoting endometrial growth and resulting in endometrial hyperplasia.

Although there are no large studies at this time that set the upper limits of the thickness of the endometrium in normal postmenopausal women, it should be thin and atrophic and less than approximately 10 mm in AP dimension (Fig 5.6).[5] It may be slightly thicker than this in patients on hormone replacement therapy.

Transvaginal sonography has a role in evaluating patients who present with vaginal bleeding. Endometrial thickening greater than 10 mm in AP dimension, in patients who are postmenopausal, usually indicates either hyperplasia or carcinoma. It can assess the amount of tissue within the endometrium and can predict in cases where there is scant endometrium, or scant cellular material, but these samples might be insufficient for diagnosis. Certainly, one can predict the relative amount of tissue that will be retrieved through dilation and curettage by the appearance of the endometrium on TVS. By measuring the endometrium in length, AP dimension, and width, one can estimate endometrial volume (Fig 5.4**E**).

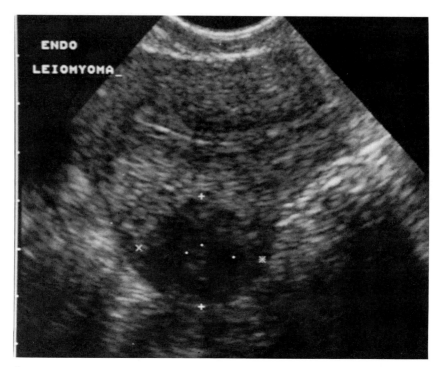

A

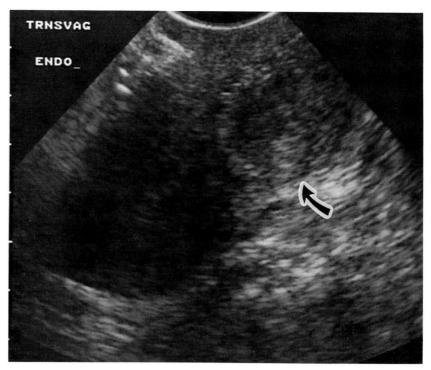

B

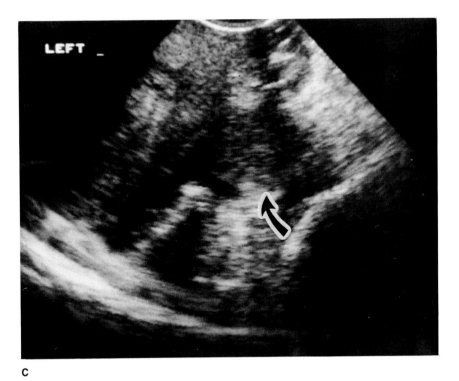

C

Figure 5.5 Leiomyoma. (**A**) Intramural fibroid (between cursors) separate from the endometrium. (**B**) Cervical fibroid (arrow). (**C**) Subserosal pedunculated fibroid (arrow).

Transvaginal sonography is not a screening procedure for these patients, since the evaluation of these patients needs to be based on a histopathologic diagnosis. However, TVS can supply information concerning the relative amount of endometrial hyperplasia. Sonographic images of endometrial thickening may result from hyperplasia but actually represent polyps over 5–10 mm. Since these are usually compressed, however, individual polyps may not be discernable with TVS. When surrounded by fluid or blood, however, the individual polyps may be discerned (Fig 5.6**F**).

Transvaginal sonography often detects thickened endometria in patients being evaluated for an adnexal mass. If the endometrium is over 10 mm in AP dimension or over 5–10 cc in volume, an endometrial biopsy may be indicated, especially if there is a history of bleeding since hyperplasia is a known precursor to carcinoma.[6]

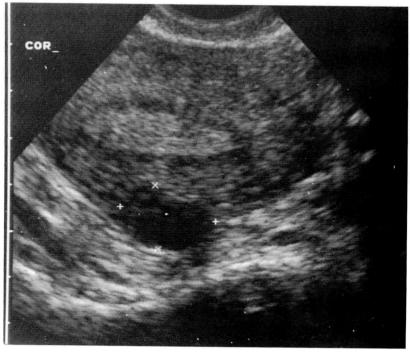

A

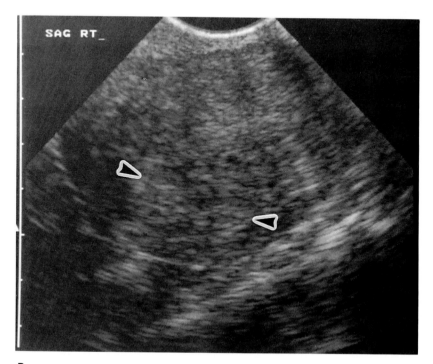

B

Figure 5.6 Endometrial hyperplasia/adenomyosis/polyps. (**A**) Thickened endometrium in a patient with endometrial hyperplasia. A small intramural fibroid is also present. (**B**) Adenomyosis causing increased echogenicity of the myometrium. (**C**) Polyps (arrows) in a hyperplastic endometrium. (Courtesy of Ellen Mendelson, MD.) (**D**) Hyperplastic endometrium in a patient with polycystic ovaries and several anovulatory cycles. (*continued*)

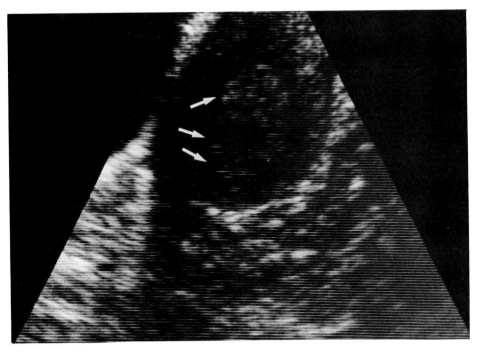

C

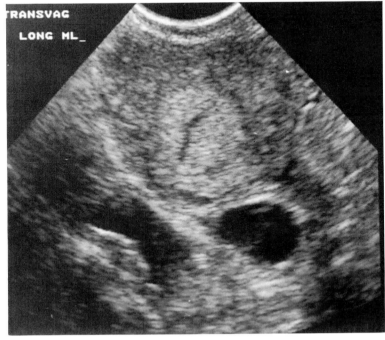

D

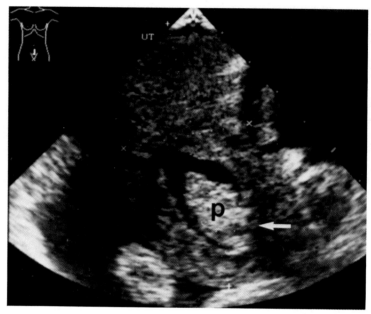

E

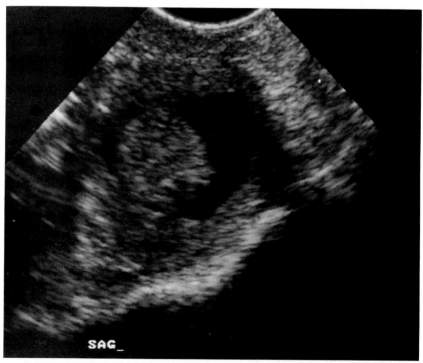

F

Figure 5.6 (*continued*) (**E**) The atrophic uterus (6.5 × 3.2 × 2.8 cm) of a 53-year-old patient is surrounded by pelvic fluid (ascites). The cavity is filled with fluid outlining a 2 × 1.2 × 1.4 cm polypoid structure (p) emerging from the upper anterior wall (arrow). The anterior wall is not outlined and seems to be contiguous with an irregular mass. Pathology revealed a benign polyp. (**F**) Papillary serous endometrial carcinoma appearing as an irregular polypoid mass within the uterine lumen.

Endometrial Neoplasms

Transvaginal sonography has a role in assessing the depth of invasion in patients with histologically proven endometrial carcinoma.[7] The extent of invasion can be detected in most cases and classified into superficial, intermediate, or deep, depending on the extent of the tumor invasion relative to thirds of myometrial distances (Fig 5.7**A,B,C,D**).

Most endometrial tumors are echogenic, even though less differentiated tumors may be hypoechoic (Fig 5.7**B,C**). Difficulties arise in tumors that are exophytic or may stretch the myometrium but not invade it. Microscopic invasion is also not detectable, and preexisting conditions such as leiomyoma and adenomyoma may make it difficult to precisely delineate the extent of myometrial invasion.

Other Conditions

Transvaginal sonography can also evaluate patients with suspected adenomyosis. In this condition, there is a spectrum of sonographic findings from absolutely normal sonographic appearances to echogenic myometrium due to multiple adenomyomas (Fig 5.8**A**). Endometritis may also demonstrate an echogenic pattern and thickening of the endometrium.

One should also realize that retained mucous secretions can simulate the appearance of endometrial thickening. Peritoneal implants to the uterine serosa from tuberculosis or gynecologic malignancies (Fig 5.8**B**) may also be seen, particularly if surrounded by fluid (Fig 7.4).

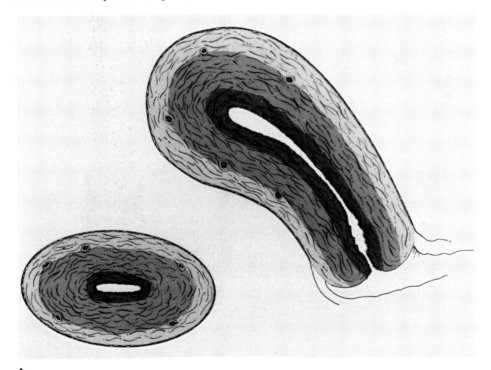

A

Figure 5.7 TVS of endometrial carcinoma with accompanying gross specimen. (**A**) Diagram showing superficial, intermediate, and deep myometrial layers relative to the arcuate vessels as determined by TVS. (*continued*)

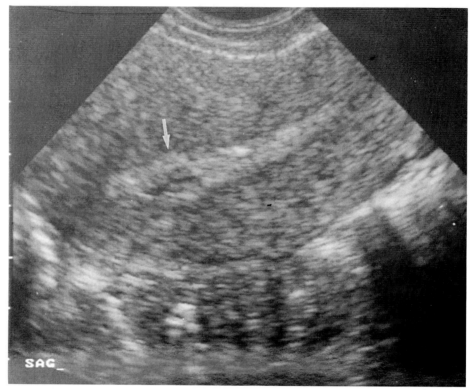

B1

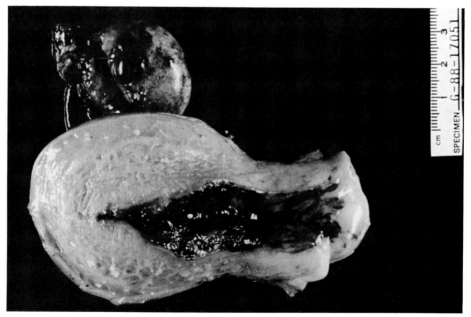

B2

Figure 5.7 (*continued*) (**B**) Superficial myometrial invasion. (1) TVS. (2) Specimen.

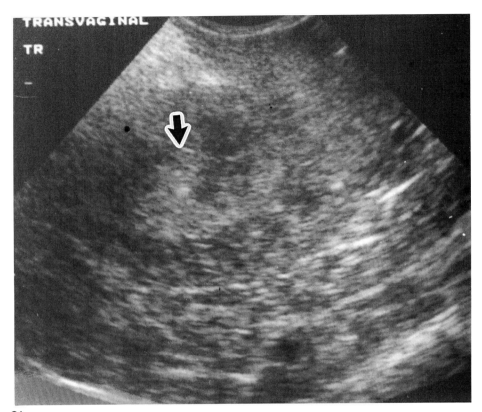

C1

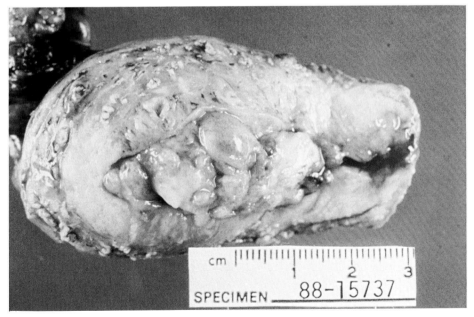

C2

Figure 5.7 (*continued*) (**C**) Intermediate myometrial invasion (arrow). (1) TVS. (2) Specimen.

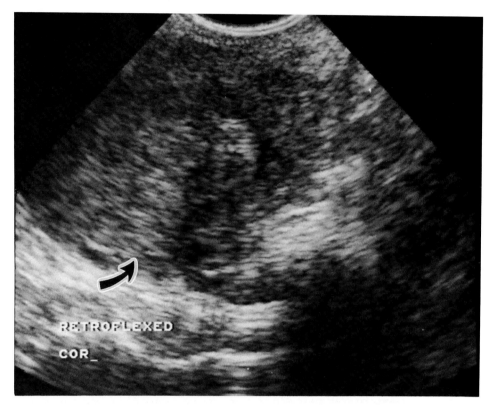

D1

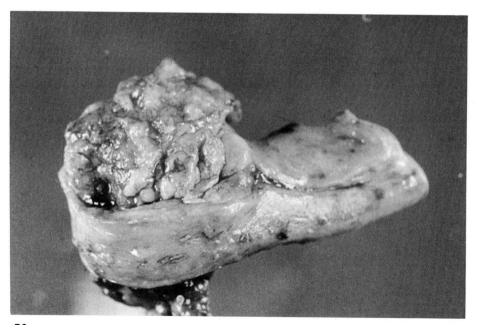

D2

Figure 5.7 (*continued*) (**D**) Deep myometrial invasion (arrow). (1) TVS. (2) Specimen.

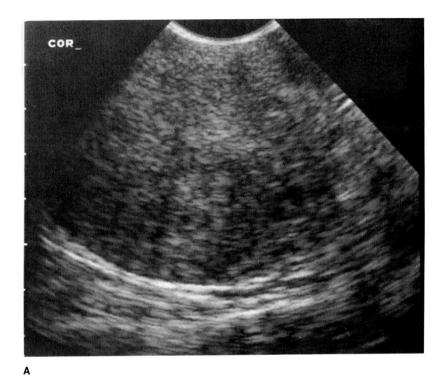

A

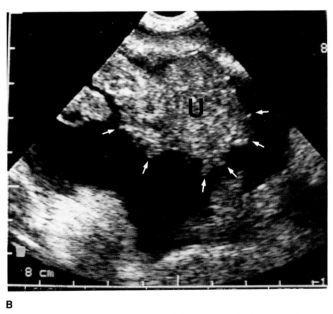

B

Figure 5.8 Miscellaneous uterine disorders. (**A**) Adenomyomatosis appearing as diffuse disruption in the myometrial texture. (**B**) Ascites in a patient with tuberculotic peritonitis. Note the irregular surface of the uterus (u) "floating" in the fluid. The irregular uterine surface may result from the fibrin deposits (arrows) prevalent in this disease. No direct visual proof could be obtained in this case.

SUMMARY

Transvaginal sonography is the diagnostic modality of choice for evaluating most uterine disorders. It is particularly useful in identifying the exact location and size of leicmyoma and other uterine tumors.

REFERENCES

1. Mendelson EB, Bohm-Velez M, Joseph N, Neiman HL: Endometrial abnormalities: evaluation with transvaginal sonography. AJR 1988;150:139–142.
2. Scholtes MCW, Wladimiroff JW, van Rijen HJM, Hop WCJ: Uterine and ovarian flow velocity waveforms in the normal menstrual cycle: a transvaginal Doppler study. Fertil Steril 1989;52: 981–985.
3. Lyons EA, Gallard G, Zheng X-H, Levi CS, Lindsay DJ: Contractions of the inner myometrium in fertility (abstract). Radiology 1989;173(P):114.
4. Friedman AJ, Barbieri RL, Benacerraf BR, Schiff I: Treatment of leiomyomata with intranasal or subcutaneous leuprolide, a gonadotropin-releasing hormone agonist. Fertil Steril 1987;48:560–564.
5. Goldstein SR: The post menopause. (In preparation).
6. Ferenczy A: Endometrial hyperplasia and neoplasia: a two disease concept. In: Berkowitz RL, Cohen CJ, Kase NG, eds. Obstetric Ultrasonography/Gynecologic Oncology. New York: Churchill Livingstone, 1988:197–213.
7. Gordon AN, Fleischer AC, Reed GW: Depth of myometrial invasion in endometrial cancer: preoperative assessment by transvaginal ultrasonography (Gynecol Oncol, in press)
8. Osmers R, Völksen M, Schauer A: Vaginosonography for early detection of endometrial carcinoma? Lancet 1990;335:1569–1571.

CHAPTER 6

The Fallopian Tubes

Ilan E. Timor-Tritsch, MD
Shraga Rottem, MD, DSc
Nathan Lewit, MD

Ultrasonic evaluation of the fallopian tubes presents one of the greatest challenges for the sonographer. Regardless of the technology applied, only gross pathology may be recognized and described. The available literature regarding the use of sonography in tubal diagnosis is scarce and limited to the description of tubal pregnancy and the gross, fluid-filled tubes. It was the clinician's responsibility to translate the sonographic report of a "fluid-filled adnexal mass" into a practical clinical diagnosis. The list of differential diagnoses could not usually be shortened substantially on the grounds of such a sonographic report.

The main reasons for the inability to see the normal tube or to partially view the fluid-filled tube are multiple. First, and probably most important, is the use of 3.5 or 5.0 MHz transducers. These transducers achieve adequate sound penetration when applied through the abdominal wall and the distended bladder; however, a price is paid in terms of resolution for the adequate penetration and relatively low attenuation that are achieved.

Because of the physical limitations of the 3.5 and 5.0 MHz transducers, axial and lateral resolution is limited to a relatively coarse outline of the general pelvic anatomy and pathology. This is even more the case if the delicate tubal anatomy and pathology are considered.

Second, the normal fallopian tube is a poor sonic reflector itself, devoid of clear interfaces (eg, fluid/tissue) that would produce a clear organ outline. It may now be easier to understand why transabdominal sonography does not produce sufficiently clear images of the healthy or the diseased fallopian tube.

It also may now seem more logical that a transvaginal probe using a higher-frequency transducer crystal should overcome the above-mentioned limitations. The sound wave, on its way to the closer pelvic organs (in this case the tubes), would be less attenuated; therefore, because of the higher frequency employed, an image with a higher-frequency resolution is obtained.

THE NORMAL TUBE

The healthy fallopian tube usually cannot be imaged unless some type of surrounding fluid is present. Such "contrasting" fluid may be the following:

1. The normal serous pelvic fluid present in a significant number of healthy women[1] amounting to several milliliters (Fig 6.1).

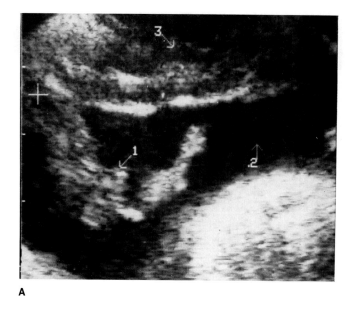

A

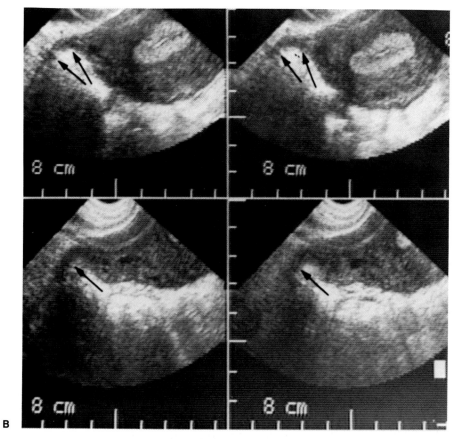

B

Figure 6.1 (**A**) The distal end of the normal left tube (1), freely floating in fluid (2), below the uterus (3). The patient complained of pelvic pain. (**B**) The first 1–2 cm of the right tube (the proximal end) at the cornual area of the uterus is depicted (arrows).

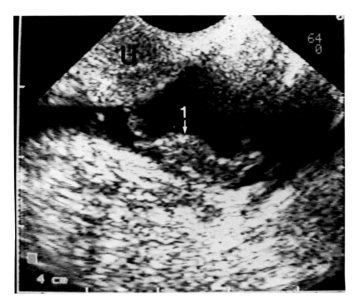

Figure 6.2 Clearly seen is the ampullar part of the left tube (1) surrounded by fluid in the pelvis; u = uterus.

2. Follicular fluid released at midcycle through the ovulation process, reaching 4–10 mL; therefore, at times of presumed ovulation or shortly thereafter the chances of detecting the ampullar part (Fig 6.2) and the fimbrial end (Fig 6.3) are increased.
3. Blood in various quantities.
4. Ascitic fluid usually produced by a neoplastic, obstructive, vascular, or other rare condition.
5. The products of an exudative or infectious process (Fig 6.4).

Sometimes, however, the proximal end of the tube, which is its fixed end, can be seen and "followed" for about 1 or 2 cm until it is "lost" within the adnexal echoes (Fig 6.1**B**).

If the patient is being examined in a slightly reversed Trendelenburg position, advantage can be taken of even the minute amount of fluid that will be pooled in the pelvis. Fluid, as previously mentioned, is the best acoustic interface for tubal imaging.

A recent study[1] pointed out that regardless of ovulation inhibition, a small amount of pelvic fluid was found in female patients in the reproductive years. This fluid increased in volume at and immediately after midcycle.

If detected, the tube presents as a tortuous echogenic structure about 1 cm wide; however, on the screen its width may vary along its entire length because of the two-dimensional scanning plane "cutting through" different parts of the "undulating" tube (Fig 6.2). The tubal lumen can be discerned only if it is filled with fluid, and when enough fluid is present, the fimbrial end of the tube may be seen (Fig 6.3). Pathological amounts of pelvic fluid enable imaging of the normal or abnormal salpinx. If the tube is detected, longitudinal and serial cross sections should be made by rotating the probe around its longitudinal axis. One advantage of the transvaginal probe is the possibility of measuring the uterus, the ovaries,

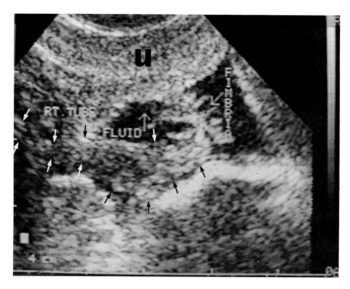

Figure 6.3 The same patient as in Fig 6.2. Below the uterus (u), surrounded by a physiological amount of fluid in the Douglas space, the right tube, including the ampullar part with the delicate fimbrial end, is imaged.

and the tube with a push–pull motion of the probe. This light pressure may move the tube into various positions to improve imaging.

The *affected tube* is diagnosed by examining its wall, luminal contents, and adherence to its surroundings.

The *tubal wall* may be evaluated if its lumen is filled with contrasting fluid. If, in addition, free fluid coats the salpinx, the wall will be even better defined.

An *acute* disease such as an inflammatory process or tubal gestation usually leads to thickening of the wall (Figs 6.5–6.8). During this acute stage the longitudinal endosalpingeal folds can be visualized (Figs 6.7 and 6.8). A tortuous hydrosalpinx is shown in Fig 6.6; this uniformly thickened wall with a total flattening of the endosalpinx may represent a transition to the *chronic* hydrosalpinx, which is characterized by a stretched, thin wall (Fig 6.9). Speculation had it that they were the remnants of the longitudinal endosalpingeal folds of the diseased mucosa. The diagnosis of hydrosalpinx was documented in these cases by laparoscopy.

The *lumen* of the tube is seen if it has been outlined by fluid or other contrasting material (eg, blood or a gestational sac). It is reasonable to suggest that if the lumen of the tube is brought into view and is distended, a pathological salpinx is present.

The *contents* of the tube may be sonolucent, possibly serous (Figs 6.7–6.9), or more uniformly echogenic fluid (with low-level echogenicity) such as a mucous or purulent fluid (Fig 6.5).

Blood clots may fill the tubal cavity, and after scans of several patients with ruptured tubal pregnancies, it would appear that blood clots in the tube present a complex and more difficult diagnostic task.

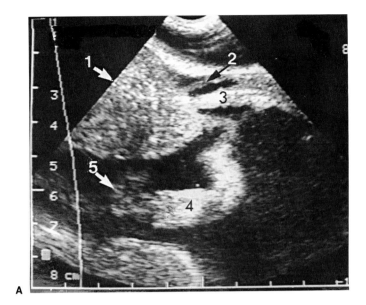

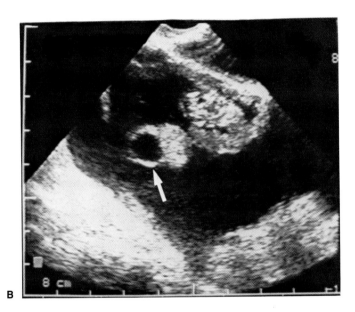

Figure 6.4 (**A**) Massive ascites outlines the uterus (1), round ligament (2), broad ligament (3), and left tube (4) with fimbrial end (5). (**B**) In the same patient, the left tube is imaged. A small 1 cm morgagnian cyst is seen at the fimbrial end (arrow).

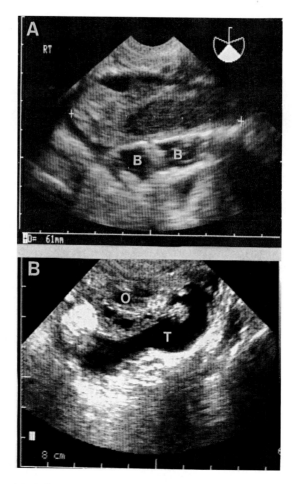

Figure 6.5 Acute pelvic inflammatory disease with pyosalpinx. (**A**) Longitudinal section of the right tube containing fluid with low-level echogenicity (pus). Behind the thick-walled tube: loops of bowel (B). (**B**) The tubo-"ovarian complex" is seen on this image taken of the cross section of the same tube. The complex was tender when touched with the probe. T = tube; O = ovary.

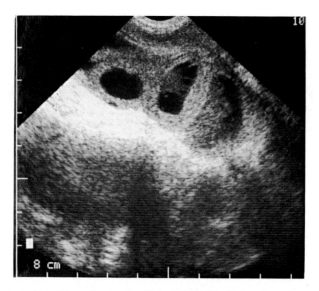

Figure 6.6 Cross section of three loops of a dilated, fluid-filled tube. Its walls are thickened. The patient was known to have occluded tubes and, at the time of the scan, had a tubal pregnancy in the contralateral tube.

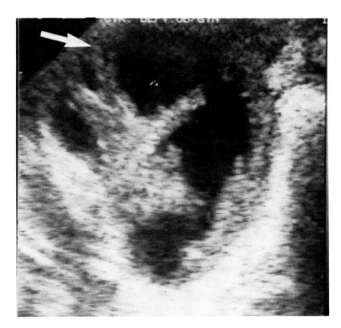

Figure 6.7 An occluded, dilated, fluid-filled sactosalpinx is evident. Some of the folds of the endosalpinx are still present. The distal end is marked with an arrow.

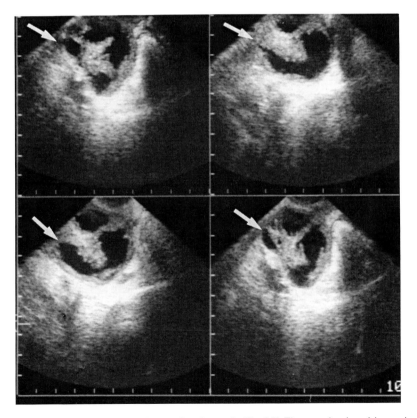

Figure 6.8 Serial cross sections of the tube shown in Fig 6.7. The proximal end is marked by arrows.

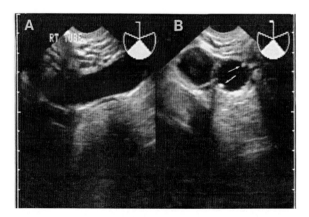

Figure 6.9 (A) Behind the cross section of the uterus (U) the longitudinal section of the right and the cross section of the left tube are seen. Both are filled with sonolucent fluid. **(B)** This longitudinal section of the right tube demonstrates the whole length of the fluid-filled right fallopian tube. The wall is about 2–3 mm thick.

An unruptured *gestational sac*, with or without active embryonic heartbeats, is relatively easy to recognize by transvaginal sonography because of the natural fluid/tissue contrast created by the fluid-filled sac (see Chapter 14).

Mobility of the tube may be determined by attempting to move, displace, and even change the position of the tube (or the adjacent ovary) with a push–pull motion of the probe under direct observation on the scope. If no adhesions are present, a free sliding movement of the pelvic organs will be appreciated. This procedure is called the "sliding organs sign" and is described in Chapter 3. A chronically affected salpinx usually shows the same picture on repeated TVS examinations.

INFLAMMATORY PROCESSES OF THE TUBE

Two entities are of importance and therefore are mentioned:

1. Inflammatory processes of the tube are the hydrosalpinx or the pyosalpinx, dilated, fluid-filled, sometimes club-shaped structures (Figs 6.5, 6.7, 6.9). As said before, their walls may be thin or thick according to the chronicity of the tubal disease.
2. Inflammatory processes of the tube and the ovary, namely the *tubo-ovarian complex* and the *tubo-ovarian abscess* (TOA) are both adnexal or adnexal and cul-de-sac conglomerates.

The experience with transvaginal imaging of the pelvis led us to the observation that these are phases in the formation of the TOA. The term *tubo-ovarian abscess*, was and is still used to describe the acute pelvic inflammatory process. This usually has an impressive clinical picture consisting of severe lower abdominal pain, usually aggravated during menstrual periods, dysmenorrhea, dispareuria, dysfunctional uterine bleeding secondary to involvement, poor function of the ovaries, palpable adnexal masses, and infertility. The process is invariably bilateral. If the pathologic features are considered, there are steps in its propagation and in arriving at the final stage, the pelvic abscess.

First, during the acute phase there is distinct inflammation of the tubal mucosa. The wall of the tube becomes thick and edematous and a large amount of purulent exudate fills the lumen, some spilling into the cul-de-sac. If the tubes become occluded—both at the fimbrial and at the cornual end—mucus and inflammatory secretions will fill the tubes, leading to a hydrosalpinx or pyosalpinx. Sometimes the tubes become convoluted and resemble the glass retorts of chemistry laboratories; hence the name *retort tubes* (see Fig 6.8). Because of the mounting pressure resulting from the increasing amount of fluid the walls of the tube become thinner. If the process stops at this stage, a chronic hydrosalpinx will result. Sometimes the sonolucent lumen of the tube assumes a crenated shape due to the fibrotic remnants of the endosalpingeal folds. This resembles a cogwheel (Fig 6.12); therefore, it is called *cogwheel sign.*[7]

When the distended tube and the involved, adjacent ovary have been fused, and the acute inflammatory process continues, the well-defined walls of the organs involved will break down, resulting in a tubo-ovarian abscess. The ovary is especially vulnerable at times of ovulation through the "defect" created by the corpus luteum. The purulent fluid fills the available space created by the breakdown of the tissues involved, creating the abscess in the cul-de-sac. If the process is "walled off," a chronic tubo-ovarian abscess may result.

During the first stage, the tubo-ovarian complex can be diagnosed by imaging the adnexa and by recognizing the anatomic structures involved, ie, the tube and the ovary. The tubes may appear edematous and fluid with low-level echogenicity may fill their lumen (Figs 6.10, 6.11). The complex is tender. There may not be free fluid in the cul-de-sac. If there is fluid in the pelvis the amount is usually small.

An attempt may be made to bring the pelvic mass in line with the scanning axis of the probe, and then apply gentle pressure to evoke motion-tenderness, which helps in the diagnosis.

With the above-mentioned sonographic picture, one should look for the presence of the "sliding organs sign" (see Chapter 3). If no sliding of the ovary or the uterus is observed, either in relation to each other or to the pelvic wall, adhesions must be suspected.

The next stage is the formation of the tubo-ovarian abscess. The image obtained by TVS is typical (Figs 6.13**A** and **B**). The structures involved can hardly be recognized, or cannot be recognized at all (Fig 6.13**A**). The pelvis is filled with a butterfly- or oval-shaped particulate matter containing fluid (Fig 6.13**B**). The two adnexa may show a slightly different picture, as if they were "out-of-phase," since the extent of involvement, the severity, and the pathological picture may vary considerably between the two sides. This phenomenon is depicted in Figure 6.13**A**.

If the gas-producing organisms are present the picture will reveal highly echogenic speckles within the abscess (Fig 6.13**B**). This image can be duplicated by scanning freshly obtained tap water in which the micro air bubbles create the floating high echoes.

The sonographic image of the inflammatory tubo-ovarian disease by the transvaginal probe is typical. A series of dilated, fluid-filled, round, thick-walled structures is apparent. Cross sections of the tube may show differences in size, but careful scanning in either plane will reveal the continuity of the tortuous lumen of the thick tube. The tube usually "embraces" the ovary, which loses its typical structure of stroma and follicles. Some of the ovarian follicles may still be recognized, thus enabling localization of the "ovarian part" of the tubo-ovarian disease (Figs 6.10 and 6.11).

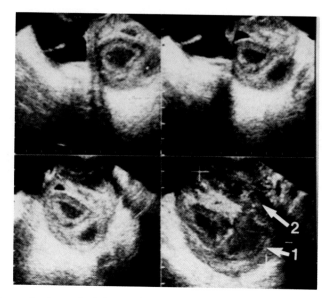

Figure 6.10 The acute phase of a tubo-ovarian abscess is shown. The tubal wall is thickened (1). The "ovarian portion," which is usually "embraced" by the dilated tube, is in the upper right of these sections (2). Pelvic fluid is evident on some of the images.

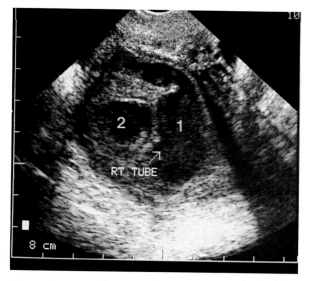

Figure 6.11 The tubo-ovarian complex is an entity easily recognized by TVS. The "tubal part" consists of the typical dilated tube (1). If the process is chronic, the wall of the tube is thin as in this picture. The "ovarian part" may show follicles or a cystic structure (2).

This tubo-ovarian conglomerate may be at its acute or its chronic stage. It also may appear as a result of recurrent flare-up in a patient with known previous pelvic inflammatory disease (PID). Spontaneous or elicited pelvic pain may be used to differentiate between acute and chronic cases of tubo-ovarian disease.

If tubo-ovarian pathology, or TOA, is diagnosed and emergency surgery is not

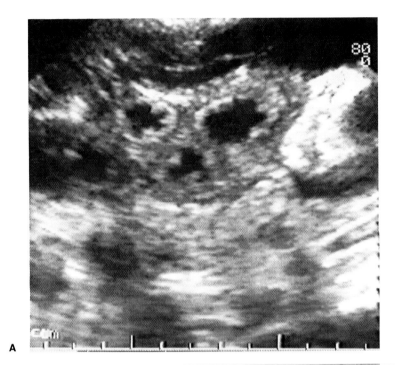

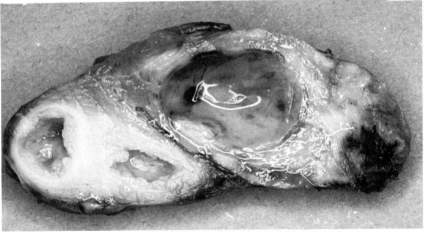

Figure 6.12 The "cogwheel" sign. (**A**) An affected, inflammatory tube is imaged. The section cuts through three loops of the tube. Note the hyperechoic protrusions of the endosalpinx into the sonolucent content rendering the cogwheel appearance. (**B**) The appearance of the specimen obtained at surgery supports the sonographic image.

considered or indicated, a series of follow-up examinations should be conducted to evaluate (a) the efficacy of conservative antibiotic treatment or (b) the appearance of a growing pelvic abscess that may need surgical intervention.

There has been speculation about the possibility of a transvaginal, ultrasound-guided fine-needle aspiration of pus for bacteriological workup, which may make early and adequate therapy possible.

The possibility of using TVS in diagnosing tubal disease was discussed by Lauder et al.[4]

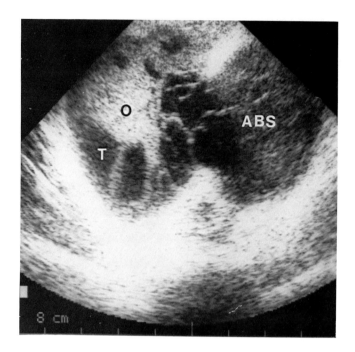

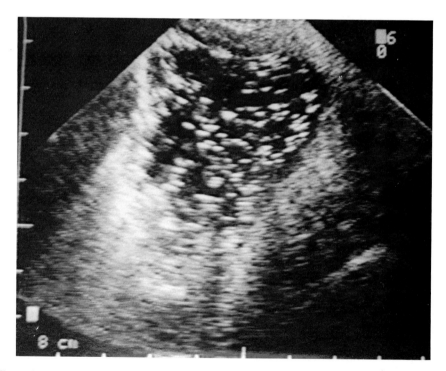

Figure 6.13 (**A**) This image illustrates the stages in the formation of tubo-ovarian disease. On the right, the ovary (O) and tube (T) are still discernible. On the left side, the tissue boundaries and the anatomy have broken down. The abscess (ABS) is evident. (**B**) Image of a pelvic abscess. The tubal or ovarian structures cannot be demarcated. A large abscess resulting from rupture of a TOA was found at surgery. The hyperechoic speckles result from gas formation in the abscess.

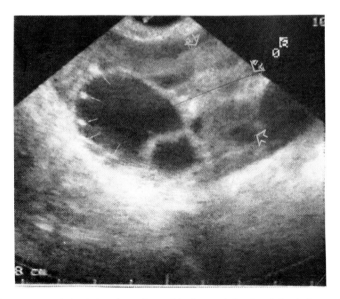

Figure 6.14 Carcinoma of the tube. An enlarged tortuous fallopian tube is imaged. The distal part (left side of picture) shows a hydrosalpinx (small arrows point to typical "cogwheel" sign). The proximal portion of the "solid" 0.3 × 3 cm mass (over arrows).

TUBAL PREGNANCY

Tubal pregnancy is widely discussed in Chapter 14 and is mentioned here only because of its typical place in the list of tubal pathologies. Tubal pregnancy should always be suspected and, if possible, ruled out using multiple clinical, laboratory, and sonographic means.

MALIGNANCY OF THE TUBE

Of all gynecological cancers, this entity is the rarest malignancy of all (0.1–0.5%), with adenocarcinoma the most common type. However, other cell types have been reported. The malignancy has a predilection for women of low parity and the average age with this at the diagnosis is 55.

The attributed symptom and sign is a lower abdominal pain, relieved by the vaginal discharge of relatively large amounts of brownish colored fluid. This cancer behaves similar to the ovarian malignancies and spreads along lymphatics, draining the ovaries. Its picture by TVS was reported by Hinton et al,[5] Mertz,[6] and Rottem et al,[7] and is comprised of an adnexal mass with mixed echogenicity (Fig 6.14). The normal ovary was seen adjacent to the mass. The diagnosis in most cases was made after the surgical specimen was examined by the pathologist.

DIFFERENTIAL DIAGNOSIS OF TUBAL IMAGING

Differential diagnoses regarding the sonographic appearance of the salpinx require the following considerations:

1. A larger-than-average *ovarian follicle* possibly presenting as a dilated chronic hydrosalpinx. Its location in the ovary and adjacent to other smaller follicles, as well as its changing size through the menstrual cycle, makes the diagnosis simple.

2. A small *ovarian cyst,* which may mimic a thin-walled, distended hydrosalpinx. A carefully performed scan will invariably detect ovarian tissue as an integral part of this cystic ovary.
3. *Encapsulated fluid* in the pouch of Douglas presenting as hydrosalpinx or pyosalpinx. One should look for a contiguous tubal wall, which is not present in cases of peritoneal inclusion cysts.

In summary, the importance of TVS in tubal workup is one of its major strengths. It is the opinion of the authors, based on the outstanding ability of TVS to visualize a pathological or normal tube, that there has been a major breakthrough in pelvic sonography of the female patient.

Imaging of *tubal pathology* seems relatively simple to perform with the transvaginal probe, because most tubal lesions are connected with the presence of fluid (eg, blood or inflammatory fluid) around and in the fallopian tubes. As discussed in previous chapters, this fluid serves as excellent "sonographic contrast material" for good imaging and diagnosis. On the other hand, imaging of a *normal salpinx* depends on the presence of the normally occurring free pelvic fluid. There is the possibility of selecting a midcycle day for the scan or placing the patient in a slightly reversed Trendelenburg position, but the obvious limitations preclude consistent imaging of the healthy tube.

Transvaginal sonography employing a higher-frequency transducer probe produces images with high resolution, opening realistic possibilities for a more reliable and clinically more meaningful diagnostic workup of the fallopian tube.

REFERENCES

1. Davis FA, Gosink BB: Fluid in the female pelvis: cyclic patterns. J Ultrasound Med 1986;5:75.
2. Timor-Tritsch IE, Rottem S. Transvaginal ultrasonographic study of the fallopian tube. Obstet Gynecol 1987;70:424–428.
3. Clarke-Pearson DL, Dawood MY: Green's Gynecology Fourth Edition. Boston, Little, Brown and Company, 1990.
4. Lander IM, Hill MC, Cosco FE, Kator NN: Adnexal and cul-de-sac abnormalities: transvaginal sonography. Radiology 1988;166:325–332.
5. Hinton A, Bea C, Winfield AC, Entman SS: Carcinoma of the fallopian tube. Urol Radiol 1988;10:113–115.
6. Merz E: Sonographische Diagnostik in Gynecologie und Geburtshilfe. Georg Thieme Verlag Stuttgart, New York, 1988.
7. Rottem S: Unpublished data.

CHAPTER 7

Ovarian Pathology

Shraga Rottem, MD, DSc
Ilan E. Timor-Tritsch, MD

INTRODUCTION

Ovarian tumors are a matter of great concern because of their malignant potential and the limited ability to safely distinguish between benign and malignant neoplasms prior to surgery. Ovarian malignant neoplasms cause more deaths than any other female genital tract malignancy. Each year, 19,000 women in the United States and 3500 in the United Kingdom die from ovarian cancer.

Due to a paucity of early and specific symptoms, the disease had spread beyond the ovaries in 73–80% of the cases when detected.[1-4]

The relationship between five-year survival and disease stage is well known.[5,6]

A late diagnosis by traditional techniques is probably the main reason for the poor prognosis,[7,8] which may be only slightly improved by aggressive surgery and the new therapeutic regimens.

However, when checkups are performed, *negative examinations* may have positive psychological effects in women with normal findings. In a Swedish study, feelings and attitudes toward ultrasound ovarian screening for early detection of ovarian cancer in risk groups were evaluated on the visual analogue scale.[9] The large majority (92%), were satisfied with the information given at the examination, and 74% felt calm afterward. Most women (88%) wanted to be examined on a regular basis, many found the examination important (82%), and nobody was overly anxious. Short-term effects of this type of screening seem to be overwhelmingly positive in women with normal findings. Long-term effects of the screening are not yet known.

When screening patients at risk for cancer, one may expect that the detection of *positive findings* would lead to an improved outlook. However, there have been no studies showing that the stage of the ovarian cancer at the time of diagnosis in patients at risk changes significantly from those without risk.

Detection of ovarian carcinoma at an early stage was for the most part considered a coincidence, regardless of the modality employed (ie, pelvic bimanual examination, serum markers, imaging, cul-de-sac cytologic washing).[10]

Ovarian tumors present with more facets than all female genital tumors together. This great diversity makes *macroscopic diagnosis* of the resected specimen in most cases inaccurate even with the naked eye. For example, in pre- and postmenopausal women, epithelial ovarian neoplasms account for at least 50% of benign ovarian tumors and 85% of primary malignant tumors. Malignant gonadal stromal and germ cell tumors are less frequent in this age group. In younger women, functional, epithelial, and benign germ cell cysts prevail.[5,11]

The serous cell carcinomas are the most common epithelial cancers. These tend to be larger than 14 cm in more than 50% of the cases, and at the time of diagnosis 3.9% are less than 5 cm in diameter.[5,11,12] The majority are composed of multilocular cysts with multiple papillary masses and solid nodules sometimes obliterating the cystic cavities. About 8% are solid adenocarcinomas without cystic elements. Benign serous cysts usually have no papillary masses on their inner surfaces. On the other hand, a smooth inner surface does not guarantee a benign nature.[12,13]

Tumor growth on the outer surface can be seen in almost half of the carcinomas, but this is also true in almost 10% of the benign lesions. Mucinous benign cysts tend to be larger, but size alone does not indicate malignancy.

The capsular surface is usually smooth, but firm mural nodules are common, and a few have intracystic papillae. Mucinous adenocarcinomas are usually cystic (approximately 76% multilocular and 24% unilocular).[12]

Other epithelial ovarian tumors also present a spectrum of cystic, solid, and papillary components.[12,13]

Germ cell and gonadal stromal tumors, benign and malignant, are usually solid.[12,13]

The dermoid cyst, which is a benign germ cell tumor, usually presents multilocular fluid with sebum, fat, hair, and teeth, making its benign nature quite easy to evaluate macroscopically.[13]

Functional ovarian cysts are by definition non-neoplastic cysts (eg, follicular or lutein cysts). They are always monolocular with smooth inner and outer surfaces. These cysts, usually less than 5–6 cm in diameter, are common in young women. Observation of spontaneous regression is the proof of their benignity.[5,13]

In certain early stages of ovarian tumors, even the *histopathological evaluation* is difficult and equivocal, depending on multiple sections of the tumor and on the skill of the pathologist.[12,13]

When a disease presents with so many macroscopic (and microscopic) characteristics, it would be unfair to expect a histological diagnosis when using ultrasonography.

Ultrasonography of the normal ovaries was first reported in 1972.[14] A large amount of literature was dedicated to the ability of the ultrasonographic method for early detection of ovarian cancer. Over the years it became evident that *transabdominal sonography* (TAS) provided a partial, but certainly not the entire, answer to this problem.

The later approach, employing *transvaginal sonography* (TVS), seemed more promising in ovarian imaging and for the evaluation of gynecological pathology.[15,16,17]

Employing this basic knowledge in dealing with ovarian cancer, we know that (1) this is an important disease with a high cumulative lifetime incidence (1.4% of all females will develop it over their lifetime); (2) it is a serious disease and the leading cause of death in women suffering a gynecological malignancy; and (3) treatment has not significantly changed the course of the disease in the last ten years. However, for patients who underwent surgical staging and were found to have stage 1a or 1b disease with well or moderately differentiated histologic features, the five-year survival was excellent (≥90%).[18]

In this chapter, we will provide the reader with the current procedures for screening of ovarian cancer, and thus, it may serve as background for understanding the available tools to detect this intractible disease.

The second aim of the chapter is to critically evaluate TVS, a promising new tool, not only for its ability to characterize ovarian lesions, but also for its potential ability to be used as the most powerful screening tool for early detection of ovarian cancer.

DIAGNOSTIC–SCREENING TECHNIQUES

There is a basic difference between *diagnostic* and *screening procedures*. The *diagnostic* algorithm is aimed at finding a disease or faulty organ in an individual who presents with symptoms or abnormal laboratory tests. *Screening* means the active search for disease amongst apparently healthy individuals who are sufficiently at risk for the diseases, in this case the *ovarian cancer*. The following diagnostic and screening techniques for ovarian cancer can be considered:

Vaginal Examination (Pelvic Bimanual Examination)

The chances for detecting ovarian cancer at an early stage by pelvic bimanual examination are extremely low. Insufficient information for the patient leads to unjustified patient reassurance based on pelvic bimanual examination performed during yearly checkups.

Andolf et al[18a] reported on 37 false negative findings in 194 women with pelvic pathology, of them 13 had ovarian tumors (3.5%). Ovarian cysts of 4 to 6 cm were missed in 7 cases while 6 cases of solid ovarian tumors were equally distributed as less or more than 3 cm. Lundberg et al found a very low prospective detection rate of ovarian masses.[19]

Enlargement of the ovaries in elderly women was considered pathological by Barber et al,[20] who called this the "post menopausal palpable ovary syndrome" (PMPO). For years, oophorectomy was recommended when PMPO was detected.[21]

Pelvic bimanual examination under anesthesia, laparoscopy, and laparotomy were liberally employed to establish that there were no ovarian masses present in patients at risk for ovarian carcinoma presenting with pelvic pain. Since pain is a subjective feeling not always caused by organic disease of the ovaries, the above-mentioned diagnostic procedures will usually reveal normal ovaries.[22–24]

Many women will be reassured by the examining physician regarding the presence or absence of ovarian pathology on the basis of palpatory findings alone. The impression of a bimanual examination of an ovary consists of transformation of palpatory signals originating at the mechanical receptors situated on the fingertips into conceptual images by the brain. *However, this "finger-tip transducer" creates only a partial picture image impression of the outer shape of the ovary.* The palpating finger does not penetrate beneath the surface of the ovary itself. In a significant number of women nonideal conditions such as obesity or previous pelvic surgery will further compromise the role of the palpation. Picking up signals from Paccini terminations and transforming them into conceptual images *aim to serve as a method* for the detection of gynecological pathology generally and for the detection of ovarian pathology particularly. It seems that we ask for the impossible to be done.

Cul-De-Sac Cytology Washing

The method of instillation and aspiration of fluid into the cul-de-sac for cytologic studies was originally proposed in the sixties, and was reproposed ten years ago. With the exception of the positive evaluation of Zylberberg,[25] the method fails to give conclusive answers to the question of pelvic malignancies,[26] and detects only disseminated cancer.[10,27]

Radiological Methods

Radiological methods such as Computerized Tomography (CT), and Magnetic Resonance Imaging (MRI) may be used at the time when ovarian tumors have already been diagnosed. Tumor spread can be detected by CT especially if located in spaces such as paravaginal, peritoneal or retroperitoneal.[28] CT and MRI may not recognize enlarged lymph nodes or peritoneal implants smaller than 2 cm.

Using MRI, adnexal structures, normal or abnormal, can be recognized[29] and imaging tumors as small as 0.5 cm is possible.[30] However, MRI is not cost effective, is time consuming, and, therefore, its use is impractical for screening. Computerized tomography has a low yield and radiation exposure. It may be useful in the diagnostic process when ultrasound suggests cancer of the ovary, but it seems to be inadequate for screening.[31]

Radioimmunoscintigraphy

Surface antigens may reflect the qualitative difference between the cancer cell and normal cells. Antibodies directed toward one of these surface antigens can be labeled with a radioactive isotope, given to the patient intravenously, and then monitored using a gamma camera. The test may help in the case of tumor recurrence or a residual tumor after first-line therapy,[32] but it is unlikely that a healthy population can be screened by this method.

Serum Markers

A variety of antigens expressed by tumors have been investigated in ovarian cancer. One of them, *CA 125,* is elevated above the level of 30 U/ml in 80–85% of clinically presenting ovarian cancers.[33-41] However, concentrations may be higher in cases of pelvic inflammatory disease and endometriosis. On the other hand, CA 125 levels may be lower sometimes, even in patients with residual tumors detected by second-look operations. The antigen is not found in the sera of patients with borderline tumors or mucinous ovarian cancers. However, another antigen, *CA 19-9,* has been found to be elevated in 87.5% of all mucinous malignancies.[42]

Sensitivity of high levels of CA 125 for Stage I disease is less than the 50% achieved for those women presenting with symptoms; therefore, CA 125 is unlikely to be used for screening.

Another antigen, *NB/70K,* has been detected in 50% of all ovarian cancers including early stages.[43,44]

Carcinoembryonic antigen (CEA) is elevated in 30–40% of all ovarian cancers, though seldom in early stages and unspecific. In contrast, *alpha-fetoprotein (AFP)* and *human chorionic gonadotropin (HCG)* are usually only elevated in ovarian cancers such as endodermal sinus tumors and cell tumors with trophoblastic elements.[10,45]

Placental alkaline phosphatase has been elevated in 17–50% of all ovarian cancers.[46]

Fibrin degradation products (FDP) have been found to be elevated in sera of patients with malignancies, but also in benign conditions such as thrombosis and renal disease, and after physical exercise.[47]

By using a combination of markers, a higher sensitivity of ovarian cancer detection may be achieved, but this would significantly increase its false positive rate. This is a relevant disadvantage when screening for ovarian cancer, a disease with a relatively low incidence since it may increase the chances of unnecessary surgical procedures.

As opposed to this, given the heterogenic nature of ovarian tumors, the detection of a highly sensitive tumor-associated antigen is a utopian prospect.

The reader will find a new attempt to distill the essence of the conception, birth, growth, and future direction of tumor markers in gynecologic oncology in a recent review.[47a]

Ultrasonography

Role of Transabdominal Sonography in Ovarian Diagnosis

Real-time sector transducer probes have been preferred for pelvic sonography over B-mode and linear transducer probes by most authors.[10,48–51] This route was preferred because of the sector scanner's ability to reach pelvic structures "hidden" by the symphysis or located deeper in the pelvis. The characteristics to be sought are the smoothness of the inner cystic wall, inner and outer nodularity of cysts, septa, exact sequences of solid and cystic components, and inner content of ovarian cysts.

A short review of TAS in pelvic imaging will illustrate its achievements in diagnosing ovarian tumors.

Lawson, in a series of 251 pelvic masses, showed an accuracy of 91% in determining the existence, size, location, and consistency of pelvic lesions.[51] Deland et al[52] predicted ovarian cancer by TAS in 13 of 14 patients. Only one of 38 ovarian tumors with a pure cystic pattern was malignant. In contrast, more than 70% of tumors with complex or solid patterns were malignant. Exact tumor size was predicted in about 90%.

Meire et al[53] showed a good correlation between sonography and pathology. In 23 women, all cystic masses *smaller than 5 cm* proved to be benign. In women in whom the cysts were *unilocular* but larger than 5 cm, 17 of 19 were benign, but in women in whom the cysts were larger and *multilocular*, 16 of 17 were malignant. Seven of 8 patients with *thick septa* and 15 of 18 with solid nodules had malignant ovarian tumors. Requard et al[54] tried to evaluate ascitic, peritoneal, omental, and lymph node spread of ovarian cancer and to characterize gross appearance of pelvic masses. Gross appearance was predicted accurately by sonography in 26 of 31 cases. The false negative for predicting spread was high: 75% for lymph nodes, 80% for omental and peritoneal spread, and 16% for ascites. There were no false positive cases.

Campbell et al[55] proposed sonographic criteria for diagnosis of ovarian neoplasia in menopausal women, in whom every palpable ovary is by definition suspect for a malignancy. The sensitivity and specificity of their results were not established.

An encouraging report by Andolf et al[56] has shown the potential value of transabdominal ultrasonography for the detection of ovarian cancer in women attending an outpatient clinic.

The use of sonography prior to second-look laparotomy, which used to be a well-established procedure, was evaluated by Sonnendecker and Butterworth, who reported a high inaccuracy with this diagnostic tool.[57]

Wicks et al[58] showed that in clinically suspicious disease, sonography had 95% sensitivity as opposed to 20% in unsuspected disease. Specificity was 92% and 100%, respectively. Ovarian volume was suggested by Sample in 1977,[59] to correlate with the endocrinological status of the patient. The problem was the volume changes from puberty through pregnancy and postmenopause. Nomograms were compiled for ovarian size as a function of the life cycle and the menstrual cycle itself.[60] This volume calculation depends heavily on exact ovarian measurements.

An enlarged ovary is not necessarily a pathological one, but ovarian tumors, or polycystic ovaries, are associated with an increase in ovarian size in the overwhelming majority of cases.

Since the long-term prognosis for patients with ovarian tumors and, more specifically, for patients with ovarian carcinoma, has been correlated with the extent of their resection, sonographic evaluation of tumor size may play an important role in patient care.

More recently, Campbell et al assessed the value of ultrasonography as a screening procedure for early ovarian cancer.[61] In this study each of 5429 self-referred women without symptoms underwent three annual screenings to detect grossly abnormal ovaries or nonregressing masses. The rate of false positive results was 2.3%. The specificity was 97.7% and the predictive value of positive results on screening was 1.5%. It was not possible to differentiate between the ultrasonic appearance of early malignant and benign tumors. The odds that a positive result on screening indicated the presence of an *ovarian tumor*, any *ovarian cancer*, or *primary ovarian cancer* were about 1 to 2, 1 to 37, and 1 to 67, respectively. The authors proposed transabdominal ultrasonography to screen women without symptoms for persistent ovarian masses (early ovarian cancer included) and suggested that the rate of false positive results would be lower if transvaginal sonography were employed. This last statement, however, was not tested in the study itself.

O'Brien et al,[62] who evaluated transabdominal ultrasonography in the initial assessment of the gynecological patient in 1984, found that this technique is even inferior to clinical evaluation. The impact of TAS on the gynecological practice was significantly lower than its impact on the obstetrical practice.

Before the development of the new transvaginal probes, TAS was only able to differentiate the normal from the abnormal pelvis. This fell short of the expectations of the gynecologist and gyneco-oncologist.

DEVELOPING THE CRITERIA FOR TRANSVAGINAL ULTRASONOGRAPHIC DIAGNOSIS OF OVARIAN PATHOLOGY

Ovarian scanning using the transvaginal probe may be more time-consuming than the transabdominal approach for one major reason: when scanning with the abdominal probe, a general view of the whole pelvis is rapidly achieved even by the beginner. Orientation and localization of the ovaries is quick, but it has severe drawbacks regarding image quality, which affects its diagnostic potential.

Finding the ovary with the transvaginal probe sometimes means a step-by-step search until the familiar image of the ovary appears on the screen. However, once the ovary is identified, thanks to the superb resolution, structures of less than 1 mm can be magnified and interrogated to discriminate between normal and abnormal findings.

The criteria for transvaginal ultrasonographic diagnosis of the normal and abnormal ovarian pathology are presented.

The Normal Ovary

The normal ovary is relatively easy to detect. In the reproductive years, it is "disclosed" by sonographic "markers," ie, the follicles or the corpus luteum, as well as by the clear sound interface created by the smooth surface and dense ovarian tissue (Fig 7.1). It is usually found above and medially, overlying the hypogastric vein. Because of its mobility, the healthy, normal-size ovary may change its location in the pelvis during transvaginal scanning. Normal amounts of pelvic fluid sometimes help outline the ovary.

If abdominal or pelvic fluid (ascites or blood) is present, the ovary is easily found by TVS. The description of normal-appearing ovaries (Fig. 7.2) constitutes valuable sonographic information for the gynecologist and the gyneco-oncologist.

The difficulty in imaging the ovaries in the postmenopausal years arises from a combination of factors such as disappearance of the follicles, shrinkage of the ovary, and decreased pelvic fluid to provide an acoustic interface (Fig 7.3). The decreased elasticity of the vagina limits the maneuverability of the probe.

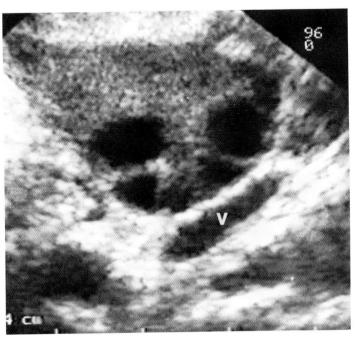

Figure 7.1 Transvaginal sonographic image of a normal ovary with follicles—its sonographic markers. V = hypogastric vein.

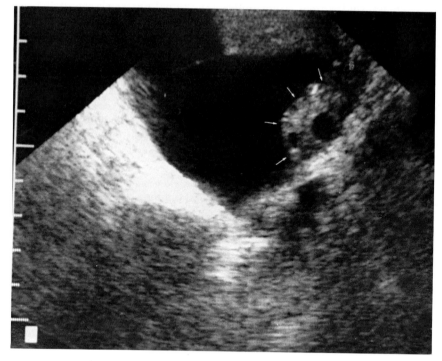

Figure 7.2 Ascitic fluid clearly outlines a normal ovary (arrows) defined by several follicles.

Sometimes the ovaries cannot be detected even after considerable time invested in the search. The application of color flow may enhance their detection by imaging the ovarian artery leading to the detection of the ovary itself. The percent of nondetected ovaries is higher in postmenopausal patients at a time when it would be most informative. There is a conundrum about the clinical meaning of this. Can this patient be reassured of the fact that her pelvis does not contain ovarian cancer? This in fact was done and is done all the time if the palpatory examination is negative.

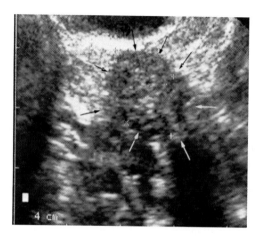

Figure 7.3 A small ovary (arrows) of a postmenopausal woman. No follicles are seen.

One view is that normalcy can only be so called if the ovary was found, imaged, and seems to be normal by criteria agreed upon. An opposing view holds that the high resolution of the transvaginal probes would detect a very small lesion if it were present. The detection rate would increase if the lesion had a sonolucent fluid compartment. Therefore, if the transvaginal sonographic examination is negative, there is a sound reason to reassure the patient. One study seems to support this view. Rodriquez et al[63] imaged by ultrasonography 85 of 104 ovaries in postmenopausal women scheduled for gynecology surgery unrelated to adnexal disease. The 19 ovaries that were not seen (18%) were atrophic at surgery with no evidence of disease. More data are needed to employ this concept of "negative TVS imaging result" clinically.

If hysterectomy had been performed, the ovaries are more difficult to locate. because of the bowel, which is filling the available space left by removal of the uterus. In this case, they can be situated anywhere in the pelvis. Using the second "abdominal hand" to displace the interfering loops of bowel can be very helpful.

Scanning the Patient With Ascites

Certainly by the time patients with ascites are evaluated, one of the first questions is whether the pathological condition arises from an ovarian tumor or is related to a nongynecological disorder (eg, hepatic, etc.).

A small quantity of fluid helps in the transvaginal ultrasonographic imaging of organs or lesions in this area, creating a fluid–tissue interface.

When a large amount of fluid is present, such as in ascites, the near field findings, such as pelvic peritoneal seedings of a tumor, are clearly outlined and ovarian pathology also may be revealed (Fig 7.4**A** and **B**). If the ovaries appear normal at the TVS scan, one may consider other reasons leading to ascites. However, in many cases of huge ascites both uterus and ovaries may be pushed toward the abdominal wall, beyond the focal length of the vaginal probe.

When to Scan for Ovarian Pathology

Scanning for ovarian problems during the second half of the cycle in nonpill users may reveal large corpus luteum cysts or supposed functional cysts. The final diagnosis may incur the need for rescanning of the patient during the first half of the next cycle. Therefore, during the reproductive years, it is recommended that scanning for ovarian problems be scheduled at the end of the menstrual period (with the exception of women using an estrogen/progesteron compound).

On the contrary, when there is a question of an ovarian mass during the perimenopausal years, it is worthwhile to schedule the scanning during the midcycle period. The small chance of finding follicles during this period improves the probability of detecting a normal ovary, which becomes a problem at this age.

However, where there are strong clinical indications for performing scanning, the examination should not be postponed in either of the two above examples.

Functional Disorders

Before menopause, the dynamic nature of the ovary should be considered. Two common entities emphasizing the changing ovarian function are described below.

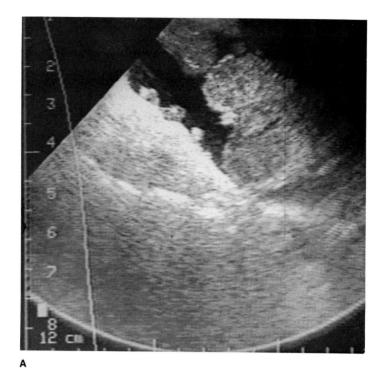

A

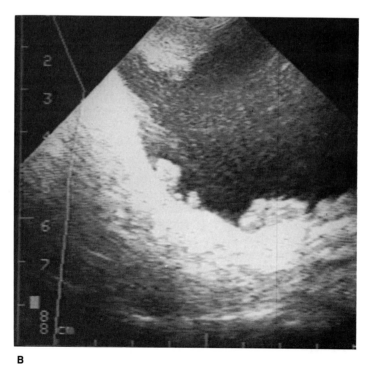

B

Figure 7.4 Two images of a 63-year-old patient diagnosed with stage III ovarian carcinoma. (**A**) Irregular tumors surrounded by ascites, and three nodular 0.75 cm structures adhering to the pelvic floor. (**B**) More of the pelvic peritoneal seeding of the tumor, outlined by ascitic fluid.

Functional Simple Cysts

These are always solitary, measuring up to 6–7 cm in diameter. Transvaginal sonography plays an important role in ruling out presence of any lesions such as irregularities in the content of the walls. Decrease in size may occur spontaneously and can be best detected by scanning the patient at day 5–10 of the next cycle. Hormonal suppression regimen can also be tried and its effect monitored by TVS.

Corpus Luteum Variants

At the time of ovulation, blood vessels are "severed" and intrafollicular bleeding occurs. The image of the corpus luteum (CL) changes almost from hour to hour and is a reflection of the natural process of bleeding, clot formation, retraction and reabsorption. Together with changes in the shape of the cyst, the dynamics of clot formation present the CL in the most bizarre fashion ever seen in a single entity. The clot may appear as an echogenic, scalloped structure, a "cavernous structure," an irregularly echogenic area, a multilocular mass, an echogenic core with "spikes," branching out to the periphery, or a fine mesh-like texture (Fig 7.5**A–F**). The CL indeed is the most fascinating structure in the female pelvis. It can mimic a number of pathologies such as neoplasia, ectopic gestation, a degenerating fibroid, etc. One should always try to identify the normal ovarian tissue around it for correct diagnosis. Followed by serial scanning, it decreases in size and blends into the normal ovarian tissue. Occasionally in the nonpregnant state, the corpus luteum may persist longer than its expected life span. In such cases, an abnormal growth may be observed, forming a corpus luteum cyst. The corpus luteum cyst may rupture, thus making the sonographic diagnosis extremely difficult. However, the free blood and blood clots can be easily seen in the pelvis.

The Polycystic Ovary

The polycystic ovary has a typical sonographic appearance[64–66] and is recognized as a larger or normal ovary of spheric shape, hosting multiple small (less than 10 mm) immature follicles crowded along its surface. This is called a "beads-on-a-string" appearance. If the patient is hormonally stimulated, the image of the polycystic ovary is even more evident and resembles the "stained glass window" shape. The above-mentioned features are shown in Fig 9.4**B** and **C**.

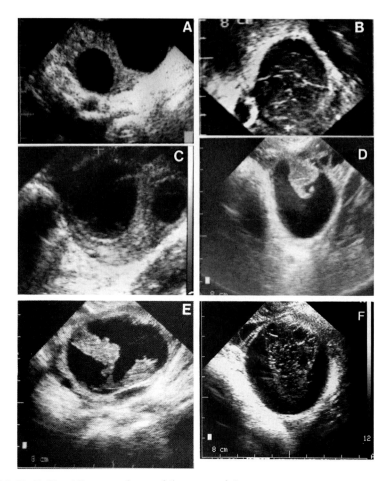

Figure 7.5 (A–F) Six of the many faces of the corpus luteum.

Criteria for Transvaginal Ultrasonographic Diagnosis of Ovarian Lesions

The role of transabdominal ultrasonography in detecting and locating pelvic masses and differentiating between ovarian and other tumors has been previously described. A significant overlap exists in many echo patterns seen in benign and malignant ovarian neoplasms. By using the transvaginal probe, particularly if it is equipped with a high-frequency crystal, pelvic structures can be scrutinized and measured at a precision of 1 mm. This high degree of accuracy prompted several studies on the correlation between ultrasonographically detected ovarian lesions and histopathological reports of ovarian neoplasias.

Three different centers (probably among many others) are conducting independent studies to characterize ovarian pathology by means of TVS. A pilot study performed at the Department of Obstetrics and Gynecology at the Rambam Medical Center showed that transvaginal sonography can identify and classify the ovarian lesions as follows[67]:

> **1.** *Septations:* these structures cross a liquid phase as echogenic bridges measuring from 0.5 mm to more than 1 cm (Fig 7.7).

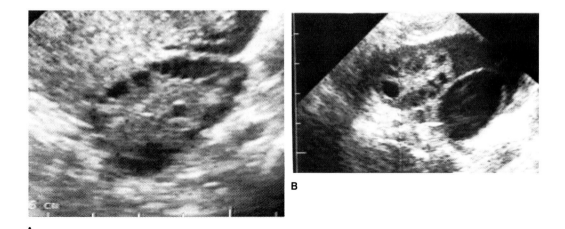

A

B

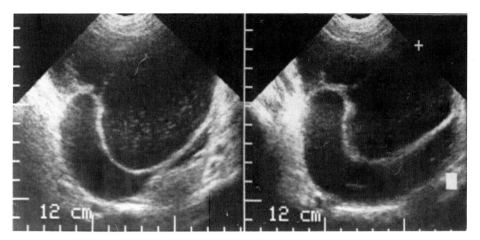

C

Figure 7.6 Three images of polycystic ovaries. (**A**) A normal-size ovary with very small peripheric follicles. (**B**) Peritoneal fluid provides high-quality images of two distinct entities: a normal-size ovary with very small follicles and a paraovarian cyst. (**C**) Small follicles are crowded at the surface of an enlarged spherical polycystic ovary.

Figure 7.7 Septations within a fluid-containing ovarian cyst; note the low-level echogenicity of the fluid. This was a luteoma.

2. *Papillae:* echogenic formations protruding into the liquid phase, measuring from 5 mm to more than 2 cm, but not occupying more than 25% of the space of the mass (Fig 7.8**A–C**).

3. *Daughter cysts:* embracing semicircular echogenic structures protruding into the liquid phase (Fig 7.9). The distance between the ends of the cyst is less than 1 cm, and they should not have interstructural contingency.

4. *Loculations:* embracing semicircular or circular echogenic structures protruding into the sonolucent content with interstructural contingency or measuring more than 1 cm between the two ends in case of a solitary structure (Fig 7.10**A–C**).

5. *Liquid phase:* intratumoral sonolucency of low-level echogenicity or completely sonolucent (Fig 7.11**A–C**).

6. *Solid lesion:* formation occupying more than 25% of the space of the mass (Fig 7.12**A,B**).

Combinations of lesions can also be detected (Fig 7.13**A,B**).

Subsequently, 904 patients were referred to transvaginal sonography for ruling out ovarian pathology.[68] Referral was based on positive findings on pelvic bimanual examination or on anamnestic risk. In the 904 patients referred, 360 ovaries presented one or more lesions at the transvaginal scan. Of these, 242 were followed by TVS until the findings resolved. Eight patients had no surgery due to their poor general conditions. In the remaining 90 patients who underwent surgery, 120 tumors were found. Ninety-nine of them were of ovarian origin: 78 were

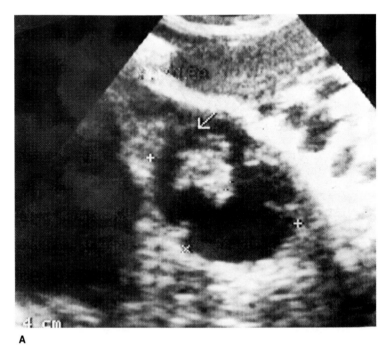

A

Figure 7.8 Papillary protrusions in three malignant tumors. (**A**) A normal-size postmenopausal ovary. The arrow points at a small papillary structure on the inner surface of a 1.8 × 1.5 cm cyst. Adenocarcinoma was the pathological diagnosis. (**B**) Low-level echogenic fluid fills an 8 × 7 cm ovarian cyst. Two of many papillary structures (P) on the inner surface of ovarian adenocarcinoma. (**C**) Small and large papillae in an ovarian cyst surrounded by ascites. The pathological report was ovarian adenocarcinoma.

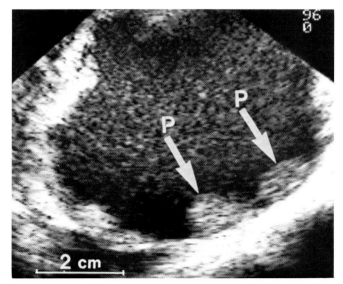

B

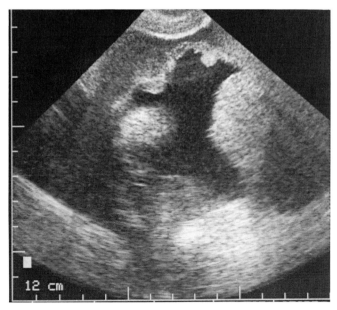

C

Figure 7.8 (*continued*)

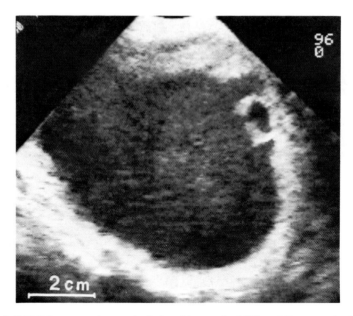

Figure 7.9 A 7 × 8.5 cm ovarian cyst. A daughter cyst of 0.8 × 0.5 cm protrudes into the echogenic fluid.

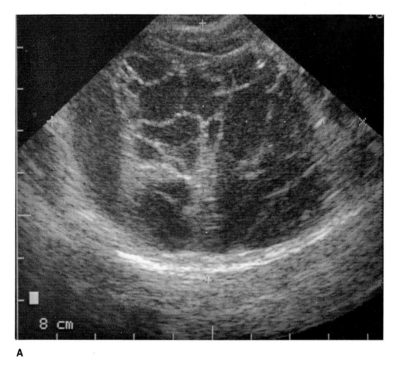

A

Figure 7.10 Three multilocular cysts show the intricate web of septa and echo-free fluid; all were subjected to pathological examination. (**A**) Benign cystadenoma. (**B**) Cystadenocarcinoma. (**C**) Dermoid cyst.

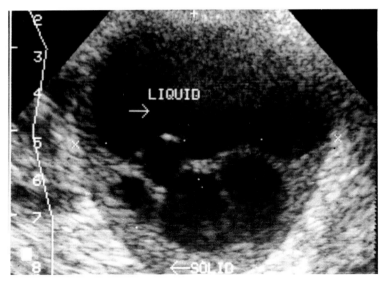

B

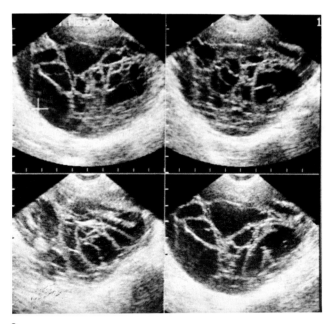

C

Figure 7.10 (*continued*)

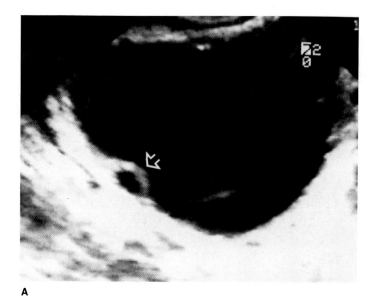

A

B

Figure 7.11 Three ovarian cysts with different echogenicity. (**A**) Sonolucent fluid in a benign cystoadenoma (arrow points at a daughter cyst. Note that the echogenicity of the fluid does not change by increasing the gain.). (**B**) Echogenic fluid in a dermoid cyst (the arrow points at a daughter cyst; an A-mode cursor is seen in the middle of the picture). (**C**) Large bilateral ovarian endometrioma scanned with a 5 MHz transvaginal probe. Note the uniformly echogenic thick blood contents (verified at operation) of the cysts. The uterus (u) and the bilateral involvement are shown.

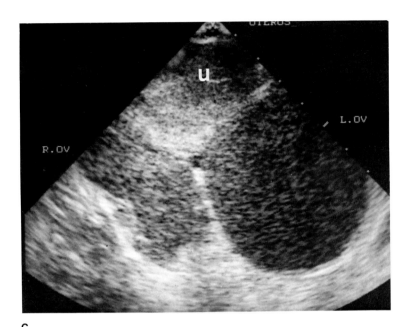

C

Figure 7.11 (*continued*)

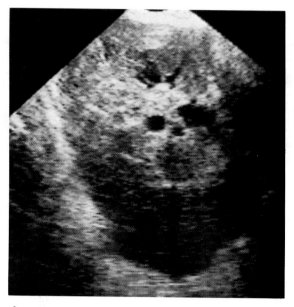

A

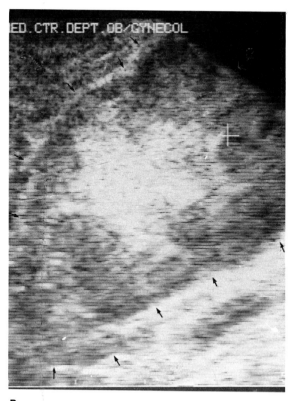

B

Figure 7.12 Solid lesions in two ovarian tumors. (**A**) A 6 × 4 cm solid tumor with mixed echo-genicity. The pathology was granulosa cell tumor. (**B**) A solid, germinal 6 × 4.5 cm tumor in a 67-year-old patient. The highly echogenic "core" is surrounded by a lower echogenic peripheral region. No Graafian follicles can be seen at this age.

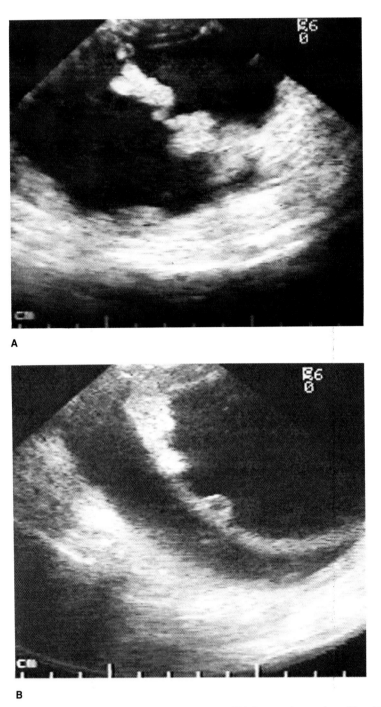

A

B

Figure 7.13 Two combinations of lesions are shown. (**A**) Thick septation and papillae. (**B**) Septation, papillae, and a daughter cyst.

benign and 21 were malignant. There were two cases of false positive diagnosis: a peritoneal inclusion cyst and a pelvic lymph node granuloma. There was one false negative case where an ovarian fibrothecoma was misdiagnosed as an intraligamentary myoma.

Transvaginal ultrasonographic findings based on the above criteria were compared to pathological findings using the computerized Statistical Analysis System (SAS). The six ultrasonographic criteria mentioned above were used as explanatory variables. Statistically significant correlation was found between ovarian malignancy and the following sonographic ovarian lesions:

1. Solid ovarian lesions ($P < 0.001$)
2. Presence of papillae ($P < 0.001$)
3. Presence of septa ($P < 0.003$)
4. Presence of papillae and septa ($P < 0.001$)

The significance of the *absence* of lesions such as papillae and or septae was also evaluated. This study proved that TVS can predict the nature of an ovarian neoplasm better than any other noninvasive test as it correlates significantly with histopathological reports.

In the aforementioned study, 4 of the 21 malignant tumors (19%) were less than 5 cm in their mean dimension. This study indicates that TVS practically eliminates most of the pitfalls reported when using TAS and with the improvement of skill and technique, we anticipate even a smaller number of errors in the future.

The results experienced in this study indicate that TVS was the most efficient means for detecting ovarian tumors (even of very small size). Its high resolution enables more detailed scrutiny of the lesions and provides information to characterize the ovarian pathology. TVS had a better predictive value for tumor detection than other noninvasive procedures.

To objectively characterize and describe the extrauterine pelvic pathology seen through transvaginal sonography, the group from Columbia Presbyterian Medical Center undertook a study.[69] The purpose of this study was to discriminate between benign and malignant entities using comparable and reproducible criteria. All laparotomies performed for gynecological indications, for a period of $2\frac{1}{2}$ years, were collected from the pathology registry. Ultrasonography files were reviewed and those patients who had undergone TVS within 1 mo before surgery were included. All the vaginal sonograms were reviewed, blinded to the pathology and to the original sonographic interpretations. A scoring system was developed which took into consideration the inner wall structure, the wall thickness, the presence and thickness of the septa, and, finally, the echogenecity of the lesion. Values of 1–5 were given to each of the four above-mentioned variables. One hundred forty-three cases with complete records qualified, but 16% of the patients were postmenopausal and the rest were premenopausal. Two hundred eighty-one ovaries were analyzed. Seventy-eight percent of the ovaries in the premenopausal group were imaged whereas only 62% of the postmenopausal ovaries were detected. Sixty-nine of the 280 ovaries were not seen at sonography in 15 bilaterally and in 39 unilaterally. In all these cases, the normal relationship among the pelvic organs was distorted by extraovarian pathology or by a large contralateral ovarian mass which was correctly described. An ovarian mass larger than 5 cm by TVS was associated with a 2.5 times greater chance of malignancy. There were 13 patients with *malignant lesions*. Of 26 ovaries in this group, 20 were affected by malignancy and 6 were normal. Only one single ovary was missed that contained a small adenocarcinoma. However, in this case the contralateral malignancy in the ovary was correctly identified. More important results of this group were: (1) The echogenicity was other than sonolucent in almost all cases. (2) The inner wall was never smooth. (3) The wall was thin in only one case (a borderline cyst adenoma). On the others the wall was thick or the lesion mostly solid. (4) More than half of the ovaries had septa from which more than one-half were thick.

Dermoids: There were 24 dermoids in 23 patients. They were all identified except one which was described as a cul-de-sac mass requiring intervention.

Endometriomas: There were 22 patients with 30 endometriomas. All of them had thin walls and almost all had contents with low-level echogenicity and a slightly echogenic core.

Simple cysts: There were 29 cysts in 21 patients. Only one was missed because of a contralateral large dermoid which was correctly diagnosed. All were thin-walled, contained sonolucent fluid, and had no papillary lesions.

Corpora lutea, hemorrhagic cysts, and *cystoadenomas* were all seen (n = 6, 5, and 6, respectively). All of them had low scores. Finally, *cystoadenofibromas* and *fibrothecomas* (n = 6 and 6, respectively) were all detected and had low scores.

The most important achievement in this trial to characterize ovarian lesions by TVS was the fact that only one true false negative occurred out of 20 ovaries with cancer. However, even in this case, the contralateral diseased ovary was correctly identified, and the patient was subjected to surgery. As the results were evaluated, it became obvious that the best discriminatory power was achieved using the described four variables together.

The likelihood of the ratio of cancer based on the lesions smaller and larger or equal to 5 cm was estimated. Introduction of the "size" parameter in our scoring system would not have improved the sensitivity because of the large number of benign lesions greater than 5 cm. Therefore, the specificity would have further decreased.

Pathology found outside the ovaries contributed to the complexity of the transvaginal images. From the study it was clear that other lesions such as subserous myomas, adhesions, and hydrosalpinges may be read as ovarian pathology with a high score unless correctly differentiated from the ovaries.

The results of this study clearly indicated that using TVS exclusively, the presence of malignancy could be predicted in each case. In addition, false positive cases did reveal benign lesions at laparotomy which would have warranted surgery. The scoring system was found to be explicit and reproducible. Its efficacy using the transvaginal route only, without complementary abdominal scanning, yielded results slightly superior to previously reported abdominal–vaginal or abdominal studies.

Bourne et al[70] presented a prospective study to screen for ovarian cancer in a high-risk group of symptomatic women. A scoring system was developed in which scores of 0 to 3 were seen in the categories of texture (solid = 3, monocystic = 1, multicystic = 2), loculations (unilocular = 0, multilocular = 1), outline of the cysts (irregular = 2, regular = 0), and also on the basis of anechoic (0), randomly echoic (2) and uniformly echogenic (1) appearance.

They observed the benign cystic lesions scored from 2 (simple cysts) to 5.5 (endometriomas and dermoids), whereas malignant lesions scored higher.

Fleischer et al[71] examined the ovaries of 30 postmenopausal patients by TVS prior to surgery. Mean age was 61 (55–92). The presence, size, and sonographic texture (not fully specified or categorized) of the ovaries were noted and compared to the resected pathologic specimen. A serum CA 125 determination was also performed. In this study both ovaries were detected 60% of the time. At least one ovary was detected 80% of the time. The size of the normal sonographically imaged ovary was 2.2 ($\pm$0.7) $\times$ 1.2 ($\pm$0.3) $\times$ 1.1 ($\pm$0.6) cm with a volume of 2.6 $\pm$ 2.0 ml. The ovaries not detected by TVS were 0.7 $\pm$ 0.4 cm. Four cysts ranging from 0.5 to 3.5 cm were found and confirmed pathologically. TVS missed a 6 cm dermoid, a 0.8 cm sertoli tumor, a 1 cm leiomyoma, and a 2 cm cystoadenoma. They concluded that TVS can accurately delineate the ovaries in most, but not all, postmenopausal women. Some pathologic lesions will not be detected. In their judgment, TVS in combination with CA 125 analysis has a significant potential for detecting early ovarian carcinoma.

According to Granberg et al,[72] the probability that unilocular tumors less than 10 cm in diameter and without papillary formations are malignant is low, irrespective of the woman's age.

Changes in Intraovarian Impedance to Flow by Color Doppler Ultrasonography

Transvaginal color Doppler imaging for the assessment of pelvic pathology was first described by Kurjak et al (see also Chapter 17).[73] One of the possible applications of this recent development is to assess whether changes in the intraovarian vasculature or blood flow impedance can be used to identify potentially malignant masses.[74]

Absence of intratumoral neovascularization and the resulting high pulsatility index can be used to exclude the presence of invasive primary ovarian cancer and therefore reduce the rate of false positive results from the screening procedure using conventional ultrasonography. Preliminary data suggest that color Doppler ultrasonography may be used to discriminate between benign and malignant ovarian lesions at an early stage of tumorgenesis. This in turn may reduce the rate of false positive results of an ultrasonography-based screening procedure.

DISCUSSION

It is natural that the technique of *pelvic bimanual examination* is the first one to be discussed. For centuries this was not only the "always" in the diagnosis of female gynecological disorders, but also the first to be done.

Gynecological practice undoubtedly depends on this examination. However, until now, there were no studies reporting encouraging results on the screening for early detection of ovarian cancer at palpation.

The role of *abdominal ultrasonography* for the diagnosis of ovarian tumors was extensively discussed during the last two decades. Two statements can summarize this era:

1. TAS was an acceptable method for differentiating the normal from the abnormal pelvis.
2. Once an ovarian mass was detected, the method rarely allowed for distinction between the ultrasonic appearance of the early malignant and benign tumors.

In our opinion, the last statement questions the validity of TAS as a screening procedure for early ovarian cancer, as recently suggested.[61] Other techniques reviewed in this chapter may provide additional information to TAS and PV but are impractical for screening.

Before analyzing the potential role of TVS as a procedure to improve the outlook of ovarian cancer, we would like to refer to one of the latest reports of Campbell et al.[61] The objective of their eight-year study was to assess the value of TAS in a screening procedure for early ovarian cancers. Their conclusion, after performing 15,977 scans in 5479 self-referred women without symptoms, was that ultrasonography can be used to screen for persistent ovarian *masses,* including early ovarian cancer. This study could not identify any morphological characteristics or patterns that could be used to differentiate between ovarian tumor-like conditions and tumors, or between benign and early malignant tumors.

The term *mass,* or *maza* in Greek, is a quantity or aggregate of matter, usually of considerable size, or an expanse or bulk with massive effect. By using the transvaginal probe, particularly if equipped with a high-frequency crystal, pelvic structures can be scrutinized and measured at a precision of 1 mm.

Therefore one may switch from the term ''mass'' to the term ''lesion,'' an abnormal change in the structure of an organ or part due to disease.

The studies from Rambam Medical Center, Kings College, and Columbia Presbyterian Medical Center presented the following conclusions.

1. *TVS has a high detection rate of ovarian tumors* with very few false negative and false positive results.
2. *TVS detects tiny ovarian lesions* with a precision heretofore not known, regardless of the ovarian or mass size.
3. *A malignant tumor can be predicted* in most cases by correlating a sonographic score originating from the presence or absence of single or a combination of several TVS characteristics.
4. The accuracy of TVS alone in predicting the malignant nature of a tumor yields results superior to previously reported abdominal studies.

The latest development, *color Doppler,* is a technique simple to use, and the results are displayed clearly.[73] The facility to resolve small changes in vascularity, and thus measure changes in impedance to flow within the ovary, is perhaps the most exciting development. *Recognition of angiogenesis as a reference point for malignant change within the ovary* may prove to be a highly significant parameter.[74] Given that the neovascularization is an obligate event in malignant change, this may enable us to observe the earliest stages in ovarian oncogenesis.

Factors promoting or inhibiting angiogenesis have been investigated, the growth and progression of tumors being dependent on the process of vascular supply. A new platelet-derived factor that stimulates endothelial cell growth and chemotaxis in vitro and angiogenesis in vivo has been recently identified.[75]

An inhibitor or angiogenesis, which is produced by cells when they are capable of expressing an active cancer-suppressing gene, has also been discovered.[76] The loss of this inhibitor activity occurs concomitantly with expression of angiogenesis and tumorigenesis.

Ovarian cancer, unlike breast cancer, has no good prognostic factors for *predicting biological behavior of the tumor* or eventual clinical outcome in patients afflicted with the disease. Clinical stage has some predictive value, but the vast majority of ovarian cancer patients have spread the disease at initial diagnosis, which makes this factor less useful in most patients. The histologic grading (determination of the degree of cellular differentiation within the tumor) has been used with some success. However, as with other malignancies, the histologic grading of ovarian cancers suffers from a lack of standardization and considerable observer-related variability.

A new tool for predicting the prospects of ovarian cancer patients is the study of a proto-oncogene, the HER-2/new, that appears in multiple copies in tumors from women who are more likely to suffer a relapse and die early.[77]

At this time, *in the lack of other practical and effective screening devices*, the authors consider *high-frequency transvaginal sonography the most powerful tool in screening for early detection of ovarian cancer.*

Detection of stage I disease still means that up to 10^9 malignant cells may be present. By using flow data from color Doppler, in addition to conventional imaging, one may detect the neovascularization, a new early reference point for malignant changes, possibly a step before the appearance of lesions. Very early detection of ovarian cancer will soon become the golden standard in many centers. The authors believe the application of transvaginal sonography will truly reflect on the outcome of this disease.

REFERENCES

1. Silverberg H: Cancer statistics, 1983, CA-A Ca J Clin 1983;33:9–25.
2. Sigurdsson K, Alm P, Gullberg B: Prognostic factors in malignant epithelial ovarian tumors. Gynecol Oncol 1983;15:370–380.
3. Einhorn N, Nilsson B, Sjövall K: Factors influencing survival in carcinomas of the ovary. Cancer 1985;55:2019–2025.
4. Yancik R, Gloeckler RL, Yates JW: Ovarian cancer in the elderly: An analysis of surveillance, epidemiology, and end results program data. Am J Obstet Gynecol 1986;154:639–647.
5. Disaia P, Creasman W: The adnexal mass and early ovarian cancer, in Clinical Gynecologic Oncology, 2d ed. St. Louis, CV Mosby, 1984, pp 254–285.
6. Kottmeier H: Annual report of the results of treatment in gynecological cancer. Vol 18. Stockholm, Federation Internationale De Gynaecologie et D'Obstetrique, 1982.
7. Cramer DW: Epidemiologic and statistical aspects of gynecologic oncology, in RC Knapp and RS Berkowitz (eds): Gynecologic Oncology, New York, MacMillan, 1986, pp 201–202.
8. Beral V: The epidemiology of ovarian cancer, in Sharp F, Soutter WP (eds): Ovarian Cancer—The Way Ahead. Chichester, Wiley, 1987;21–31.
9. Andolf E, Jorgensen C, Underberg N, Ursing I: The psychological effects of ultrasound screening for ovarian carcinoma in women with normal results. Submitted to Psycho Obstet Gynecol, 1989.
10. Smith L: Detection of malignant ovarian neoplasms: a review of the literature. 1. Detection of the patient at risk; clinical, radiological and cytological detection. Obstet Gynecol Surv 1984;39:313–328.
11. Disaia P, Creasman W: Advanced epithelial ovarian cancer, in Clinical Gynecological Oncology, 2d ed. St. Louis, Mo. CV Mosby, 1984, 286–360.
12. Hart W: Pathology of malignant and borderline epithelial tumors of ovary, in Coppleson M (ed): Gynecologic Oncology. London, Churchill Livingstone, 1981, 633–654.
13. Scully R: Atlas of Tumor Pathology. Tumors of the Ovary and Maldeveloped Gonads. Bethesda, Armed Forces Institute of Pathology, 1979.
14. Kratochwil A, Urban G, Friedrich F: Ultrasonic tomography of the ovaries. Ann Chir Gynaecol 1972;61:211–214.
15. Schwimer SR, Lebovic J: Transvaginal pelvic ultrasonography. J Ultrasound Med 1984;3:381–383.
16. Timor-Tritsch IE, Rottem S: Transvaginal Sonography. New York, Elsevier, 1988.
17. Timor-Tritsch IE, Bar-Yam Y, Elgali S, Rottem S: The technique of transvaginal sonography with the use of 6.5 MHz probe. Am J Obstet Gynecol 1988;158:1019–1024.
18. Young RC, Walton LA, Ellenberg SS, et al.: NEJM 1990;332:1024–1028.
18a. Andolf E, Jorgensen C: A prospective comparison of clinical ultrasound and operative examination of the female pelvis. J Ultrasound Med 1988;7:617–620.

19. Lundberg WI, Wall JE, Mathers JE: Laparoscopy in evaluation of pelvic pain. Obstet Gynecol 1973;42:812–816.
20. Barber HRK, Graber EA: The PMPO syndrome. Obstet Gynecol 1971;38:921–923.
21. Barber HRK: Ovarian cancer: diagnosis and management. Am J Obstet Gynecol 1984;150:910–916.
22. Gido-Frank L, Gordon T, Taylor HC: Pelvic pain and female identity. Am J Obstet Gynecol 1960;79:1186.
23. Jeffcoate TNA: Pelvic pain. Br Med J 1969;3:431.
24. Parsons L, Sommers SC (eds): Pelvic Pain in Gynecology, 2d ed. Philadelphia, W.B. Saunders, 1978.
25. Zylberberg B, Salat-Baroux J, Ravina JH, Demarcourt V, Dormont D: Cancer de l'ôvaire: intrêrêt de la ponction du Douglas et du dosage d l'antigène carcino-embryonnaire dans le liquide pêroto-nêal. J Gynecol Obstet Biol Reprod 1982;11:365–370.
26. Popkin DR: Early diagnosis of ovarian cancer. Can Med Assoc J 1979;120:1106–1108.
27. Joppi M, Pezzini MB, Tapparelli E: Washing puncture of pouch in early diagnosis and follow-up of ovarian tumors. Eur J Gynecol Oncol 1982;III:I:60–63.
28. Fleischer AC, Walsh JW, Jones HW, Shaff MI, James AE: Sonographic evaluation of pelvic masses. Method of examination and role of sonography relative to other imaging modalities. Radiol Clin North Am 1982;20:397–412.
29. Dooms GC, Hricak H, Tscholakoff D: Adnexal structures: MR imaging. Radiology 1986;158:639–646.
30. Fishman-Javitt MC, Lovecchio JL, Stein HL: Imaging strategies for MRI of the pelvis. Radiol Clin North Am 1988;26:633–651.
31. Lewis E: The use and abuse of imaging in gynecologic cancer. Cancer 1987;60:1993–2009.
32. Symonds EM, Perkins AC, Pimm MV, Baldwin RW, Hardy JG, Williams DA: Clinical implications for immunoscintigraphy in patients with ovarian malignancy: a preliminary study using monoclonal antibody 791T/36. British J Obstet Gynecol 1985;92:270–276.
33. Bast RC, Siegal FP, Runowicz C, Klug TL, Zurawski VR, Schonholz D, Cohen CJ, Knapp RC: Elevation of serum CA 125 prior to diagnosis of an epithelial ovarian carcinoma. Gynecol Oncol 1985;22:115–120.
34. Crombach G, Zippel HH, Wurz H: Erfahrungen mit CA 125, einem Tumormarker fur maligne epitheliale Ovarialtumoren. Geburtshilfe Fraunheilkd 1985;45:205–212.
35. Schröck R, Hafter R, Graeff H, Schmid L: Die simultane Bestimmung von CA 125 und D-Dimer im Plasma and Aszites beim Ovarialkarzinom. Onkologie 1985;5:260–262.
36. Einhorn N, Bast RC, Knapp RC, Tjernberg B, Zurawski VR: Preoperative evaluation of serum CA 125 levels in patients with primary epithelial ovarian cancer. Obstet Gynecol 1986;67:414–416.
37. Kaeseman H, Caffier H, Hoffmann FJ, Crombach G, Wurz H, Kreienberg R, Möbus V, Schmidt-Rhode P, Sturm G: Monoklonale Antikôrper in Diagnostik und Verlaufskontrolle des Ovrialkar-zinoms. CA 125 als Tumormarker. Klin Wochenschr 1986;64:781–785.
38. O'Connell GJ, Ryan E, Murphy J, Prefontaine M: Predictive value of CA 125 for ovarian carcinoma in patients presenting with pelvic masses. Obstet Gynecol 1987;70:930–932.
39. Heinonen PK, Kallioniemi OP, Koivula T: Comparison of CA 125 and placental alkaline phosphatase as ovarian tumor markers. Tumori 1987;73:301–302.
40. Brioschi PA, Irion O, Bischof P, Bader M, Forni M, Krauer F: Serum CA 125 in epithelial ovarian cancer: a longitudinal study. Br J Obstet Gynecol 1987;94:196–201.
41. Di-Xia C, Schwartz PE, Xinguo L, Zhan Y: Evaluation of CA 125 levels in differentiating malignant from benign tumors in patients with pelvic masses. Obstet Gynecol 1988;72:23–27.
42. Fioretti P, Gadducci A, Ferdeghini M, Bartolini T, Fontana V, Facchini F: Preoperative evaluation of CA 125 and CA 19-9 serum levels in patients with ovarian masses. Eur J Gynaec Oncol 1988;4:291–294.
43. Knauf S: Clinical evaluation of ovarian tumor antigen NB/70K: monoclonal antibody assays for distinguishing ovarian cancer from other gynecologic disease. Am J Obstet Gynecol 1988;158:1067–1072.
44. Knauf S, Taillon-Miller P, Helmkamp BF, Bonfiglio TA, Beecham JB: Selectivity for ovarian cancer of an improved serum radioimmunoassay for human ovarian tumor associated antigen NB/70K. Gynecol Oncol 1984;17:349–355.
45. Rubin SC, Lewis JL: Tumor antigens in ovarian malignancy. Clin Obstet Gynecol 1986;29:693–704.
46. Vergote I, Onsrud M, Nustad K: Placental alkaline phosphatase as a tumor marker in ovarian cancer. Obstet Gynecol 1987;69:228–232.

47. Astedt B, Svanberg L, Nilsson IM: Fibrin degradation products and ovarian tumours. Br Med J 1971;4:458–459.

47a. Daunter B: Tumor markers in gynecologic oncology 1990;39:1–15.

48. Garrett W: Ultrasound, in Coppleson M (ed): Gynecologic Oncology. London, Churchill Livingston, 1981, pp 254–257.

49. Bernadino M, Dood G: Imaging of the pelvic contents in the female oncologic patient. Cancer 1981;48:504–510.

50. Nash C, Alberts D, Suciu T, et al: Comparison of B-mode ultrasonography and computed tomography in gynecologic cancer. Gynecol Oncol 1979;8:172–179.

51. Lawson T, Albarelli J: Diagnosis of gynecologic pelvic masses by gray scale ultrasonography: analysis of specificity and accuracy. Am J Roentgenol 1977;128:1003–1006.

52. Deland M, Field A, Van Nagell J, et al: Ultrasonography in the diagnosis of tumors of the ovary. Surg Gynecol J Obstet 1979;18:346–348.

53. Meire H, Farrant P, Gulta T: Distinction of benign from malignant ovarian cystology ultrasound. Br J Obstet Gynecol 1978;85:893–899.

54. Requard K, Mettler F, Wicks J: Preoperative sonography of malignant ovarian neoplasms. Am J Radiol 1981;137:79–82.

55. Campbell S, Goessens L, Goswamy R: Real time ultrasonography for determination of ovarian morphology and volume. Lancet 1980;1:425–426.

56. Andolf E, Svolenius E, Astedt B: Ultrasonography for early detection of ovarian carcinoma. Br J Obstet Gynecol 1986;93:1286–1289.

57. Sonnendecker E, Butterworth A: Comparison between ultrasound and histopathological evaluation in ovarian cancer patients with complete clinical remission. J Clin Ultrasound 1985;13:5–9.

58. Wicks J, Mettler F, Hilgus R, et al: Correlation of ultrasound and pathologic findings in patients with epithelial carcinoma of the ovary. J Clin Ultrasound 1984;12:397–402.

59. Sample W, Lippe B, Gyepes M: Gray scale ultrasonography of the normal female pelvis. Radiology 1977;25:477–483.

60. Queenan J, O'Brien G, Baris L, et al: Ultrasonic scanning of ovaries to detect ovulation in women. Fertil Steril 1980;34:99–105.

61. Campbell S, Bhan V, Royston P, Whitehead MI, Collins WP: Transabdominal ultrasound screening for early ovarian cancer. Br Med J 1989;299:1363–1367.

62. O'Brien WF, Buck DR, Nash FD: Evaluation of sonography in the initial assessment of the gynecologic patient. Am J Obstet Gynecol 1984;149:598–602.

63. Rodriguez HM, Platt LD, Medearis AL, Lacardia M, Lobo RA: The use of transvaginal sonography for evaluation of postmenopausal ovarian size and morphology. Am J Obstet Gynecol 1988;159:810–814.

64. Swanson M, Sauerbrei EE, Cooperberg PL: Medical implication of ultrasonically detected polycystic ovaries. JCU 1981;9:219–222.

65. Parisi L, Tramonti M, Casciano S, et al: The role of ultrasound in the study of polycystic ovarian disease. JCU 1982;10:167–172.

66. Nicolini U, Ferrazzi E, Bellotti M, Travaglini P, Elli R, Scaperrotta RC: The contribution of sonographic evaluation of ovarian size in patients with polycystic ovarian disease. J Ultrasound Med 1985;4:347–351.

67. Rottem S, Levit N, Thaler I, Yoffe N, et al: Classification of ovarian lesions by high frequency transvaginal sonography. JCU 1990;18:359–363.

68. Rottem S, Lewit N: Transvaginal sonography versus histopathology of ovarian tumors. Submitted for publication.

69. Sassone M, Artner A, Westhoff C, Warren W, Timor-Tritsch IE: Transvaginal sonographic characterization of ovarian pathology: evaluation of a new scoring system to predict ovarian malignancy. Submitted for publication.

70. Bourne T, Campbell S, Whitehead MI, Collins WP: Transvaginal ultrasound screening for ovarian cancer in a high risk group. Presented at The Third World Congress on Vaginosonography in Gynecology, June 14–17, 1990, San Antonio, Tex.

71. Fleischer AC, McKee MS, Gordon AN, et al: Transvaginal sonography of postmenopausal ovaries with pathologic correlation. Presented at The Third World Congress on Vaginosonography in Gynecology. June 14–17, 1990, San Antonio, Tex.

72. Granberg S, Nortrom A, Wikland M: Tumors in the lower pelvis as imaged by vaginal sonography. Gynecologic Oncology 1990;4:229.

73. Kurjak A, Zalud I, Iurkovic D, Alfirevic Z, Miljan M: Transvaginal color Doppler for the assessment of pelvic circulation. Acta Obstet Gynecol Sound 1989;68:131–135.

74. Bourne T, Campbell S, Steer C, Whitehead MI, Collins WP: Transvaginal colour flow imaging: a possible new screening technique for ovarian cancer. Br Med J 1989;299:1367–1375.
75. Ishikawa F, Miyazono K, Hellman U, et al: Identification of antiogenic activity and the cloning and expression of platelet derived endothelial growth factor. Nature 1989;338:557–561.
76. Rastinejad F, Polverini PJ, Bouck NP: Regulation of the activity of a new inhibitor of angiogenesis by a cancer suppressor gene. Cell 1989;56:345–355.
77. Slamon DJ, Godolphin WG, Jones LA, Holt JA, et al: Studies of HER-2/new photo-oncogen in human breast and ovarian cancer. Science 1989;244:707–712.

CHAPTER 8

Transvaginal Ultrasound of the Lower Urinary Tract

Martin Quinn, MRCOG

BACKGROUND

Vaginal ultrasound, with the appropriate equipment, is a new technique for imaging the lower urinary tract.[1] New endoprobes with reduced dimensions and enhanced specifications, permit direct imaging of the bladder neck and proximal urethra during provocative maneuvers such as a cough or Valsalva maneuver. A positive diagnosis of "genuine" stress incontinence (GSI), and the objective assessment of the anatomic effects of suprapubic operations, may be simply achieved without discomfort to the patient.

Urinary incontinence occurring on two or more occasions per month affects 3–8% of women aged 18–65 in the United Kingdom.[2] The most common cause is GSI occurring on its own or in association with detrusor instability.[3] A proportion of patients have isolated detrusor instability that should be differentiated from GSI since the treatment of the two conditions differs markedly. At present there are many techniques available to investigate a complaint of urinary incontinence but no consensus over an optimal, or minimal, sequence of investigation. Many clinicians still rely on a history supported by clinical evidence of urinary leakage concurrent with a cough, although the concern remains that cough-induced urinary leakage associated with DI may be confused with that associated with GSI. Where urodynamic investigations have become established, filling cystometry is used to exclude detrusor instability in patients with a history of stress leakage, thereby establishing a diagnosis of GSI.[4] Videocystourethrography (VCU) is a radiological assessment of the bladder outlet that may be used to provide positive evidence of GSI since leakage of contrast medium may be imaged directly.[5] Pad testing,[6] urethral electrical conductance measurements,[7] urethral pressure profilometry,[8] and neurophysiological techniques[9] may be helpful in selected cases or as research techniques, but do not figure in the management of most patients with a complaint of urinary incontinence. The primary disadvantages of urodynamic investigations are that they are invasive and require established facilities to perform and interpret the investigations.[10]

Many radiological techniques have been used to image the lower urinary tract using both x-ray and ultrasound. The reference standard for the diagnosis of GSI is widely held to be VCU, where the bladder and urethra are indirectly outlined by the contrast medium.[5,11] Leakage of contrast media concurrent with a cough establishes a diagnosis of GSI through urethral catheterization, and exposure to x-rays is a significant disadvantage of the procedure. Prior to the development of the cine-radiography techniques necessary for VCU, the bladder and urethra were outlined by contrast media and a metallic bead-chain, respectively, and static films taken before and after a Valsalva maneuver, although this was neither sensitive nor specific for the diagnosis of GSI.[12] The anatomical consequences of different suprapubic operations on the position of the bladder neck were observable with BCUG, since it was fixed in a retropubic position with the appropriate operation.

Many ultrasound approaches to the lower urinary tract have been described, with different authors suggesting abdominal, perineal, rectal, and vaginal routes.[1,12–15] Abdominal and perineal scanning have been restricted by the low frequency of ultrasound transducers that have limited resolution deep in the pelvis and intervening structures that interfere with image production (the pubic symphysis cavitary and pubic rami). With the technical improvements of recent generations of endoprobes, high-resolution images of the bladder neck and proximal urethra have been achieved by both rectal and vaginal scanning, although the vaginal route is much preferred by patients.[1] Many ultrasound descriptions of patients with urinary incontinence have been limited to the descent of the bladder neck with a cough or Valsalva maneuver.[15,16] Such information does not improve on that provided by BCUG in terms of the diagnosis of GSI since there is much overlap between normal and incontinent patients.[12] Ultrasound systems with enhanced technical specifications (see below) permit direct imaging of urinary leakage concurrent with a cough, ie, "genuine" stress incontinence. Opening of the bladder neck and urinary leakage occur with detrusor instability, although the nature and timing of these events differentiate them from the passive response of the continence mechanism to an increase in intraabdominal pressure in patients with GSI.[16,17]

EQUIPMENT

Successful ultrasound imaging is dependent on equipment specifications (Table 8.1). All scans in this description have been produced by a 7 MHz mechanical sector scanner with an offset field that scans through an arc of 112° over a focal range of 1–6 cm (Fig 8.1). The offset field and reduced external dimensions ensure that the appropriate anatomical field will be visualized without distortion of the

TABLE 8.1 Operating Characteristics of Vaginal Endoprobes

Characteristics	Discussion
Reduced, external dimensions High operating frequency Wide field angle Offset field High frame rate	The operating characteristics of vaginal endovaginal probes suitable for imaging the lower urinary tract at rest and during dynamic events, eg, a cough. Many endovaginal probes have a linear array format with an operating frequency of 5 MHz, reduced field angle, and an asymmetric transducer containing a fixed array of piezoelectric crystals. Such equipment is not suitable for imaging the lower urinary tract since it does not provide sufficient resolution and may generate distortion of the anatomical features because of the increased size of the transducer.

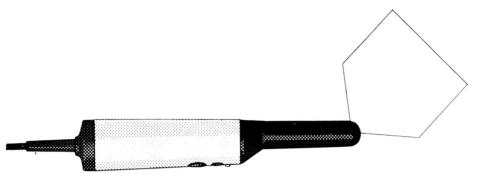

Figure 8.1 The endovaginal probe is a mechanical sector probe (Bruel & Kjaer 8537) with an external diameter of 18 mm. It has an operating frequency of 7 MHz and scans through an arc of 112° over a focal range of 1–6 cm. The offset field and reduced external dimensions ensure the appropriate anatomical field (Fig 8.2) without distortion of the anatomical features.

anatomical features. Dynamic events require a frame rate of 16–20 frames per second to obtain adequate resolution of the effects of a cough on the continence mechanism. Imaging of the lower urinary tract may be obtained with linear array systems, although their principal disadvantage is the relatively bulky, asymmetrical shape of the transducer that may distort the anatomic features.

Complete assessment of the incontinent patient includes history, examination, and ultrasound scanning in both recumbent and sitting positions with a full bladder. Scanning in the recumbent position familiarizes the examiner with the technique and the interrelationship between the symphysis pubis and the bladder neck. Examination in the sitting position on an adapted commode is necessary to establish a specific diagnosis of GSI.

TECHNIQUE

After a full explanation of the technique, the patient is placed in the dorsal, recumbent position similar to that for digital, vaginal examination. The endoprobe is lubricated with coupling gel, placed in the middle finger of a sterile, disposable plastic glove, and relubricated before being placed 1–2 cm within the introitus. Rotation of the endovaginal probe around its longitudinal axis identifies a midline sagittal plane in which the lower half of the symphysis pubis, the bladder neck, and the urethra may be imaged (Fig 8.2). After transfer to the sitting position, the endoprobe is relubricated and introduced by the patient herself, where it is held in the appropriate imaging plane by the examiner. Opening of the bladder neck and proximal urethra with urinary leakage concurrent with a cough establishes a diagnosis of GSI. The examination is completed by voiding to completion so that the bladder volume may be recorded.

Potential disadvantages of this technique include distortion of the anatomical features and significant prolapse of the anterior vaginal wall, which renders accurate observations difficult. Distortion of the anatomical features by the endovaginal probe is avoided by the reduced external dimensions and offset field, though the precise effect on the adjacent tissues is visible throughout the examination, and any undesirable effects may be avoided by reorientation of the endoprobe. Moderate or severe prolapse of the anterior vaginal wall prevents ultrasound examination in the sitting position though scanning in the recumbent position may be possible.

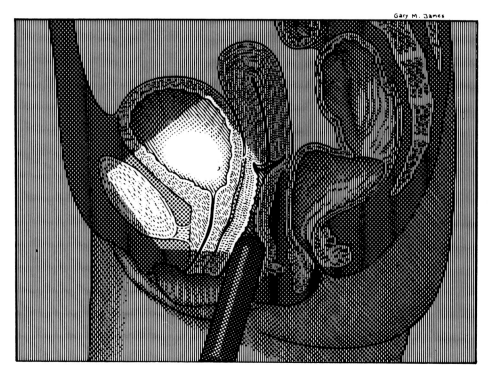

Gary M. James

Figure 8.2 The anatomical field is a sagittal section of the anterior pelvis in the plane of the symphysis pubis. The important landmarks are the inferior border of the symphysis pubis and the bladder neck that may be imaged in both recumbent and sitting positions.

THE ULTRASOUND FEATURES OF THE LOWER URINARY TRACT

The ultrasound images of the lower urinary tract depend on the varying acoustic impedances of the constituent tissues that include urine, muscle, cartilage, ligament, and bone (Figs 8.3 and 8.4). Stored urine appears as a hypoechoic feature (Fig 8.3**A**) whereas cortical bone has a dense, hyperechoic appearance (Fig 8.4). In all scans, the longitudinal axis of the patient extends from the top left corner of the scan (head) to the bottom right corner (feet) due to the offset field of the transducer.

The Symphysis Pubis and Pubic Ramus

The symphysis pubis appears as a dense, uniform, hyperechoic feature since it is composed of cartilage (Fig 8.3**B**) and appears in the same midline plane as the urethra. Adjacent to the symphysis, the pubic ramus may be imaged by rotating the endoprobe into an oblique plane to demonstrate the hypoechoic appearance of the trabecular bone of the pubic ramus that has a dense, hyperechoic inferior border of cortical bone (Fig 8.4). The distinction between the two structures is important since the symphysis pubis defines a sagittal, midline plane that is a fixed reference point in the area of interest.

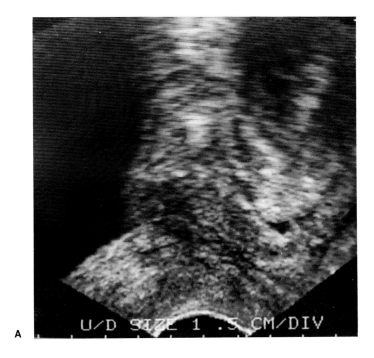

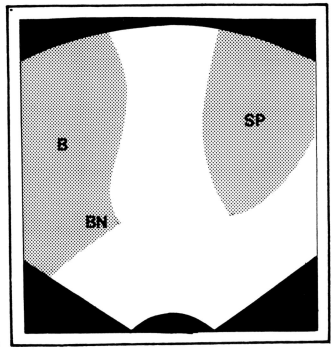

Figure 8.3 (A and B) The bladder (B) appears as a hypoechoic feature on the left side of the scan due to the reduced, acoustic impedance of the stored urine. The symphysis pubis (SP) has a dense, hyperechoic appearance and remains in a fixed position during a cough or Valsalva maneuver. The urethra passes from the bladder neck (BN) beneath the inferior border of the symphysis pubis, toward the right bottom corner of the scan. In the resting position, the walls of the urethra are opposed, and its course is distinguished by the acoustic appearances of this adjacent blood supply. The position of the tip of the endoprobe is indicated on the inferior border of the scan so that any distorting effect may be avoided by reorientation of the endovaginal probe.

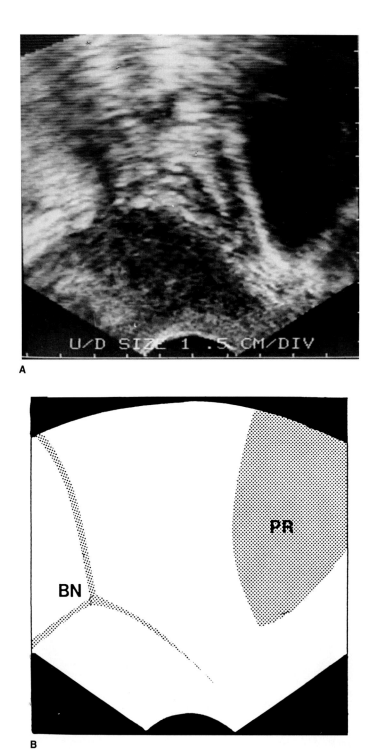

Figure 8.4 (A and B) This is the same patient as in Fig 8.3, with emptied bladder, the urethra in similar position, and with the endoprobe in an oblique plane. The pubic ramus (PR) appears as a hypoechoic feature with a dense, inferior border due to the respective acoustic properties of trabecular and cortical bone. The appearances contrast markedly with those of the symphysis pubis that is only visible in a sagittal, midline plane. BN = bladder neck.

The Bladder and Urethra

The position of the bladder is defined by the hypoechoic appearances of the stored urine. From a radiological standpoint the "bladder neck" refers to the junction of the stored urine and the urethra that may, or may not, correspond to functional and histological definitions. In the normal situation, the urethra is a collapsed tube without lumen whose ultrasound appearances are produced by the adjacent vascular supply (Figs 8.3 and 8.4). Urethral catheterization will confirm the course of the urethra, though this has rarely been necessary.

In patients without urinary incontinence, provocative maneuvers have little or no effect on the ultrasound appearance of the continence mechanism. Minor posterior or inferior displacement of the bladder neck and proximal urethra may occur, though there is neither opening of the bladder neck nor urinary leakage. A Valsalva maneuver produces downward displacement of the lower urinary tract, though the inferior excursion appears to be limited by an intact, anterior, suspensory mechanism.

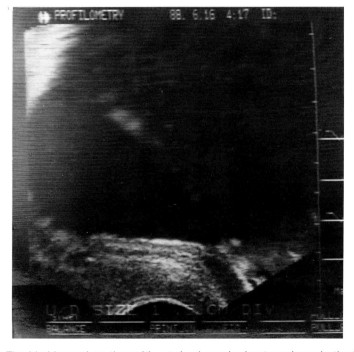

Figure 8.5 The bladder and urethra with a twin-channel microtransducer in the bladder and urethra. One transducer is in the bladder on the distal tip of the catheter and the other is in the proximal urethra. Conventional urodynamics may be performed using the ultrasound technique to image the lower urinary tract simultaneously.

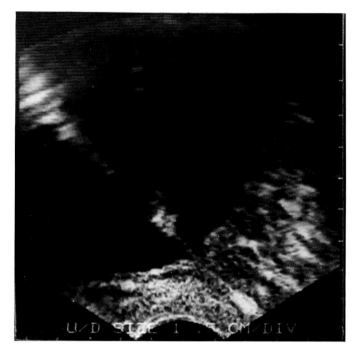

Figure 8.6 A similar scan with a urethral electric conductance catheter in the urethra. The twin electrodes are positioned 1–2 mm apart on the catheter and are clearly visible at rest and during provocative maneuvers.

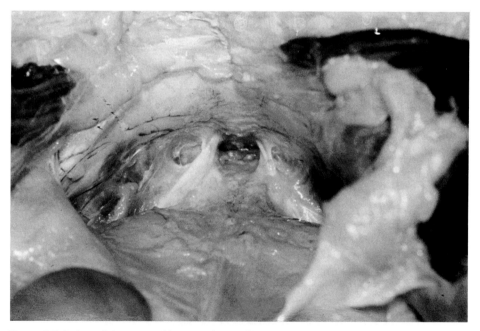

Figure 8.7 A view of the retropubic space in a nulliparous patient showing the superior surface of the bladder, pubovesical ligaments (also called the posterior limb of the pubourethral ligaments), symphysis pubis, and iliopectineal ligaments. The pubovesical ligaments comprise part of an expansion in the prevesical space that connects the anterior surface of the bladder, the levator ani, and the posterior surface of the pubic ramus.[22]

The Pubovesical Ligaments

The anterior suspensory mechanism of the bladder neck and its role in the support of the bladder neck have been controversial topics for over 40 years.[18-20] Recent, innovative work has improved our understanding of the precise anatomical relationships of this area.[20,21,22] The pubovesical ligaments (formerly termed the posterior pubourethral ligaments) may be consistently demonstrated as a broad band of hyperechoic material extending from the posterior surface of the pubis to the anterior surface of the bladder on either side of the midline (Figs 8.7 and 8.8). This view is an oblique section of the tendineus fascia and the precervical fascia, all having a common insertion in this region. Attenuation of these structures is frequently observed in parous patients, though complete disruption of the anterior suspensory mechanism is only observed on rare occasions following traumatic vaginal delivery.

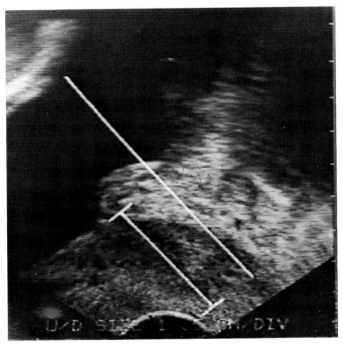

Figure 8.8 The pubovesical ligaments appear as dense, echogenic bands extending from the posterior surface of the pubis to the anterior surface of the bladder on either side of the midline. From a functional point of view, they are ideally placed to support the bladder neck and the proximal urethra close to the posterior surface of the pubis, and restrict downward displacement associated with a cough or Valsalva maneuver.

THE ULTRASOUND FEATURES OF URINARY INCONTINENCE

In the resting position, there are no specific differences in the position of the bladder neck, relative to the inferior border of the symphysis pubis, between patients with and without urinary stress incontinence. As a group, the mean position of the bladder neck is lower in patients with GSI compared to a matching group of parous patients without urinary symptoms; but there is considerable overlap between the two groups. Scanning in the sitting position during a series of coughs is a sensitive and specific technique for the differentiation of patients with urinary stress incontinence.[17] Opening of the bladder neck and proximal urethra with urinary leakage concurrent with a cough establishes a diagnosis of GSI, whereas in patients without urinary symptoms, there is little or no effect on the continence mechanism (Fig 8.9). From a practical standpoint, the important issue is to distinguish patients with GSI and cough-induced detrusor instability (DI). Urinary leakage associated with GSI is an immediate consequence of a sufficient increase in intraabdominal pressure, whereas that associated with DI results from an active event occurring at a clear interval after the cough (Fig 8.10).

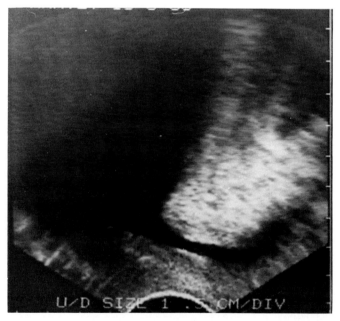

Figure 8.9 Genuine stress incontinence. Opening of the bladder neck and proximal urethra, with urinary leakage concurrent with a cough, establishes a diagnosis of GSI. The freeze-frame shows urine in the proximal and mid-urethra; however, the appearances of GSI are better observed in dynamic images at the time of the examination.

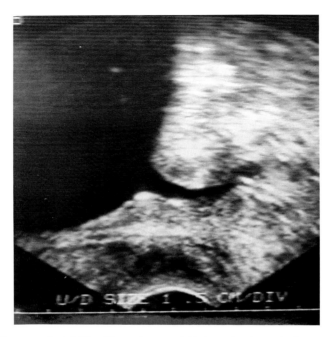

Figure 8.10 Detrusor instability. The nature and timing of urinary leakage associated with cough-induced detrusor instability permit differentiation from GSI. The leakage is associated with an active process including an increase in intravesical pressure and a clear interval between the cough and subsequent urinary loss.

Comparison Between Vaginal Ultrasound and Urodynamic Investigations in the Diagnosis of "Genuine" Stress Incontinence

A prospective comparison between vaginal ultrasound and urodynamic investigations has been undertaken to evaluate the effectiveness of the new technique in the diagnosis of GSI.[17] Urodynamic investigations were undertaken in 124 patients prior to evaluation by vaginal ultrasound on a subsequent occasion, without knowledge of the preceding results. Urodynamic studies included some or all of the following investigations: history, physical examination, frequency–volume chart, filling and voiding cystometry, urethral pressure profilometry, and video-cystourethrography (see Table 8.2). At the appointment for vaginal ultrasound,

TABLE 8.2 Urodynamic Investigations

Patient Breakdown	Discussion
124 patients had filling and voiding cystometry 80 patients had urethral pressure profilometry 23 patients had video-cystourethrography	Urodynamic investigations, in addition to clinical history, physical examination, and frequency–volume chart, in a group of patients undergoing urodynamic evaluation prior to comparison with vaginal ultrasound.

history was taken before the scanning in recumbent and sitting positions was undertaken. Of the group of 124 patients, 99 of the 124 had a final urodynamic diagnosis that included GSI, and 25 of the 124 were normal, or had pure DI. Discordance occurred between the two techniques in 9 of the 124 patients, giving vaginal ultrasound a sensitivity of over 90% in the diagnosis of GSI compared with the reason for discordance in the final urodynamic diagnosis. The reason for discordance in the majority of cases was that the patient presented with relatively minor symptoms of stress incontinence, eg, stress leakage while playing tennis or some similar vigorous exercise, and the urodynamic diagnosis was determined by the absence of detrusor instability during filling cystometry. The ultrasound appearances showed downward displacement of the bladder neck and proximal urethra during provocative maneuvers, though the opening of the bladder neck and proximal urethra with concurrent urinary leakage could not be demonstrated since the magnitude of the stress that produced the leakage was not reproducible in the testing situation. All patients having GSI associated with abnormal urethral pressure profilometry or an abnormal VCU had unequivocal ultrasound appearances of GSI. These results demonstrate vaginal ultrasound to be a simple and sensitive technique for the diagnosis of GSI, though filling cystometry may be required to objectively demonstrate the absence of detrusor instability in patients with relatively minor symptoms of stress incontinence or in those patients in whom an objective diagnosis of detrusor instability was required.

THE ANATOMICAL CONSEQUENCES OF SUPRAPUBIC OPERATIONS FOR "GENUINE" STRESS INCONTINENCE

Suprapubic operations for GSI have been increasingly popular due to the improved results over vaginal operations.[23] Of the operations in common usage, colposuspension,[24] needle suspension,[25] and sling operations[26] comprise the majority of procedures. Each operation achieves its effect by elevation and/or support of the bladder neck. There are distinctive anatomical effects associated with a successful outcome (Figs 8.11 and 8.14). Variations in surgical technique are common, though there are few controlled studies over the medium and long term in patients with either primary or recurrent stress incontinence are few.[27,28] Persistent postoperative symptoms include a range of gynecological and urological symptoms (Table 8.3). The etiology of urological complaints, with irritative symptoms that include frequency and urgency, has not been explained with traditional investigations, though it is frequently said that "suprapubic surgery worsens detrusor instability in patients with combined GSI and DI." At the same time, it is clear that a successful operation alleviates both problems in many patients.[23] Vaginal ultrasound has provided an insight into this paradox, and, in so doing, raised questions as to the merit of identifying the cause of irritative symptoms in patients with demonstrable GSI prior to suprapubic surgery.[17]

Previously, the anatomical effects of suprapubic operations have been demonstrated by bead-chain cystourethrography. This is a cumbersome procedure requiring urethral catheterization and exposure to x-rays. The results of BCUG are of limited value since the important anatomical landmarks, ie, the bladder neck and proximal urethra, may only image indirectly by instilling contrast media into the bladder and outlining the urethra with a metallic bead-chain. Vaginal ultrasound is an objective and reproducible technique for determining the position of

TABLE 8.3 Urological Complications After Colposuspension

Complications	Discussion
"Early" recurrent stress incontinence	Urological complications after colposuspension
"Late" recurrent stress incontinence	include a variety of urinary problems that may be
Frequency–urgency syndrome	detected with vaginal ultrasound.
Persistent stress incontinence	

the bladder neck relative to the fixed reference point of the inferior border of the symphysis pubis. This technique is particularly suitable for the assessment of the anatomical effects of different suprapubic operations (Figs 8.11–8.14). With the patient in the recumbent position, and the endoprobe maintained in a horizontal plane with a spirit level fixed to the needle biopsy, the inferior border of the symphysis pubis may be reliably imaged in a sagittal midline plane. Having identified this fixed reference point, the urethrovesical junction (or bladder neck) may be imaged both pre- and postoperatively by minor rotation of the endoprobe around its longitudinal plane. In the preoperative patient, the bladder neck is identified in the same sagittal plane as the inferior border of the symphysis pubis, though after suprapubic surgery it may be positioned in a parasagittal plane. Observer variation is low since the bladder neck is maintained in a fixed position by the supporting sutures after a successful colposuspension or needle-suspension operation.[17] Two series of patients have been studied following colposuspension

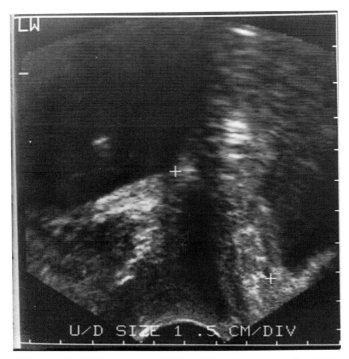

Figure 8.11 Successful colposuspension. The bladder neck has been elevated to a fixed, retro-pubic position with the urethra almost parallel to the posterior surface of the pubis. The resolution of the ultrasound image permits the hyperechoic features of the nonabsorbable nylon sutures to be distinguished in the vaginal fornices and at their insertion on the iliopectineal ligament.

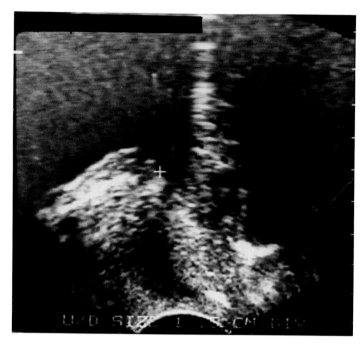

Figure 8.12 Frequency–urgency syndrome. This postoperative scan of a colposuspension shows the vaginal fornices indenting the trigone of the bladder. The supporting sutures have been placed inaccurately (too close to the vaginal vault), resulting in the trigone being suspended on a shelf of vagina.

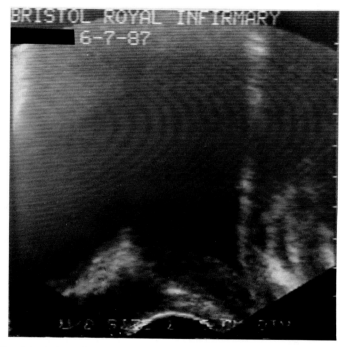

Figure 8.13 Persistent stress incontinence. The vaginal fornices are indenting the bladder base posterior to the trigone, ie, the supporting sutures have been placed at the vaginal vault. There has been no elevation/support of the bladder neck, and the patient has persistent stress leakage.

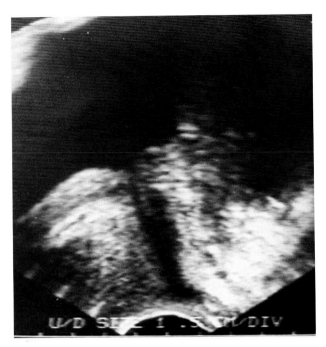

Figure 8.14 Successful bladder neck needle-suspension. The bladder neck has been supported in a high, retropubic position similar to that after colposuspension. Scanning in an oblique plane on either side of the midline enables the integrity of the supporting sutures to be established.

and needle-suspension operations, respectively. In both series the operations were performed by both gynecologists and urologists using similar techniques, and the results were not related to the seniority or specialty of the surgeon.[17]

Colposuspension

Burch (1961) described this variation of retropubic urethropexy when he secured the vaginal fornices to the ipsilateral, iliopectineal ligament.[24] The bladder neck was elevated, and supported in its new position by a shelf of vaginal tissue posterior to the urethrovesical junction. This operation produced a more secure supporting mechanism than traditional urethropexy, as described by Marshall–Marchetti–Krantz, where paraurethral tissues are secured to the periosteum of the pubis *directly*.[32]

Over 60 patients have been assessed with vaginal ultrasound after colposuspension. Successful symptomatic and urodynamic results are associated with elevation and support of the bladder neck in its new position (Fig 8.11). Unsuccessful results produced a range of ultrasound appearances that were often associated with inaccurate placement of the supporting sutures. Persistent, or worsening, irritative symptoms of frequency and urgency are caused by the vaginal shelf indenting the trigone (Fig 8.12), whereas persistent stress incontinence occurs when the supporting sutures are inadvertently placed closer to the vaginal vault, causing indentation of the bladder base, which neither elevates nor supports the bladder neck (Fig 8.13). Recurrent stress incontinence occurs in two situations:

(1) in the immediate postoperative period as a result of primary failure of the supporting sutures; and (2) in the perimenopausal patient when, after a successful colposuspension some years previously, together with evidence of intact supporting sutures by digital vaginal examination, recurrent stress incontinence occurs as a result of a degree of laxity of the supporting tissues. Subsequent bladder neck needle-suspension, with the sutures tied securely posterior to those of the original colposuspension, has been successful in three out of four patients.

Bladder Neck Needle-Suspension Procedures

Many variations of needle-suspension operation have been described, though the aims of each variation appear to be similar to those of colposuspension, ie, elevation and support of the bladder neck in a fixed, retropubic position. Overall results vary from 91% in a series that did not include objective evaluation of the operation,[25] to almost half this success rate.[33] Many reports describe an early significant failure rate, though subsequent failures may also occur after a prolonged symptom-free interval.

Over 30 patients have been scanned following needle-suspension operations.[17] Approximately one-third sustained early, recurrent stress incontinence associated with one or both sutures cutting through the supporting tissues. Unilateral suture failure occurred in three patients, and on each occasion continence was not maintained by the single supporting suture. Irritative postoperative symptoms were not a feature of the operation.

CONCLUSIONS

Confirmation of a diagnosis of urinary stress incontinence will remain a controversial issue since there is no single investigation that will detect the condition in every patient. Some clinicians will adhere to history and physical demonstration of stress leakage though this may be difficult to arrange in a busy clinical setting. Others will operate a selective policy with urodynamic investigations being reserved for those patients with a mixed history or urinary leakage and irritative symptoms. The diagnosis of GSI will continue to be made by the exclusion of detrusor instability using twin-channel filling cystometry, since the technique is well established and the equipment is widely available. Extensive urodynamic investigations, including urethral pressure profilometry and videocystourethrography appear to be unnecessary in the majority of cases and might be reserved for a minority of patients or research protocols. Vaginal ultrasound provides a simple, noninvasive technique for the diagnosis of GSI that is acceptable to patients, and it is a technique easy to acquire by interested clinicians. Its clinical application may be enhanced by the ability to reliably detect the effects of detrusor instability on the continence mechanism during simple, provocative maneuvers, such as a series of coughs or simple bladder filling, though appropriate controlled studies are yet to be completed.

Accurate and reproducible observations of the anatomical consequences of suprapubic operations will assist in the diagnosis of persistent, postoperative symptoms and permit the comparison of the anatomical effects of different types of surgical procedures. The observation that postoperative, irritative symptoms may be produced by inaccurate placement of sutures at colposuspension, and may bear no relationship to the presence of preoperative detrusor instability, emphasizes the importance of determining the presence or absence of GSI in patients with mixed symptoms. If the patient is shown to have the condition and surgery is indicated, there is little value in determining the presence or absence of DI since an accurate colposuspension will cure both GSI and DI in the majority of cases.

Vaginal ultrasound with the appropriate equipment is a new technique for imaging the lower urinary tract. It has significant advantages over conventional x-ray techniques and other routes of delivering ultrasound. Information from this technique will improve our management of patients with urinary symptoms and our understanding of the pathophysiology of the lower urinary tract. Further evaluation of its role in the detection of the effects of detrusor instability on the continence mechanism is required. Vaginal ultrasound, in this present format, will not replace all aspects of conventional urodynamic testing, but a reduction in the number of patients requiring extensive, invasive testing should be anticipated.

REFERENCES

1. Quinn MJ, Beynon J, Mortensen NM, Smith PJB: Transvaginal endosonography in the assessment of urinary stress incontinence. Brit J Urol 1988;62:414–418.
2. Thomas TM, Phymat KR, Blannin J, Meade TW: Prevalence of urinary symptoms. Brit Med J 1980;281:1243–1245.
3. Hilton P: Urinary incontinence in women. Brit Med J 1987;299:455–460.
4. Enhorning G: Simultaneous recording of intravesical and intraurethral pressure. Acta Chirurgica Scandinavica (suppl) 1961;276.
5. Bates CP, Whiteside CG, Turner-Warwick R: Synchronous cine/pressure/flow cystourethrography with special reference to stress and urge incontinence. Brit J Urol 1970;42:714–723.
6. Sutherst J, Brown M, Shawer M: Assessing the severity of urinary incontinence in women by weighing perineal pads. Lancet 1981;1128–1129,1981.
7. Plevnik S: Urethral electric conductance, in Drife JO, Hilton P, Stanton SL (eds): Micturition (pp. 111–127). Springer Verlag, 1990.
8. Hilton P, Stanton SL: Urethral pressure measurement by microtransducer. I. An analysis of variance; II. An analysis of rotation variations, in Sundin T, Mattiasson A (eds): Proceedings of the 11th annual meeting of the International Continence Society, Lund, Sweden, 1981, p 69.
9. Kirby RS, Eardley R: Role of electrophysiological studies, in Drife JO, Hilton P, Stanton SL (eds): Micturition (pp. 143–151). Springer Verlag, 1990.
10. Stanton SL: What is the place of urodynamic investigations in a district general hospital? Brit J Ob Gyn (editorial) 1983.
11. Versi E, Cardozo L: Perineal pad weighing versus videographic analysis in genuine stress incontinence. Brit J Ob Gyn 1986;93:364–366.
12. Green T: Development of a plan for the diagnosis and treatment of urinary stress incontinence. Am J Obstet Gynecol 1962;83:632–648.
13. Bhatia NN, Ostergard DR, McQuown D: Ultrasonography in urinary incontinence. Urology 1987;29:90–94.
14. Gordon D, Pearce M, Norton P, Stanton SL: Comparison of ultrasound and lateral chain urethrocystography in the determination of bladder neck descent. Am J Obstet Gynecol 1989;160:182–186.
15. Richmond D, Sutherst JR, Brown MC: Screening of the bladder base and urethra using linear array transrectal ultrasound scanning.
16. Koelbl H, Bernaschek G, Deutinger J: Assessment of female urinary incontinency by introital sonography. J Clin Ultrasound 1990;18:370–374.
17. Quinn MJ: Vaginal ultrasound and urinary stress incontinence, in Drife JO, Hilton P, Stanton SL (eds): Micturition. Springer Verlag, 1990, pp. 129–142.
18. Zacharin RF: The suspensory mechanism of the female urethra. J Anat 1963;97:423–427.
19. Milley PS, Nicholls DH: The relationship between the pubourethral ligaments and the urogenital diaphragm of the female urethra. Anat Rec 1970;170:281–283.

20. Delancey JOL: Pubovesical ligament: a separate structure from the urethral supports (pubourethral ligaments). Neurourol Urodynam 1989;8:53–61.
21. Delancey JOL: Correlative study of paraurethral anatomy. Obstet Gynecol 68:91–97.
22. Delancey JOL: Anatomy of the urethral sphincters and supports, in Drife JO, Hilton P, Stanton SL (eds): Micturition. Springer Verlag, 1990, pp. 3–16.
23. Stanton SL, Cardozo L: Results of the colposuspension operation for incontinence and prolapse. Br J Ob Gyn 1979;86:693–697.
24. Burch JC: Urethrovaginal fixation to Cooper's ligament for correction of stress incontinence, cystocele and prolapse. Am J Obstet Gynecol 1961;117:805–813.
25. Stamey T: Endoscopic suspension of the vesical neck, in Stanton SL, Tanagho E (eds): Surgery of Female Incontinence. Springer Heidelberg, 1980;ch. 7, pp. 77–90.
26. Hohenfellner R, Petrie R: Sling procedures, in Stanton SL, Tangho E (eds): Surgery of Female Incontinence. Springer-Verlag, New York, 1980.
27. Gillon-Stanton SL: Long term follow-up of surgery for urinary stress incontinence in elderly women. Br J Urol 1984;56:478–481.
28. Kirby RS: Assessment of the results of Stamey bladder neck suspension. Br J Urol 1989;63:153–162.
29. Dundas D, Hilton P, Williams JE, Stanton SL: Aetiology of voiding difficulty after colposuspension. Proceedings of the 12th annual meeting of the International Continence Society, Leiden, Netherlands, 1982.
30. Galloway NTM, Davies N, Stephenson TP: The complications of colposuspension. Br J Urol 1987;60:122–124.
31. Hertogs K, Stanton SL: Lateral bead-chain urethrocystography after successful and unsuccessful colposuspension. Br J Ob Gyn 1985;92:1179–1185.
32. Krantz K: Marshall–Marchetti–Krantz procedure, in Stanton SL, Tanagho E (eds): Surgery of Female Incontinence. Springer Heidelberg, 1980, ch. 4, pp. 47–54.
33. Mundy AR: A trial comparing the Stamey bladder neck, needle suspension procedure with colposuspension for the treatment of stress incontinence. Br J Urol 1983;55:687–690.

CHAPTER **9**

The Use of Transvaginal Sonography in the Diagnosis and Treatment of Infertility

Arie Drugan, MD
Joseph Itskovitz, MD, DSc
Joseph M. Brandes, MD

INTRODUCTION

The value of ultrasound in the diagnosis and treatment of female infertility has been well established in the past decade. Monitoring of ovulation by ultrasonic evaluation of follicular size[1-6] has been further complemented by ultrasound-guided aspiration of human oocytes for in vitro fertilization (IVF) through the transabdominal[7,8] or the transvaginal[9,10] routes.

Transvaginal ultrasonography (TVS) has rapidly gained popularity for the treatment of infertility[11] as well as for general purpose imaging of pelvic organs.[12-14] The proximity of the transvaginal probe's tip to the pelvic organs allows the use of high-frequency transducers (6.5–7 MHz), improving picture resolution and resulting in a clearer and more detailed scan of the evaluated organ. In most cases, TVS can provide significant additional information when findings of transabdominal sonography (TAS) are equivocal or confusing,[15] as they may be in the obese patient. In many infertility centers, TVS is today's preferred ultrasonographic modality, since it provides (1) maximal clarity of the ovaries and follicles, uterus, and pelvic blood vessels; and (2) increased patient convenience and compliance, obviating the need of a full bladder for the examination.

In this chapter we report the experience with TVS monitoring of ovulation induction and transvaginal oocyte pickup for IVF. With increasing confidence and experience in transvaginal ultrasound-guided procedures, new clinical applications for TVS are now emerging. These will also be reviewed in the association of TVS and infertility.

MONITORING OF OVULATION INDUCTION

The Ovarian Cycle

Follicles can be observed on TVS at a diameter of 2–3 mm, compared with 5 mm by TAS; they reach a diameter of 10 mm approximately 6 days before ovulation. Later on, in the natural ovarian cycle, only one follicle dominates. Hackeloer et al[1,16] found that the rate of growth of the dominant follicle was linear from day 5 to ovulation, averaging 2 mm per day. The mean diameter of the preovulatory follicle

193

was 20.2 mm (range: 18 to 24 mm). They also found a linear correlation between serum estradiol level and the diameter of the preovulatory follicle.[1] These observations are in accordance with those of Baird and Fraser,[17] who demonstrated that 95% of the circulating estradiol is secreted by the growing dominant follicle. DeCherney and Laufer[18] showed that in the natural cycle, ovulation occurs within a narrow range of follicular diameters (20–25 mm). In their study, follicular size (as estimated by ultrasound) was more accurate than serum estradiol in predicting ovulation, although best results were obtained by combining both parameters.

In stimulated cycles, generally more than one dominant follicle develops and although both serum estradiol and follicular diameter seem to increase linearly, the correlation between the two is significantly lower than in natural cycles. A far better correlation is found in stimulated cycles between serum estradiol and total follicular volume, due to the existence of multiple follicles at different stages of development.[19] The value of ultrasonography in these cases is in making the decision to withhold administration of HCG when estradiol levels are apparently preovulatory but derived from multiple small follicles.[18] Premature HCG administration, when the leading follicles are smaller than 14 mm, may result in follicular atresia and a short luteal phase.[20] It is generally recommended to induce ovulation with HCG when the leading follicles are 16–18 mm in size and serum estradiol levels reach 200–400 pg/ml per each preovulatory follicle.

For the investigation of follicular development, we use the Elscint ESI 1000 sector scanner (Elscint Ltd., Israel) equipped with a 6.5 or 7.0 MHz transvaginal transducer; the technical data for the transducer are described in Chapter 1, and a detailed step-by-step description of the technique is given in Chapter 2. The examination is performed with the patient in lithotomy position, after she has emptied her bladder. The midline plane with the uterus must be imaged first. Then the ovary and its follicles are scanned, in the space between the posterolateral aspect of the uterus and the clearly recognizable iliac vessels on the lateral pelvic wall. Flow and pulsation are easily demonstrated in these vessels when observed in a longitudinal scan.

A few anatomical structures must be differentiated from ovarian follicles. These include (1) the cross section of the internal iliac artery and vein; (2) the bowel; (3) the hydrosalpinx; and (4) ovarian cysts. Blood vessels scanned in cross section can be identified by rotating the transducer scanning plane by 90°. The round structure previously observed changes to an elongated one (two parallel lines) with or without pulsation. Parts of the bowel, if studied carefully, will show peristalsis; intraluminal contents are also somewhat echogenic. A hydrosalpinx or ovarian cyst is more difficult to distinguish structurally from larger follicles. In such cases, serial daily scanning helps, since these structures (in contrast to follicles) do not grow under hormonal influence.

Several studies[13,21–24] compared transabdominal with transvaginal monitoring of ovarian follicles. The unanimous impression was that TVS gives sharper delineation of follicular borders than TAS, and that the number of preovulatory follicles estimated by TVS was in closer correlation with the number of follicles observed at laparoscopy for IVF.[21,23] This impression, which we share, is demonstrated graphically in Fig 9.1. Thus, the increased accuracy of transvaginal evaluation of the ovarian cycle, combined with increased patient comfort and simpler patient scheduling (by obviating the need for a full bladder before and during the procedure) cause TVS to be the preferred method for follicular monitoring in induced or natural cycles.

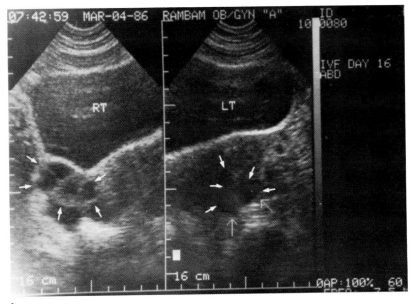

A

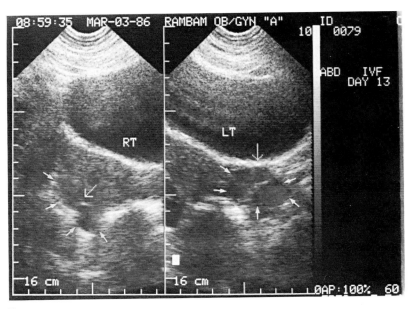

B

Figure 9.1 Comparison of views of ovarian follicles by the transabdominal/transvesical route (**A,B**) and the transvaginal route (**C,D**). Both patients' ovaries were hormonally stimulated and scanned on the day of ovulation induction.

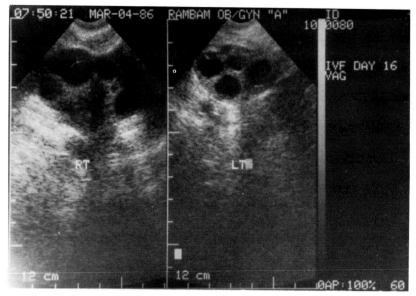

C

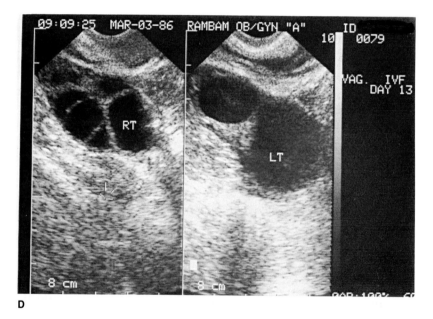

D

Figure 9.1 (continued)

Ovulatory and postovulatory events may also be followed with TVS. Ovulation—the release of antral fluid and collapse of the follicle—is followed within an hour by the development of a corpus hemorrhagicum (filling of the follicle area with echogenic material) and the collection of fluid in the cul-de-sac. The latter may be more easily demonstrated by positioning the patient in anti-Trendelenburg tilt, which allows peritoneal fluid to pool in the cul-de-sac (Fig 9.2). Accumulation

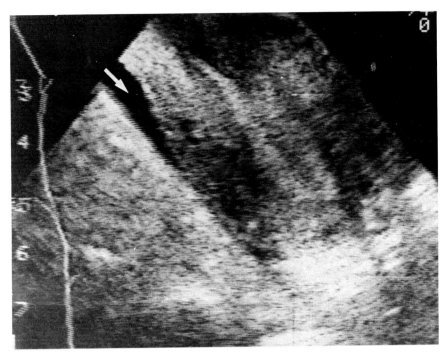

Figure 9.2 Longitudinal section of a retroverted uterus. A small amount of fluid is present in the cul-de-sac (arrow) after ovulation has taken place.

of fluid in the cul-de-sac, together with echogenic areas within, and blurring of follicular borders are accepted as ultrasonographic evidence of ovulation. It should be remembered, however, that some fluid may appear in the cul-de-sac even before ovulation, probably by transudation from preovulatory follicles. This fluid, if present, may create a tissue–fluid interface, which outlines the posterior surface of the uterus and, occasionally, the adnexa. Figures 9.3**A** and 9.3**B** show the development of the corpus luteum as seen by TVS.

Ovarian ultrasonography has also been proven useful in the diagnosis of abnormal follicular growth and development patterns, such as the luteinized unruptured follicle syndrome (LUFS) or follicles rupturing at preovulatory size.[25,26] Transvaginal scanning of the ovaries may facilitate the recognition and diagnosis of these cases. Abnormal follicular growth patterns are common in patients with luteal phase defects. In these patients, an increased incidence of follicles rupturing at a smaller than normal size has been demonstrated.[26] Patients with unexplained infertility may also show a higher incidence of abnormal follicular growth patterns.

Polycystic ovarian disease (PCOD) is a type of menstrual dysfunction characterized by chronic anovulation, inappropriate gonadotropin secretion, and hyperandrogenism. Women with PCOD commonly exhibit increased sensitivity to induction of ovulation and a tendency to ovarian hyperstimulation. The typical sonographic appearance (Fig 9.4**A**) is a somewhat enlarged ovary with a large number of small follicles (3–6 mm in size) crowded at its surface.[27] If hormonally stimulated, the ovaries assume a typical ''stained glass'' pattern resulting from the ''crowding'' of the follicles. This may be the expression of the high tension or pressure the elastic tunica albuginea is under (Fig 9.4**B, C**).

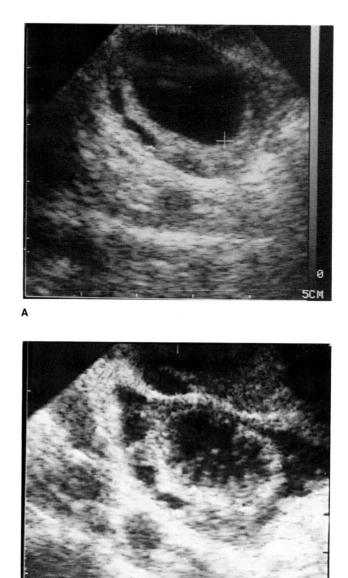

A

B

Figure 9.3 Corpus luteum formation. (**A**) Dominant follicle on day 15 in an unstimulated cycle. (**B**) Same ovary 3 days later. Note wheel–spike appearance of intrafollicular hemorrhage: corpus luteum.

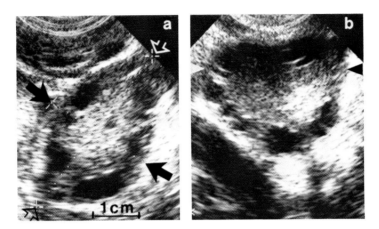

Figure 9.4A Polycystic ovary. Large, ovoid-shaped ovary with small equisized follicles (3–6 mm in size) crowded beneath the tunica albuginea. The typical beads-on-a-string appearance. (**a**) Longitudinal. (**b**) Transverse. The arrows mark the points of measurements.

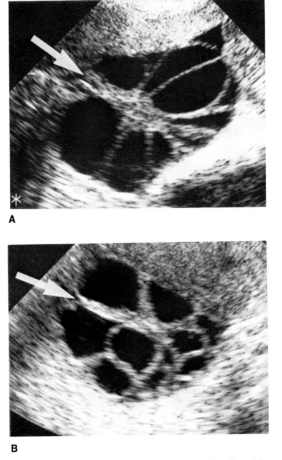

Figure 9.4B, C Two polycystic ovaries that were hormonally stimulated for ovulation induction. The arrows indicate the area of the hilus.

1. Tubo-ovarian inflammatory processes are imaged as complex adnexal conglomerates consisting of a dilated, fluid-filled tube (hydrosalpinx or pyosalpinx) in close association with a somewhat cystic, edematous ovary. Tenderness during examination may occur in the acute inflammatory phase; however, in chronic inflammatory processes, fixation of pelvic organs by adhesions is typical, and the adnexa will not "slide" when pushed with the transvaginal probe (Figs 6.5–6.13, Chapter 6).

2. Chapter 6 deals with all aspects of the acute and chronic tubo-ovarian disease. It is extremely common to reveal cystic structures considered to be part of the ovary and therefore labeled follicles. However, these "round" fluid-filled structures are the cross sections of the tortuous hydrosalpinx. By rotating the shaft of the probe the structure reveals its pear-shaped appearance. If normal stimulation of the ovaries is in progress, these structures thought to be "follicles" will of course not change their size. In Lande's series,[28] twelve patients with documented tubo-ovarian abscess were diagnosed by TAS as having nonspecific adnexal masses. Transvaginal sonography corrected the diagnosis in 8 of those patients, demonstrating tube-shaped fluid collections characteristic of pyosalpinx. Moreover, TVS added useful information in all 7 patients with disease involving the recto-uterine fossa (ie endometriosis).

   Endometrial (chocolate) cysts may involve the ovaries of the cul-de-sac. Because of their highly viscous blood filling, these cysts usually assume a spherical shape which may be altered by pressure from adjacent organs. The blood filling confers to chocolate cysts a homogenous echogenicity resembling that of dermoid cysts.

3. The sonographic characteristics of the endometrial cyst are discussed in Chapter 7.

The Endometrial Cycle

Cyclic endometrial changes in response to changing hormonal levels along the natural or stimulated menstrual cycle are easily detected with TVS. Two aspects of the endometrium appear to change progressively throughout the follicular pre-ovulatory phase: reflectivity and thickness. Smith et al[28] described reflectivity as a means of endometrial grading based on comparison of the gray-scale appearance of the endometrial texture with that of the myometrium. This work was published in 1984 and reflects the observations made by transabdominal sonography. They are mentioned here only for their historical importance and as a base for later, transvaginally obtained, observations. Four patterns of endometrial response were described:

Grade D is characterized by an almost anechoic endometrium in the presence of a prominent midline echo, which represents the endometrial canal. This endometrial pattern is commonly seen in the early to midfollicular phase.

Grade C is characterized by a solid area of reduced reflectivity and, therefore, appears darker than the surrounding myometrium. This mild but positive response to levels of circulating estradiol is typical to midfollicular phase.

Grade B endometrium is comparable in reflectivity to the surrounding myometrium, and its gray-scale appearance is indistinguishable. The initial appearance of an endometrial halo is notable. This pattern is normally seen preovulatory.

Grade A endometrium appears brighter than the myometrium and represents a favorable endometrial response to estrogens, typically seen at ovulation. The thickness of the endometrium is measured on both sides of the midline, through the central longitudinal axis of the uterine body. An endometrial thickness less than 5 mm is usually associated with the early follicular phase; in the periovulatory period the expected endometrial thickness is about 10 mm. The higher resolution and better tissue texture characterization allowed by TVS makes it the method of choice for evaluation of the endometrial response. Representative pictures are shown in Fig 9.5.

Several studies[29-35] attempted to correlate endometrial thickness and sonographic appearance with a view to the possibility of predicting implantation and pregnancy. The conclusions are, however, conflicting. Some authors[29-32] suggested that endometrial growth during ovarian stimulation and endometrial thickness at the time of oocyte retrieval were possible predictive parameters for implantation. Other studies, however, could not document a correlation between endometrial thickness and estrogen or progesterone levels or pregnancy rate.[33-35] On the other hand, the texture of the endometrium apparently has prognostic significance in association with implantation. Welker et al,[35] who examined 190 in vitro fertilization patients, detected three endometrial patterns after hormonal stimulation.

Pattern A: Homogeneous hyperechogenic.

Pattern B: Outer hyperechogenic endometrium layer and an inner hypoechoic layer.

Pattern C: The uterine cavity is distended by a contained amount of fluid.

Pattern B was the one that correlated in a positive fashion with subsequent implantation. The authors suggested that the inner layer in this pattern could be caused by the stretched glands and vessels.

In this study, no relationship could be found between the thickness of the endometrium, hormonal values, and the likelihood of implantation. Even endometrial diameters as low as 6 mm coincided with pregnancies. In Welker's study[35] a significantly higher pregnancy rate was observed in the group of patients whose endometrial pattern at oocyte retrieval consisted of an outer hyperechogenic layer and an inner hypoechogenic layer.

Gonen et al[31,32] performed two consecutive studies on the endometrial pattern in stimulated cycles and its possible predictive value for implantation.

In the first study,[31] on 108 patients, the endometrium was significantly thicker on the day before ovum retrieval in the pregnant than in the nonpregnant women, whereas the mean estradiol level did not differ between the groups.

In the second study,[32] the texture of the endometrium was graded according to its reflectivity. Three types of endometrium have been defined:

Type A: An entirely homogeneous hyperechogenic endometrium.

Type B: An intermediate isoechogenic pattern.

Type C: A multilayered endometrium consisting of prominent outer and central hyperechogenic lines with inner hypoechogenic or sonolucent regions.

Significantly more patients had multilayered endometrium (Type C) in the group who conceived than in the group who did not.

Again the thickness of the endometrium was found to be a reliable, predictive

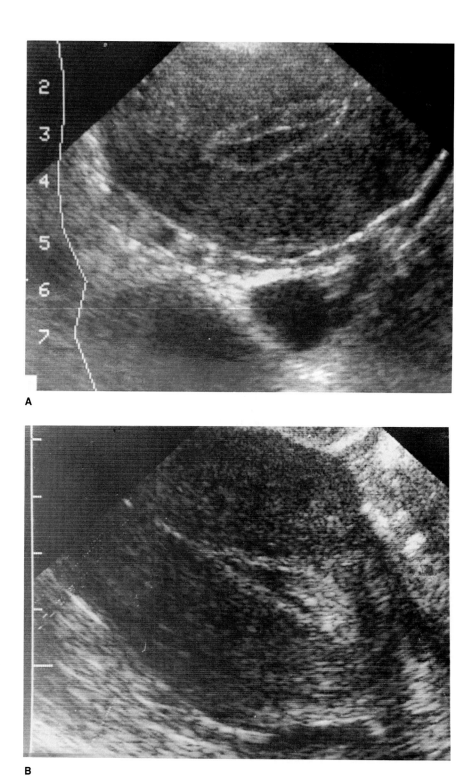

Figure 9.5 Example of a transvaginal ultrasonographic view of endometrial response. (**A**) Transverse section of uterus with endometrial response grade C. (**B**) Longitudinal section of the same uterus. (*continued*)

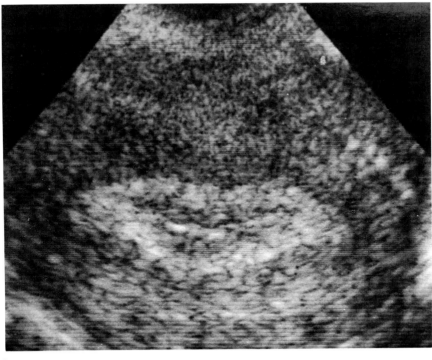

C

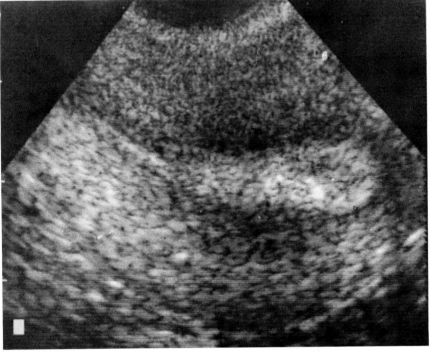

D

Figure 9.5 (*continued*) (**C**) Transverse section of a uterus with endometrial response grade A. (**D**) Longitudinal section of the same endometrium.

parameter for implantation. No pregnancy occurred when endometrial thickness was less than 6 mm on the day before ovum retrieval. Stenzik et al[36] performed vaginal Doppler flow measurements in women in the *in vitro* fertilization program. They found that the vascular resistance of uterine arteries on the day of follicular aspiration was significantly lower in women who become pregnant when compared to women who did not become pregnant.

Thus it appears that the ultrasonic evaluation of the endometrium and uterine hemodynamics, in addition to follicular measurements and hormonal values, can provide important information for the success of the in vitro fertilization program. The lack of uniform terminology is still a problem that has to be overcome.

THE CERVIX

Transabdominal ultrasonographic evaluation of the uterine cervix is possible, but a full bladder is necessary to measure cervical length and to document membrane herniation into the cervical canal.[37,38] Michaels and associates[39] showed that the development of cervical incompetence is a dynamic process, changes occurring at the level of the internal os being quite often inaccessible by routine examination. Thus, sonographic changes may be the earliest indication of incipient cervical failure.

Brown and coworkers[40] compared the yield of ultrasonographic assessment of the cervix and lower uterine segment in pregnancy by the transabdominal and transvaginal approaches. Transabdominal evaluation of the cervix was correct in 76% of cases, compared to 83% using the transvaginal route. These results suggest that the transvaginal technique should be preferred for the evaluation of the cervix and lower uterine segment in pregnancy, since this approach avoids the distortion that may be caused by a full bladder.

Transvaginal sonography may also be useful in the evaluation of placental relationship to the cervix (see Chapter 10). Because the optimal point of examining the cervix and lower uterine segment is about 2.5 cm away from the external os, slight vaginal bleeding or suspected placenta previa should not preclude the careful use of transvaginal probe even in the second or third trimester.[41]

OVARIAN FOLLICULAR ASPIRATION FOR IN VITRO FERTILIZATION

Transvaginal ultrasonographic guidance for oocyte retrieval has gained rapid popularity over laparoscopic or transvesical follicular aspiration and has become the method of choice for ovum pickup in most IVF centers.[15,42–47] Transvaginal follicular aspiration combines advantages advertised for all ultrasound-guided oocyte aspiration (avoidance of general anesthesia, decreased cycle cost, performance in an ambulatory setup) with better imaging of follicular borders and the needle tip within the follicle (Figs 9.6 and 9.7). The increased resolution and the shorter needle path afforded by the transvaginal approach minimizes the risk of perforation to bowel or major pelvic vessels; it also has obvious advantages in the obese patient or when the ovaries are fixated by adhesions deep in the cul-de-sac. In our IVF unit, transvaginal oocyte pickup has virtually replaced all other methods for follicular aspiration; laparoscopic oocyte retrieval is now reserved only for patients who need simultaneous evaluation of the pelvic anatomy.[48]

At Rambam Medical Center, patients are prepared with povidone-iodine vagi-

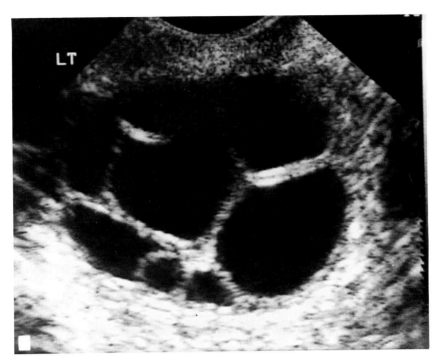

Figure 9.6 Cross section of left ovary after hormonal induction of ovulation before oocyte retrieval. Note how the high resolution of the 6.5 MHz probe enables visualization of each and every follicle with its follicular wall.

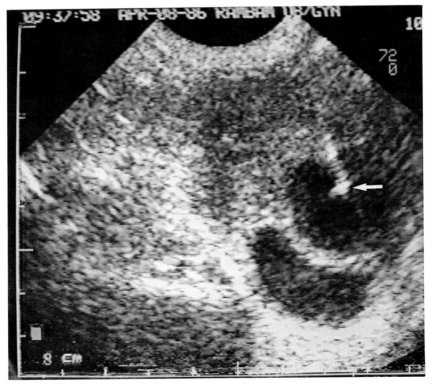

Figure 9.7 Follicular aspiration; the needle tip is seen inside the follicle (arrow).

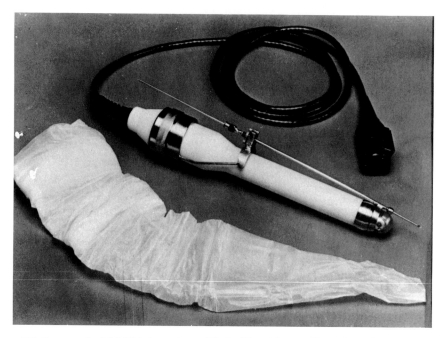

Figure 9.8 Transvaginal 6.5 MHz transducer fitted with guide, needle, and sterile probe covers.

nal suppositories on the day before and on the morning of the procedure. Systemic antibiotic prophylaxis is not used routinely in our center. For follicular aspiration, the patient is placed in the lithotomy position after the bladder has been emptied. Transvaginal ultrasound scanning of the ovaries and the cul-de-sac is repeated just before the operative procedure to rule out ovulation. Then, intravenous analgesia by pethidine hydrochloride (50 to 100 mg) and diazepam (5 to 10 mg) is given and the vagina is thoroughly cleaned again with povidone-iodine 10% solution and rinsed with normal saline. The patient is draped with sterile sheets and a sterile plastic bag is used to cover the 6.5 MHz transducer fitted with needle guide (Fig 9.8). The draped tip of the probe is covered with sterile paraffin oil, the transducer is introduced deep into the vagina and the largest diameter of the target follicle is aligned with the computer-generated biopsy line. The needle (1.6 mm outer diameter) is firmly and quickly advanced through the vaginal wall into the follicle, and fluid is aspirated under a suction pressure of 100 mm Hg, making delicate rotation movements with the needle until the aspirate becomes bloodstained. If possible, other follicles are then aspirated without withdrawing the needle. Contrary to previous experience, we do not flush the aspirated follicles because it does not increase the oocyte recovery rate. After all the follicles have been aspirated, the pelvic organs are scanned to rule out active bleeding from puncture sites.

The experience gathered by the IVF/ET Unit at Rambam Medical Center (Haifa, Israel) is shown in Table 9.1.

The transvaginal sonographically guided procedures for IVF proved to be simple, effective, and safe. Infectious complications developed in only one of our patients, which responded promptly to antibiotic therapy. Vaginal bleeding occurs occasionally, but can be controlled effectively with pressure applied to the vaginal vault. In one patient, bleeding from multiple puncture sites caused significant

TABLE 9.1 Rambam IVF Unit: Results 1987–1989

Attempted transvaginal OPU	628
Successful OPU	623 (99.2%)
Oocytes obtained	3240
Storage oocytes/attempted OPU	5.2
Fertilization rate	66%
Embryo transfer	530 (85%)
Chemical pregnancies	95
Pregnancy/OPU	15.2%
Pregnancy/ET	17.9%

OPU = oocyte pickup

decrease in hematocrit, which required intravenous fluid administration and observation. Moreover, discomfort levels caused by TVS-guided oocyte retrieval for IVF are easily managed by the majority of patients, with minimal residual effects over time.[48] Although theoretical concerns have been raised about possible adverse effects of TVS on reproductive function of human oocytes, no effect on fertilization or subsequent cleavage of the retrieved ova was demonstrated.[50] Thus, TVS can be recommended as the preferred method for monitoring of ovulation induction and follicular aspiration for in vitro fertilization and embryo transfer.

OTHER TVS-GUIDED PROCEDURES

Infertility and IVF/ET program staff should be familiar with two puncture procedures.

1. *Multifetal pregnancy reduction* to a final lower number of fetuses to improve their chances of survival; and
2. *Salpingocentesis* to needle-puncture the ectopic pregnancy, avoiding more invasive surgical interventions.

Both procedures may have to be performed on patients treated by the infertility specialist.

Both are extensively dealt with in Chapter 16 on transvaginally guided puncture procedures.

SUMMARY AND CONCLUSIONS

In modern treatment of infertility, TVS has become the method of choice for monitoring induction of ovulation and for oocyte retrieval for IVF. Better resolution, shorter needle path, and avoidance of general anesthesia are major advantages of transvaginal sonographic-guided needle procedures. With increasing experience and confidence, additional procedures, like reduction of multifetal gestations and puncture treatment of ectopic pregnancies, have also been introduced. It is expected that the expanding experience with transvaginal diagnostic as well as therapeutic procedures and increased availability of ultrasound scanners equipped with high-resolution transvaginal probes will establish TVS as an indispensable tool in the diagnosis and treatment of the infertile couple.

REFERENCES

1. Hackeloer BJ, Fleming R, Robinson HP: Correlation of ultrasonic and endocrinologic assessment of human follicular development. Am J Obstet Gynecol 1979;135:122.
2. O'Herlihy C, de Crespigny LC, Lopata A, et al: Preovulatory follicular size: a comparison of ultrasound and laparoscopic measurements. Fertil Steril 1980;32:24.
3. Renaud RL, Macler J, Dervain I, et al: Echographic study of follicular maturation and ovulation during the normal menstrual cycle. Fertil Steril 1980;33:272.
4. Fleischer AC, Daniell JF, Rodier J, et al: Sonographic monitoring of ovarian follicular development. J Clin Ultrasound 1981;9:275.
5. Kerin JR, Edmonds OK, Warnes GM, et al: Morphological and functional relations of Graafian follicle growth to ovulation in women using ultrasonic, laparoscopic and biochemical measurements. Br J Ob Gyn 1981;88:81.
6. de Crespigny LC, O'Herlihy C, Robinson HP, et al: Ultrasonic observation of the mechanism of human ovulation. Am J Obstet Gynecol 1981;139:616.
7. Lenz S, Lauritsen JG, Kjellow M: Collection of human oocytes for in vitro fertilization by ultrasonic guided follicular puncture. Lancet 1981;1:1163–1164.
8. Feichtinger W, Kemeter P: Laparoscopic or ultrasonically guided follicle aspiration for in vitro fertilization. J In Vitro Fertil Embryo Transfer 1984;1(4):244–249.
9. Gleicher N, Friberg J, Fullan N, et al: Egg retrieval for in vitro fertilization by sonographically controlled vaginal culdocentesis. Lancet 1983;2:508–513.
10. Dellenbach P, Nisand I, Moreau L, et al: Transvaginal sonographically controlled ovarian follicle puncture for egg retrieval. Lancet 1984;1:1467–1471.
11. Meldrum DR, Chetkowski RJ, Steingold KA, et al: Transvaginal ultrasound scanning of ovarian follicles. Fertil Steril 1984;42–803.
12. Schwimer SR, Lebovic J: Transvaginal pelvic ultrasonography. J Ultrasound Med 1984;3:381.
13. Schwimer SR, Lebovic J: Transvaginal pelvic ultrasonography: accuracy in follicle and cyst size determination. J Ultrasound Med 1985;4:61.
14. Trimor-Tritsch IE, Rottem S, Thaler I: Review of transvaginal ultrasonography: a description with clinical application. Ultrasound Quart 1988;6:1–34.
15. Coleman BG, Arge PH, Grumbach K, et al: Transvaginal and transabdominal sonography: prospective comparison. Radiology 1988;163:639.
16. Hackeloer BJ: Ultrasound scanning of the ovarian cycle. J In Vitro Fertil Embryo Transfer 1984;1:217–220.
17. Baird DT, Fraser IS: Blood production and ovarian secretion rates of estradiol and estrone in women throughout the menstrual cycle. J Clin Endocrinol 1974;38:1009–1015.
18. DeCherney AH, Laufer N: The monitoring of ovulation induction using ultrasound and estrogen. Clin Obstet Gynecol 1984;27:993–1002.
19. Vargyas JM, Marrs RP, Kletzki DA, et al: Correlation of ovarian follicle size and serum estradiol levels in ovulatory patients following clomiphene citrate for in vitro fertilization. Am J Obstet Gynecol 1982;144:569–573.
20. Siebel MM, McArdtle CR, Thompson IE, et al: The role of ultrasound in ovulation induction—a critical appraisal. Fertil Steril 1981;36:573–576.
21. Yee B, Barnes RB, Vargyas JM, et al: Correlation of transabdominal and transvaginal ultrasound measurements of follicle size and number with laparoscopic findings for in vitro fertilization. Fertil Steril 1987;47:828–832.
22. Gonzales JC, Curson R, Parsons J: Transabdominal versus transvaginal scanning of ovarian follicles: are they comparable? Fertil Steril 1988;50:657–659.
23. Andreotti RF, Thompson GH, Janowitz W, et al: Endovaginal and trans-abdominal sonography of ovarian follicles. J Ultrasound Med 1989;8:555–560.
24. Mendelson EB, Bohm-Velez M, Joseph N, et al: Gynecologic imaging: comparison of transabdominal and transvaginal sonography. Radiology 1988;166:321–324.
25. Janssen-Caspers HAB, Kruitwagen RFPM, Wladimiroff JW, et al: Diagnosis of luteinized unruptured follicle by ultrasound and steroid hormone assays in peritoneal fluid: a comparative study. Fertil Steril 1986;46:823.
26. Ying YK, Daly DC, Randolph JF, et al: Ultrasonographic monitoring of follicular growth for luteal phase defects. Fertil Steril 1987;48:433.
27. Orsini LF, Venturoli S, Lorusso R, et al: Ultrasonic findings in polycystic ovarian disease. Fertil Steril 1985;43:709.

28. Lande IM, Hill MC, Cosco FE, Kator NN: Adnexal and cul-de-sac abnormalities: transvaginal sonography. Radiol 1988;166:325–332.

29. Smith B, Porter R, Ahuja K, et al: Ultrasonic assessment of endometrial changes in stimulated cycles in an in vitro fertilization and embryo transfer program. J In Vitro Fertil Embryo Transfer 1984;1:233–238.

30. Glissant A, de Mouzon J, Frydman R: Ultrasound study of the endometrium during in vitro fertilization cycles. Fertil Steril 1985;44:786.

31. Gonen Y, Casper RF, Jacobson W, et al: Endometrial thickness and growth during ovarian stimulation: a possible predictor of implantation in in vitro fertilization. Fertil Steril 1989;52:446–450.

32. Gonen Y, Casper RF. Prediction of implantation by the sonographic appearance of the endometrium during controlled ovarian stimulation for IVF. J Vitro Fert Embryo Transfer 1990;7:146–152.

33. Fleischer AC, Herbert CM, Sacks GA, et al: Sonography of the endometrium during conception and nonconception cycles for in vitro fertilization and embryo transfer. Fertil Steril 1986;46:442.

34. Rabinowitz R, Laufer N, Lewin A, et al: The value of ultrasonographic endometrial measurement in the prediction of pregnancy following in vitro fertilization. Fertil Steril 1986;45:824.

35. Welker BG, Gembruch U, Diedrich K, et al: Transvaginal sonography of the endometrium during ovum pickup in stimulated cycles for in vitro fertilization. J Ultrasound Med 1989;8:549–553.

36. Stenzik K, Grab D, Sasse V, Hütter W, Rosenbusch B, Terinde R: Doppler sonographic findings and their correlation with implantation in an in vitro fertilization program. Fertil Steril 1989; 52:825–828.

37. Bowie JD, Andreotti RF, Rosenberg ER: Sonographic appearance of the uterine cervix in pregnancy—the vertical cervix. Am J Radiol 1983;140:737–740.

38. Fried A: Bulging amnion in premature labor: Spectrum of sonographic findings. Am J Radiol 1981;136:181–185.

39. Michaels WH, Montgomery C, Karo J: Ultrasound differentiation of the competent from the incompetent cervix—prevention of preterm labor. Am J Obstet Gynecol 1986;154:537–546.

40. Brown JE, Thieme GA, Shah DM, et al: Transabdominal and transvaginal endosonography: evaluation of the cervix and lower uterine segment in pregnancy. Am J Obstet Gynecol 1986;155:721–726.

41. Farine D, Fox HE, Jakobson S, et al: Vaginal ultrasound for diagnosis of placenta previa. Am J Obstet Gynecol 1988;159:566–569.

42. Feichtinger W, Kemeter P: Transvaginal sector scan sonography for needle guided transvaginal follicle aspiration and other applications in gynecologic routine and research. Fertil Steril 1986; 45:722–725.

43. Seifer DB, Collins RL, Paushter DM, et al: Follicular aspiration: a comparison of an ultrasonic endovaginal transducer with fixed needle guide and other retrieval methods. Fertil Steril 1988;49:462–467.

44. Gembruch U, Diedrich K, Welker B, et al: Transvaginal ultrasonic guided oocyte retrieval for in vitro fertilization. Hum Reprod 1988;3(suppl 2):59–63.

45. Katayama KP, Roessler N, Gunnarson C, et al: Ultrasound guided transvaginal needle aspiration of follicles for in vitro fertilization. Obstet Gynecol 1988;72:271–274.

46. Schulman JD, Dorfman AD, Jones SL, et al: Outpatient in vitro fertilization using transvaginal ultrasound guided oocyte retrieval. Obstet Gynecol 1987;69:665–668.

47. Drugan A, Timor-Tritsch IE: Transvaginal ultrasonography, in Evans MI, Fletcher JC, Dixler AO, Schulman JD (eds): Fetal Diagnosis and Therapy: Science, Ethics and the Law. Philadelphia, Lippincott Harper, 1989.

48. Itskovitz J, Boldes R, Levron Y, et al: Transvaginal ultrasonography in the diagnosis and treatment of infertility. J Clin Ultrasound 1990 (in press).

49. Shatford LA, Brown SE, Yutzpe AA, et al: Assessment of experienced pain associated with transvaginal ultrasonography-guided oocyte recovery in in vitro fertilization patients. Am J Obstet Gynecol 1989;160:1002–1006.

50. Daya S, Wicklan M, Nilsson L, et al: Fertilization and embryo development of oocytes obtained transvaginally under ultrasound guidance. J In Vitro Fertil Embryo Transfer 1987;4:338–342.

CHAPTER 10

The Use of the Vaginal Probe in the Diagnosis of Placenta Previa

Dan Farine, MD
Lawrence W. Oppenheimer, MD, MRCOG
Ilan E. Timor-Tritsch, MD

HISTORICAL BACKGROUND

The first description of placenta previa (PP) was that of Guillemeau in 1685, who explained that "The surgeon must consider if it is the child or the afterbirth which presents first."[1] However, this description went unnoted for Giffart who, in narrating a case of hemorrhage, wrote in 1730: "I can not receive as absolutely true the opinion of those authors, who say that the placenta is always attached to the fundus uteri, for in this case, as in many others, I have every reason to believe that it adhered on the internal orifice, or very near to it; and that, in dilating, the latter occasioned the separation of the after-birth, and as a consequence the hemorrhage."[2] It was Levret (1750) in France and Smellie (1751) in England who familiarized the concept of placenta previa. The management of placenta previa has always been controversial. The methods described in the 18th and 19th centuries continued to be presented and discussed in De Lee and Greenhill's textbook.[3] These methods, which are obviously contraindicated today, include:

1. Tamponade of the vagina.
2. Rupture of membranes (Puzo's operation).
3. Braxton Hicks Version: rupture of membranes, version of the fetus and traction on one leg until the fetus provides a tamponade.
4. Metreuresys: dilatation of the cervix using a water bag.
5. Willet's Forceps: an instrument resembling myoma forceps, which grasps the fetal scalp and, by pulling on it, applies it to the cervix by traction.
6. Vaginal cesarean delivery—using Duhrssen incisions.

The first cesarean delivery for placenta previa was performed in 1892, and shortly thereafter it became an accepted practice, although, even fifty years later, the vaginal approaches listed above were still practiced.

The liberal use of blood was advocated by Bill in 1927.[4] The conservative management of attempting to defer delivery until fetal viability is achieved was introduced in 1945.[5] The use of ultrasound for localizing the placenta was introduced by Gottesfeld in 1966.[6]

DEFINITIONS

There are several different definitions of placenta previa. Most classifications are based on the relationship of the location of the placenta to the internal os and were set in the times when placenta previa was diagnosed by vaginal examination. The common definitions in North America include:

1. Complete (total or central) placenta previa: the placenta completely covers the internal os.
2. Partial placenta previa: the placenta partially covers the dilating internal os.
3. Marginal placenta previa: the margins of the placenta reach the dilating internal os.
4. Low-lying placenta: the margins of the placenta are in proximity to the internal os.

In the United Kingdom, the common classifications are a *major degree of placenta previa,* in which the placenta obstructs labor (complete and significant partial placenta previa), and a *minor degree of placenta previa* (low-lying and marginal placenta previa).

STATISTICS

Placenta previa complicates 1 of every 200–250 births. The variation is dependent on the population studied (and mainly the ratio of multiparity and previous cesarean sections), and on the definition used for diagnosis (ultrasound vs. vaginal examination at birth). The incidence in nulliparas is 1 : 1,500 while it is 1 : 20 in grand multiparas.[7] There is a strong association between parity and the risk of PP, and its association with previous cesarean deliveries is even more striking.[8] The risk of PP in the presence of a previous cesarean delivery is 4–8%,[9] and up to 10% with four or more cesarean deliveries.[10]

NATURAL HISTORY

The classic presentation of a patient with placenta previa is painless bleeding, as opposed to abruptio placenta, which is accompanied by pain and uterine activity. This classic presentation is misleading since about 10% of the patients with PP do have pain or contractions and actual abruption.[7] This makes sense if we consider the fact that the clinical presentation of placenta previa with bleeding is probably the result of shearing forces on the cervix and lower uterine segment.

The initial episode of bleeding occurs prior to 30 weeks in 30% of cases; the peak incidence is around 34 weeks. About one-third of patients bleed after 36 weeks gestation and about 10% will bleed only during labor.[11]

The amount of bleeding in the initial episode is quite variable and often difficult to assess since it usually relies on the patient's history alone. Cotton et al estimated that 20% of their patients bled more than 500 ml in the initial episode.[12]

A patient with a placenta previa is likely to bleed again in a majority of cases, and in 50%, delivery is indicated within 72 hours.[12]

There is a risk of intrauterine growth retardation in nearly 20% of patients with placenta previa.[13]

DIAGNOSIS

The diagnosis is usually established after an episode of painless vaginal bleeding. Findings on physical examination which are suggestive of placenta previa include:

1. The absence of palpable uterine activity.
2. Abnormal lie of the fetus. In 35%, there is a transverse or breech presentation.[12]
3. Unengaged presenting part.
4. Placental souffle heard over the brim.

All these findings are only suggestive of placenta previa and warrant investigation with ultrasound.

Transabdominal Ultrasonographic Diagnosis

In 1966 Gottesfeld introduced the sonographic diagnosis of placenta previa.[6] This technique was immediately accepted and has become the "gold standard" for diagnosing placenta previa. Digital examination, which could induce major bleeding,[11] has become practically contraindicated and the radiologic technique of amniography has been abandoned.[14] However, traditional transabdominal sonography (TAS) does have a false positive rate of 2–6%.[15] This may lead to unnecessary hospitalization and surgery.[16] TAS has a false negative rate of 7%.[12] This rate is lower later in pregnancy and less than 2% in the third trimester.[15] The risk of a false negative examination is clinically more significant than that of false positive diagnosis since a vaginal examination may result in catastrophic bleeding.

Limitations of Transabdominal Sonography for the Diagnosis of Placenta Previa

There are several technical problems in using TAS for outlining the exact location of the placenta and its relationship to the internal os. These include the following:

1. Patient obesity often causes the placenta to be out of the focal range of the probe.[17]
2. A posterior placenta and even a lateral placenta are not always well imaged.[18]
3. The fetal head (when in the vertex position) may cast an acoustic shadow on the internal os and the placenta.[19]
4. An overdistended bladder may push the low uterine segment to a horizontal position and lead to a false diagnosis of placenta previa.[20] On the other hand, an empty bladder makes the examination more difficult as there is no acoustic window.

There are other problems besides these technical difficulties. Up to 45% of women scanned at the beginning of the second trimester seem to have a placenta previa. At term, only 10% of these women will have the same diagnosis.[21] This phenomenon has been labeled "placental migration" and is due to the stretching of the lower uterine segment. With the accuracy of TAS, the patient needs to be rescanned to ascertain the diagnosis later in pregnancy. Even then, at times, the diagnosis is difficult to establish and a "double set-up" examination may be required.[22]

These factors lead to a false positive diagnosis of placenta previa in 2–6% of women scanned in the third trimester.[15] A false positive diagnosis may lead to unnecessary restriction of activity, hospitalization, costly ultrasonic examinations and patient anxiety.[16]

Patients with "placental migration" who were diagnosed to have a placenta previa that subsequently resolved are similar to women with low-lying placentae, and are still at a high risk (45%) of antepartum bleeding, abruptio placenta, and IUGR.[23] The implications of these limitations in diagnosis are, therefore, that a patient labeled to have a placenta previa will be hospitalized for a long period until either fetal maturity is achieved or a major bleed necessitates a cesarean delivery. The patient with a false positive diagnosis of placenta previa may have an unnecessary hospitalization resulting in a cesarean delivery; whereas the patient with a false negative diagnosis of placenta previa may have bleeding following vaginal examination. These women can be saved the anxiety accompanying false diagnosis, as well as the inconvenience and cost of prolonged hospitalization.

Magnetic Resonance Imaging (MRI) and Perineal Sonography

Until recently there was no other method (besides vaginal examination) comparable to abdominal ultrasound. A recent paper indicated that *magnetic resonance imaging* (MRI) is superior to abdominal ultrasound in the diagnosis of placenta previa.[24] Even if MRI was found to diagnose placenta previa accurately, its use would be restricted by its limited availability, mostly in major medical centers, as well as its high cost. Furthermore, the experience with this technique is practically limited to one center.[24,25] The safety of a magnetic field in pregnancy has not been established.[26]

An alternative method is *perineal scanning,*[27] which overcomes several of the disadvantages of TAS; however, the distance between the probe and the internal os is too large to use the same frequency as that of TVS.

TRANSVAGINAL SONOGRAPHY (TVS) FOR THE DIAGNOSIS OF PLACENTA PREVIA

The normal anatomy of the pregnant uterus at TVS was first established (Fig 10.1). Patients with suspected placenta previa on previous sonography or patients with a bleed in either the second or third trimester were studied. TVS was performed only on a patient not actively bleeding for 24 hr. The placental location on TAS was established prior to TVS evaluation. When a placenta previa was considered, TVS was performed only by a physician familiar with this technique. TVS was performed within 24 hr following TAS, so that the methods could be compared. The results of both modalities were reported to the attending physicians. These results were compared to the location of the placenta as determined at delivery. Patients diagnosed as having placenta previa (Fig 10.2) were admitted to hospital until delivery and patients labeled as not having placenta previa were discharged 72 hr after the last bleed, with instructions to return immediately if bleeding, contractions, or pain recurred.

The main findings in our series of 77 patients[28] were as follows:

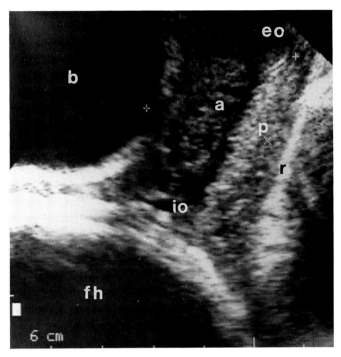

Figure 10.1 The longitudinal (sagittal) section of the normal cervix is imaged. The anterior cervical lip (a) is highlighted by the sonolucent full bladder (b). The posterior cervical lip is bordered by the hyperechoic rectum. The fetal head (fh) is well applied to the internal os (io). The normal cervical canal extends from the internal os to the external os (eo). Of course there is no placenta previa present. (Reprinted with permission from The American College of Obstetricians and Gynecologists.)[33]

1. There was no vaginal bleeding for at least 12 hr following TVS in any of the patients studied.
2. The internal os was clearly seen by TVS in all 77 cases studied and in only 54 cases (70%) by TAS.
3. TVS enabled not only delineation of the relationship of the placenta to the internal os but also the imaging of other relevant structures such as:
   a. The marginal sinus—a real-time examination using the high-frequency probe shows visible blood flow.
   b. Blood vessels in the uterus and cervix—(these vessels should not be confused with the placental marginal sinus. A thorough examination in different planes can distinguish between these vessels and the marginal sinus).
   c. Blood and blood clots—blood clots (Fig 10.3) can be easily distinguished from the placenta. Unclotted blood is less echogenic and easily demonstrable even in small quantities. Clotted blood appears echogenic.
4. When both methods ruled out placenta previa, the diagnosis was invariably confirmed at delivery.
5. Twenty-two patients were diagnosed as having placenta previa by the abdominal route and as not having placenta previa by the vaginal route. All these patients did not have placenta previa at delivery.

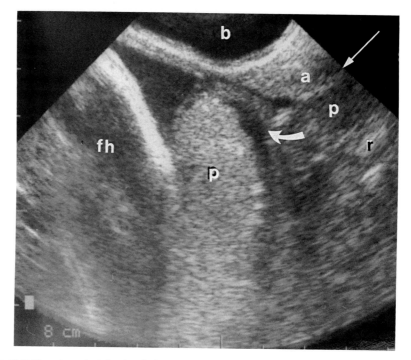

Figure 10.2 The placenta (p) extends from posterior, covering the internal os (solid white arrow). The fetal head (fh) is elevated by the placenta (b = bladder, r = rectum, a and p = anterior and posterior cervical lips). This is a sagittal scan. The direction of the cervical canal is indicated by a thin arrow. (Reprinted with permission from The American College of Obstetricians and Gynecologists.)[33]

6. Thirty patients were found to have placenta previa by both methods. At delivery, twenty of these women indeed had placenta previa and ten did not. The women who were misdiagnosed by both methods had their scans prior to 35 weeks gestation and were all diagnosed to have marginal placenta previa by TVS. These findings are compatible with the concept of cervical stretching as the explanation for ''placental migration'' in the third trimester.

7. Five women had a TVS diagnosis of placenta previa and a TAS diagnosis of no previa. All had marginal placenta previa at delivery.

The use of the vaginal probe significantly improved the accuracy of the diagnosis of placenta previa.

Table 10.1 summarizes the findings of both the sonographic methods, and the actual location of the placenta at delivery. Table 10.2 describes the rates of false positive and false negative diagnoses, and the predictability of both methods.

ADVANTAGES OF THE TRANSVAGINAL OVER THE TRANSABDOMINAL METHOD

The vaginal scanning route has several obvious advantages over the traditional abdominal route:

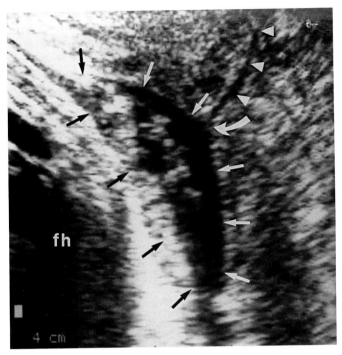

Figure 10.3 White and black arrows outline blood collection between the fetal head (fh) and the cervix. The internal os is marked by a solid arrow. The cervical canal is highlighted by arrowheads. The clotted blood is echogenic, the liquid fraction of it is sonolucent. This patient had bleeding from an anterior marginal placenta previa. (Reprinted with permission from The American College of Obstetricians and Gynecologists.)[33]

TABLE 10.1 Comparison of Transvaginal Sonography (TVS) and Transabdominal Sonography (TAS) to Location of Placenta at Birth

Ultrasound Diagnosis	No. of Cases	Diagnosis at Delivery
TAS no previa TVS no previa	20	No previa in all cases
TAS previa TVS no previa	22	No previa in all cases
TAS no previa TVS previa	5	Previa in all cases
TAS previa TVS previa	30	Previa in 20 cases No previa in 10 cases

TABLE 10.2 The Predictive Value of Transvaginal Sonography (TVS) and Transabdominal Sonography (TAS) in Diagnosing Placenta Previa

	TVS	TAS
False positive rate	29%	62% (p < 0.01)
False negative rate	0%	20% (p < 0.01)
Positive predictive value	71%	38% (p < 0.01)
Negative predictive value	100%	80% (p < 0.01)
Sensitivity	100%	79%
(p > 0.05)		
Specificity	81%	38% (p < 0.01)

1. Physical considerations:
   a. The proximity of the probe to the internal os and the placenta, which results in less signal attenuation.[17]
   b. This proximity enables the use of a higher frequency (5–6.5 MHz) resulting in better resolution.
   c. The image obtained by TVS can be magnified without loss of resolution. This enables an accurate measurement of distances (such as the distance between the internal os and the placental edge).
2. Anatomical considerations: There is no need to angle the probe to scan behind the pubic bone. The technical problems using the transabdominal approach (obesity, bladder, fetal head, posterior placenta) are nonexistent with the vaginal approach.
3. Observer bias: The diagnosis by TVS is based on measuring the distance from a clearly visualized internal os to the placental edge, and not by looking at the placenta and assuming the location of the internal os, as is often done by TAS.
4. Patient convenience: A survey revealed that the patients tolerated the procedure well and preferred it to the inconvenience of filling their bladders for TAS.[29]
5. Sonographer convenience: TVS is usually less time-consuming than TAS.
6. Diagnostic value: The accuracy of TVS is much higher than TAS (Table 2).

THE ERRONEOUS RISKS OF USING A VAGINAL PROBE

A major issue, which initially hindered the use of a transvaginal approach, was the "classic rule" of obstetrics: Any manipulation of the vagina when placenta previa is suspected is contraindicated:

> . . . The diagnosis of placenta previa rarely can be firmly established by clinical examination unless a finger is passed through the cervix and the placenta is palpated. Such examination of the cervix is never permissible unless the woman is in an operating room and preparations are made for immediate cesarean section, since even the gentlest examination of this sort can cause torrential hemorrhage. Furthermore, such an examination should not be made unless delivery is planned, for the trauma may cause bleeding of such a degree that immediate delivery becomes necessary even though the fetus is immature. . . .[30]

Two factors should be considered in this respect:

1. The vaginal probe is inserted under direct and constant imaging of its route. The relationship of the tip of the probe to the cervix is continuously assessed, as opposed to digital or speculum examinations, which are performed "blindly." If any problem, such as a dilated cervix or bulging membranes, is encountered, the probe can be kept at a distance from them.
2. The focal zone of the high-frequency probe is 2–5 cm. To achieve a clear picture, the tip of the probe must be kept 1–2 cm away from the cervix itself; therefore, no cervical contact occurs. Advancing the probe too close to the cervix will result in an image that is out of focus. To correct this the probe has to be pulled slightly outward.

LIMITATIONS OF TVS

There are several limitations of TVS that should be mentioned:

1. Like any diagnostic technique, TVS is an acquired skill. The novice should therefore not manipulate a vaginal probe in any patient suspected of having a placenta previa.
2. The vaginally operated high-frequency probe enables excellent imaging of the cervix and lower uterine segment in the third trimester. It is, however, ineffective in imaging the upper part of the uterus in the second half of pregnancy.
3. Transvaginal sonography often proves that a placenta previa "diagnosed" by the abdominal route is actually a low-lying placenta. When discovered prior to 35 weeks gestation, a diagnosis of marginal placenta previa is not predictive of the location of the placenta at birth. There were 10 such cases of false positive diagnoses (by both transvaginal and transabdominal sonography) with "placental migration" toward term. When such a diagnosis is made we recommend a repeat examination closer to term.

The sensitivity and negative predictive value of TVS in our series was 100%. The specificity, positive predictive value, and false positive rates of transvaginal scanning were twice as good as those obtained by transabdominal scanning (Table 10.2). If those cases diagnosed before 35 weeks gestation as "marginal placenta previa" are excluded, all other transvaginal diagnoses were confirmed to be correct.

This study suggests that the traditional transabdominal approach to the diagnosis of placenta previa can be improved upon. Transvaginal sonography is a safe method for diagnosing placenta previa, resulting in improved accuracy over the conventional transabdominal route. In our hands, the use of this technique resulted in less hospitalizations, fewer cesarean deliveries, and less double setup examinations.

THE DIAGNOSIS OF PATHOLOGICALLY ADHERENT PLACENTAE USING TRANSVAGINAL SONOGRAPHY

Placenta accreta, percreta, or increta are rare but serious complications of placenta previa, with a maternal death rate of 25%.[31] Placenta previa is a major risk factor for placenta accreta; it was identified in one-third of the 622 reported cases of placenta accreta. The other factors associated with placenta accreta were pre-vious cesarean section, previous curettage, and gravidity >6. As discussed above, these are also risk factors for placenta previa.

Antenatal identification of placenta increta was suggested in two case reports, in which the usual subplacental sonolucent space was missing,[32,33] and in six cases a diagnosis of placenta accreta was suggested by TAS because of abnormal blood flow patterns within the placenta.[34]

In another report,[35] 16 patients with persistent placenta previa were followed with TVS, and could be prospectively divided into two groups. In nine of the sixteen cases TVS revealed abnormal placental morphology with a peculiar pla-cental lacunar blood flow pattern, though two were lost to follow-up. The features on TVS that were suggestive of a morbidly adherent placenta in this group were:

1. Placental thickness is greater than 1 cm with multiple sonolucencies (blood lakes) (Fig 10.4).
2. Lakes (lacunae) that occupy practically all the thickness of the placenta.
3. There is pulsatile and laminar blood flow within the lacunae.

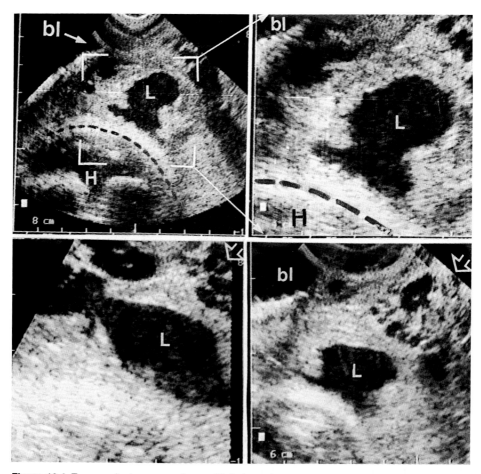

Figure 10.4 Transvaginal sonography sagittal views demonstrating the typical "swiss cheese" pattern of lucencies in an abnormally adherent placenta with lacunar flow (bl = bladder, L = lacunae, H = fetal head; the open arrows indicate the approximate location of the external os). The upper right image is an enlarged portion of the upper left image. (Reprinted by permis-sion of The C.V. Mosby Company.)[39]

4. Occasionally the borders of the placenta were not clear, and dilated vascular structures with pulsatile flow could be seen within the myometrium and the cervix.

The 6 patients with normal morphology had uneventful cesarean deliveries and revealed placenta previa. Two patients were lost to follow-up, 7 of the 8 (86%) patients with lacunar blood flow required cesarean hysterectomy. All these patients with cesarean hysterectomy had pathological evidence of placenta accreta or increta. The blood loss in the "lacunar blood flow" group (2814 ml) was significantly higher than that in the "nonlacunar flow" group (967 ml). The authors suggest that the findings of lacunar blood flow necessitate informing the patient of the possibility of placenta accreta and blood loss and the possible need for transfusion as well as surgical ligation of large arteries or cesarean hysterectomy to control blood loss. Such a pattern warrants notifying the anesthetist of the risk of excessive bleeding, obtaining enough blood for the delivery, and selecting a competent surgical team.

MANAGEMENT

The initial step in the management of a patient with second or third trimester bleeding is admission to hospital for assessment of the maternal and fetal condition. This assessment would include insertion of a large bore IV, a complete blood count, cross and type for at least two units of blood, as well as assessment of maternal vital signs and fetal well-being by fetal heart monitoring. Even suspicion of placenta previa is a contraindication to digital examination of the cervix, unless the obstetrician is ready to perform an emergency cesarean delivery.[30]

The patient who is bleeding excessively should have appropriate blood and fluid replacement and be reassessed. If the gestational age is advanced (36–38 weeks) a prompt cesarean delivery is indicated when the patient has stabilized. At earlier gestations, the aim of the treatment is to get over the initial bleeding, thus gaining time for fetal maturity. However, if the patient continues to bleed and is unstable, a cesarean delivery is indicated at an earlier gestational age.

The sonographic examination is aimed at localizing the placenta as well as assessing fetal biometry and well-being. We do not perform vaginal sonography at the time of initial bleeding, because the management is not altered at this stage by the vaginal examination, and because of possible medico–legal implications of such an examination with acute bleeding.

Once acute bleeding has settled, the patient is assessed by both TAS and TVS in order to obtain an optimal diagnosis. The examination assesses the location of the placenta in relation to the internal os as well as the border of the placental bed and the pattern of the blood flow in the placenta. A diagnosis of PP by TVS necessitates hospitalization until delivery. Patients without placenta previa undergo a speculum examination and are hospitalized for at least 72 hr following the initial bleed. Although we never manage patients with placenta previa as outpatients, such management is acceptable provided the patient is highly motivated and understands the nature of the disorder and its implications. The patient should be constantly attended by an adult and live within 10–15 min from the hospital (weather and transportation conditions permitting).[36]

Expectant management is the key for optimal results. Hematocrit should be maintained above 30, though patients' awareness of AIDS and hepatitis have made this goal less achievable.

There is controversy over the role of tocolytics in the presence of placenta previa. Cotton et al[12] reported a 66% success rate in expectant management, a protocol using tocolysis and blood transfusion, as opposed to 43%–46% in previous series using transfusions alone. Recent data cast doubt on the use of tocolysis even in the absence of maternal bleeding.[37] Betamimetics are relatively contraindicated in the presence of maternal bleeding[38] and are associated with significant maternal morbidity.[39] Therefore, we do not use betamimetics in women bleeding from placenta previa.

Optimal timing of delivery is 36–38 weeks depending on fetal well-being, fetal lung maturity, and presence or absence of maternal bleeding.[16] We recommend a repeat sonographic examination to better outline the relationship of the placenta to the internal os, thus diagnosing late placental migration. This examination also outlines the margins of the placenta for the surgeon performing a cesarean delivery and enables better counseling regarding the risk of placenta accreta.

The diagnosis of complete placenta previa at this stage is an absolute indication for a cesarean section. The diagnosis of a marginal or partial placenta previa should be discussed with the patient; in a patient with several episodes of bleeding, the standard management is either a cesarean delivery or expectant management with double setup at labor.[22] In our hands, TVS practically eliminated the requirement for, and the risk of, double setup examination.

SUMMARY

The data presented above indicate that transvaginal sonography is a safe method of diagnosis for patients with suspected placenta previa. It is superior to transabdominal sonography, being more accurate in outlining the internal os, placental edge, placental anatomy, and blood flow pattern. Transvaginal sonography is acceptable for the patient and easy for the sonologist or sonographer. Transvaginal sonography may be used as the first choice in the workup of all patients suspected of placenta previa, but should definitely complement *all* transabdominal sonographical examinations in such women. Whenever multiple lacunar structures with intensive blood flow are observed in a placenta previa, special measures should be taken in anticipation of a possible pathologically adherent placenta.

REFERENCES

1. Dunal B: L'hemorrhagie produite par l'insertion du placenta. Montpellier. 1985, p 13.
2. Cazeaux P: A theoretical and practical treatise on midwifery, 4th American ed. from the 6th French ed. Lindsay and Blakiston, Philadelphia, 1866.
3. De Lee JB, Greenhill JP: The principles and practice of obstetrics. 8th ed. Philadelphia, WB Saunders, 1943.
4. Bill A: Treatment of placenta previa by prophylactic blood transfusion and cesarean section. *Am J Obstet Gynecol* 1927;14:523.
5. Johnson HW: The conservative management of some varieties of placenta previa. *Am J Obstet Gynecol* 1945;50:248.
6. Gottesfeld KR, Thompson JH, Taylor ES: Ultrasound placentography: a new method for placental localization. *Am J Obstet Gynecol* 1966;96:538.
7. Hibbard LT: Placenta previa, in Sciarra JJ (ed): *Gynecology and Obstetrics*. Vol. 2, New York, Harper and Row, 1981.
8. Singh PM, Rodrigues C, Gupta AN: Placenta previa and previous cesarean section. *Acta Obstet Gynecol Scand* 1981;60:367.

9. Kelly JV, Iffy L: Placenta previa, in Iffy L, Kaminetzky HA (eds): *Principles and Practice of Obstetrics and Perinatology*. Vol 2. New York, John Wiley & Sons, 1981.
10. Clark SL, Kooning PP, Phelan JP: Placenta previa/accreta and prior cesarean section. *Obstet Gynecol* 1985;66:89.
11. Crenshaw C, Jones DED, Parker RT: Placenta previa: a survey of twenty years experience with improved perinatal survival by expectant therapy and cesarean delivery. *Obstet Gynecol Survey* 1973;28:461.
12. Cotton DB, Read JA, Paul RH, Quilligan EJ: The conservative aggressive management of placenta previa. *Am J Obstet Gynecol* 1980;137:687.
13. Brar HS, Platt DL, DeVore GR, Horenstein J: Fetal umbilical velocimetry for the surveillance of pregnancies complicated by placenta previa. *J Reprod Med* 1988;33:741.
14. Gordon A, Pinchen C, Walker E, Tudor J: The changing place of radiology in obstetrics. *Br J Radiol* 1984;57:891.15.
15. Laing FC: Placenta previa: False negative diagnoses. *J Clin Ultrasound* 1981;9:109.
16. D'Angelo LJ, Irwin LF: Conservative management of placenta previa: a cost-benefit analysis. *Am J Obstet Gynecol* 1984;149:320.
17. Timor-Tritsch IE, Rottem S: *Transvaginal Sonography*. New York, Elsevier Publishing Co. 1987, pp 1–13.
18. Edlestone DI: Placental localization by ultrasound. *Clin Obstet Gynecol* 1977;20:285.
19. King DL: Placental ultrasonography. *J Clin Ultrasond* 1973;1:21.
20. Williamson D, Bjorgen J, Worman M: The ultrasonographic diagnosis of placenta previa: value of the post void scan. *J Clin Ultrasound* 1978;6(1):58.
21. Wexler P, Gottesfeld KR: Second trimester placenta previa: an apparently normal placentation. *Obstet Gynecol* 1973;50:706.
22. Chervenak F, Lee Y, Hendler M, Monoson RF, Berkowitz RL: Role of attempted vaginal delivery in the management of placenta previa. *Obstet Gynecol* 1984;64:798.
23. Newton ER, Brass V, Cetrulo CL: The epidemiology and clinical history of asymptomatic mid-trimester placentae previa. *Am J Obstet Gynecol* 1984;148:743.
24. Powell MC, Buckley J, Price H, et al: Magnetic resonance imaging and placenta previa. *Am J Obstet Gynecol* 1986;154:565.
25. Powell MC, Worthington BS, Symonds EM: Magnetic resonance imaging (MRI) in obstetrics. I. Maternal anatomy. *Br J Obstet Gynecol* 1988;95:31–37.
26. Mattison DR, Angtuaco T, Long C: Magnetic resonance imaging in obstetrics and gynecology. *Contemp Obstet Gynecol* 1987;29:48–81.
27. Jeanty P, d'Alton M, Romero R, Hobbins JC: Perineal scanning. *Am J Perinatol* 1986;3:289.
28. Farine D, Fox HE, Jacobson S, Timor-Tritsch IE: Is it really placenta previa? *Eur J Obstet Gynecol* May 1989;31(2):103–108.
29. Slavik T: Transvaginal sonography: The technician view. JUM 1988;7:214.
30. Pritchard JA, MacDonald PC, Gant NF: *Williams Obstetrics*, 17th ed. Norwalk, Conn., Appleton-Century-Crofts, 1985, p 409.
31. Fox H: Placenta accreta, 1945–1969. *Obstet Gynecol Survey* 1972;27:475.
32. Tabsh KMA, Brinkman CR III, King W: Ultrasound diagnosis of placenta increta. *J Clin Ultrasound* 1982;10:288.
33. Cox SM, Carpenter RJ, Cotton DB: Placenta percreta: ultrasound diagnosis and conservative surgical management. *Obstet Gynecol* 1988;72:452.
34. Mendonca LK: Sonographic diagnosis of placenta accreta: presentation of six cases. *J Ultrasound Med* 1989;8:166.
35. Guy GP, Peisner DB, Timor-Tritsch IE: Ultrasound evaluation of uteroplacental blood flow patterns of abnormally located and adherent placentas. *Am J Obstet Gynecol* 1990;163:723–727.
36. Silver R, Depp R, Sabbagha RE, Dooley SL, Socol ML, Tamura RK: Placenta previa: aggressive expectant management. *Am J Obstet Gynecol* 1984;150:15.
37. King JF, Grant A, Keirse MJ, Chalmers I: Beta-mimetics in preterm labour: an overview of the randomized controlled trials. *Br J Obstet Gynaecol* 1988;95:211.
38. Creasy RK: Preterm labor and delivery, in Creasy RK, Resnik R (eds): *Maternal Fetal Medicine—Principles and Practice: Tocolysis and Bleeding*, 2d ed. Philadelphia, WB Saunders, 1989, p 488.
39. Katz M, Robertson PA, Creasy RK: Cardiovascular complications associated with terbutaline treatment for preterm labor. *Am J Obstet Gynecol* 1981;139:605.

CHAPTER 11

Sonoembryology

Ilan E. Timor-Tritsch, MD
Zeev Blumenfeld, MD
Shraga Rottem, MD, DSc

INTRODUCTION

High-resolution transvaginal probes enable us to study early gestations in greater detail than ever before. The term *sonoembryology* was suggested[1,2] to reflect the ability of these new probes to focus on small structures and organs in the embryonic and fetal periods. If the traditional nomenclature is followed, then sonographic examination of the conceptus up to 9 weeks should be called *sonoembryology* and after the ninth week *sonofetology*. The term embryo (embruon) means "to grow" in Greek; fetus is defined as "offspring" in Latin. These terms were artificially designated to the conceptus to distinguish between two stages in development: embryo until the ninth week of gestation, fetus thereafter. These terms are usually used interchangeably, not only in daily communication between health professionals, but also in the literature (eg, "appearance of the *fetal pole*"—referring to weeks 6–7 of the gestation at which time it should still be called *embryonic pole*). We see no reason to use the terms "sonoembryology" and "sonofetology" to distinguish between imaging the pregnancy before and after 9 weeks. Lately, the term "transvaginal ultrasound *embryography*" has also been employed.[3] The term "sonoembryology" will be used here to describe the technique of detailed structural examination of the conceptus until it reaches the early second trimester. To understand and appreciate the images produced by a high-frequency transvaginal transducer probe, it is necessary to review several aspects of early embryological development. This short review is limited to a discussion of relevant highlights considered important in understanding some of the structures observed during scanning of early gestation.

CHRONOLOGY OF DEVELOPMENT

Preimplantation Period

In the rhesus monkey and in the human, the embryo reaches the uterus as a morula of about 16 cells still covered by the zona pellucida.[4] The early uterine morula in the human is about 0.1 to 0.2 mm in diameter,[4] a fact that must be appreciated if the events of implantation, ie, the attachment of the embryo to, and its embedment in, the endometrium, are to be understood. On the fourth or fifth day after ovulation, when the primate morula enters the uterine cavity, the endometrium is in the luteal phase and is approximately 5 mm thick. Its glands are actively secreting, and the walls are, therefore, covered by a film of mucus.[4] The morula is carried into the film of uterine secretion by the ciliary current from the uterine tube and lies free in it for the next 4 to 5 days. The mucosal surface is roughened by irregular depressions, most of which represent the openings of endometrial glands. These gland mouths may be wider than the diameter of the morula. The blastocyst may become lodged in or between these depressions as the first step in the attachment and implantation process. During this period, the morula loses its zona pellucida and develops into a spherical blastocyst, consisting of an outer layer of trophoblastic cells surrounding an inner fluid-filled blastocyst cavity and an inner cell mass. Also during this time, because of the absorption of fluid into its cavity from the uterine secretions, the blastocyst expands to a diameter of about 0.24 mm, but there is no increase in cytoplasmic substance. The oxygen and nutrient material required by the embryo at this very early stage are derived from the endometrial secretions. Until this point, no signs of pregnancy can be seen in any kind of sonographic examination.

Peri-implantation Period

The blastocyst has already attached and been partially implanted by 7–8 days after ovulation. The mode of early attachment of the human ovum is probably similar to that of the rhesus monkey, but the process commences at an earlier date. By the tenth or eleventh day postovulation, the human ovum becomes embedded in the endometrial stroma, partly because of the earlier attachment and partly because of the greater activity of the invading trophoblast. The stroma shows edema and congestion, which may result from the action of some substances produced by the implanting trophoblast and which may partly explain the degeneration of the uterine epithelium overlying this edematous stroma. Still, the edema and thickening of the endometrium observed on ultrasound examination are not yet diagnostic of pregnancy. This congested and edematous stroma provides nutritive material for the trophoblast, which now thickens rapidly at the region of contact where it differentiates into two layers: the original, inner, cellular *cytotrophoblast* or Langhans' layer, and the outer *syncytiotrophoblast* layer covering the cytotrophoblast and forming the layer of actual contact with the maternal tissues. The defect in the uterine epithelium caused by penetration of the ovum is gradually closed by a coagulum of fibrin and by proliferation of the adjacent epithelium. This method of embedment is called interstitial implantation, and at its completion the ovum lies in the superficial part of the stratum compactum, projecting slightly into the uterine lumen. After implantation of the blastocyst, the endometrium is called decidua and is divided into three topographically distinct portions depending on its relationship to the blastocyst: decidua capsularis, decidua basalis, and decidua parietalis (Fig 11.1**A, B**). The blastocyst normally implants in the endometrium of the uterine body, most frequently on its upper posterior wall. Because of this location, the transvaginal transducer probe is in closer proximity to the embryo than the transabdominal scanner.

The trophoblast is not uniformly developed over the surface of the implanted blastocyst, being thicker on its deep aspect (ie, toward the decidua basalis) than on its superficial aspect (decidua capsularis). This is probably due to the poorer supply of nutrients to the trophoblastic cells nearer the uterine lumen, and may be recognized on transvaginal sonography by the thicker trophoblast on the deep aspect of the gestational sac, the future placenta.

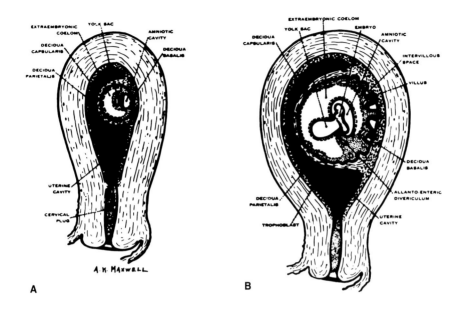

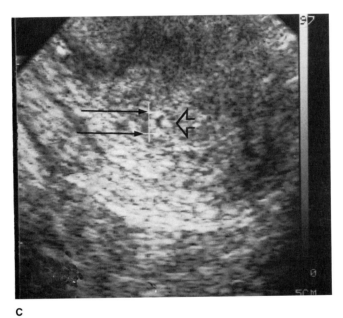

Figure 11.1 Diagrammatic representation of 5-week (**A**) and 6-week (**B**) embryos. Note the relationship among the decidua parietalis, decidua capsularis, and decidua basalis. (**C**) A normal 4-week 4-day intrauterine pregnancy. Only the gestational sac (open arrow) can be seen with TVS at this early stage. The gestational sac is only 4 mm in diameter (between long arrows).

(continued)

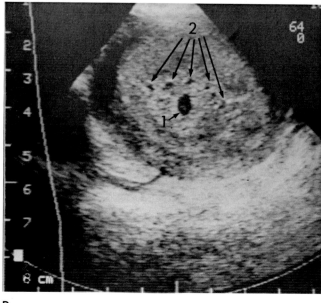

D

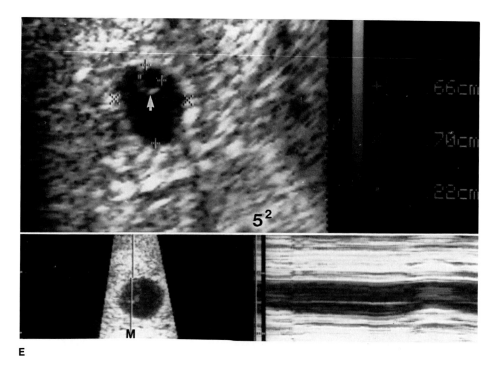

E

Figure 11.1 (*continued*) (**D**) Normal 5-week 0-day intrauterine pregnancy. The first structure that can be seen within the gestational sac is the yolk sac (1). Note the lacunar intervillous spaces (2) at this stage (as in Figs 11.1**B** and 11.2). (**E**) A 5-week 0-day chorionic sac measuring 6.6 × 7.0 mm with a 2.2 mm yolk sac (arrow). Embryonic pole is not seen. No fetal heart activity was detected by M-mode sweep (M). (Reprinted with permission of C.V. Mosby Company.)[19] (Figures 11.1**A** and 11.1**B** are reproduced from Human Embryology[4] by permission of The Macmillan Press Limited.)

After the morula has become a blastocyst, a primitive yolk sac (Fig 11.2) lined by a single layer of trophoblastic cells forms. This layer of trophoblastic cells proliferates inward toward the primitive yolk sac (Fig 11.2), forming the extraembryonic mesoderm, and outward toward the uterine epithelium.[5,6] The primitive yolk sac decreases considerably in size. In the inner cell mass of the blastocyst, the amniotic cavity forms (Fig 11.1**A, B**). Within the extraembryonic mesoderm, another cavity—the extraembryonic coelom—forms (Fig 11.3), and this progressively surrounds the primitive yolk sac (Figs 11.3 and 11.4). The extraembryonic coelom eventually surrounds the amniotic cavity, and, from that time, the remaining yolk sac is called the secondary yolk sac. The amniotic cavity and the secondary yolk sac are connected to the trophoblast by the connective stalk that prefigures the umbilical cord. At these stages the size of the gestation is below the resolution of the high-frequency transvaginal probes.

At about the fourth gestational week (since the last menstrual period [LMP]), the germinative layer, located between the amniotic cavity and the secondary yolk sac, progressively differentiates to produce the fetus (Fig 11.5). The outer aspect of the extraembryonic coelom is contained within the original trophoblastic layer, which proliferates on one side of the implantation to form the placenta and on the other side to form the chorionic membrane. The portion of the chorionic membrane opposite the implantation adherent to the decidua capsularis separates the virtual uterine cavity from the extraembryonic coelom (Figs 11.1, 11.3, and 11.4). With the growth of the fetus and its amniotic cavity, the secondary yolk sac is squeezed by the amniotic cavity against the extraembryonic coelom. The yolk sac (Fig 11.4) now decreases in size and is connected by the vitelline duct through the connective stalk to the fetal abdomen. The anatomic features of the developing fetus, starting with the fetus and moving outward (Figs 11.1, 11.3, and 11.4), are the amniotic fluid, the amnion, the extraembryonic coelom, the decidua capsularis, the uterine cavity, the decidua parietalis, and the myometrium.[6]

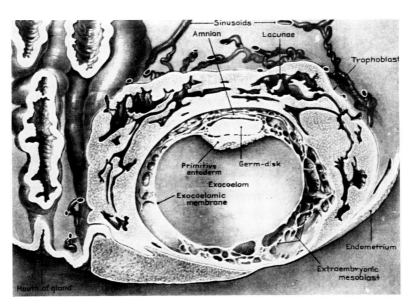

Figure 11.2 Day 11 of embryonic development (after ovulation). Note the primitive yolk sac, the extraembryonic mesoderm, and the lacunae at the depth of the implantation site of the gestational sac. (Reproduced by permission of The Macmillan Press Limited, from Human Embryology.[4])

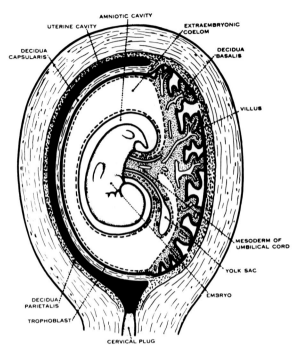

Figure 11.3 Diagrammatic representation of a 6-week embryo. Note the amniotic cavity surrounded by the extraembryonic coelom, and the intervillous spaces in the early placenta. (Reproduced by permission of The Macmillan Press Limited, from Human Embryology.[1])

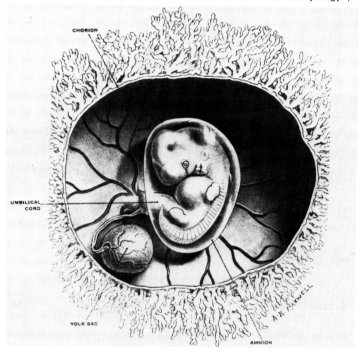

Figure 11.4 A 5½-week embryo. Note the relationship of the yolk sac and yolk stalk to the umbilical cord. Once the amniotic sac grows to encompass and obliterate the extraembryonic coelom, the yolk sac is incorporated into the umbilical cord and is only rudimentary. (Reproduced by permission of The Macmillan Press Limited, from Human Embryology.[1])

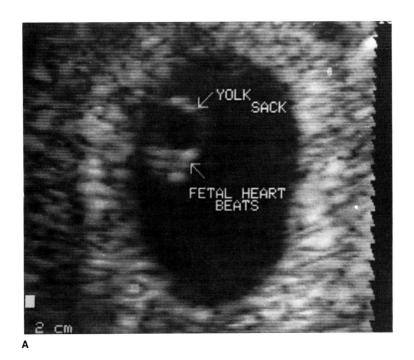

A

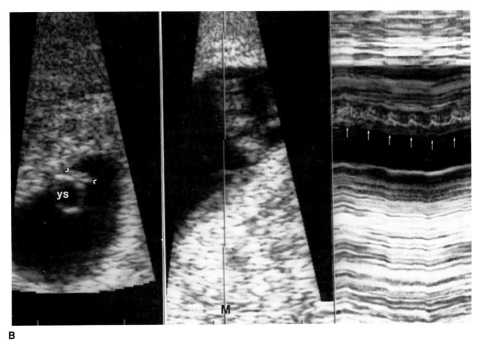

B

Figure 11.5 (A) A 6-week 1-day intrauterine pregnancy. Note the yolk sac which at this early stage is larger than the embryo. The gestational sac measures 16 × 12 mm. At this early stage, fetal heartbeats can be detected by TVS at the place marked. **(B)** One way to document embryonic heartbeats is to apply an M-mode cursor (M) and observe the small deflections of the echoes (arrows). The CRL is 3.5 mm; the gestational age is 6 weeks and 2 days (ys = yolk sac). (Reprinted with permission of C.V. Mosby Company.)[19]

Development of the Fetal Circulation

During implantation, maternal blood comes into direct contact with the trophoblastic syncytium lining the lacunae.[4] This blood is a new source of nutrition for the embryo and its membranes. With this source of nutrition established only a fraction of a millimeter from it, the embryo itself rapidly differentiates. At 5 weeks after LMP, transvaginal sonography is able to detect and clearly show lacunar formations at one pole of the implanted gestation. These lacunar structures show distinct flow and, as seen in Figure 11.6**D**, they form a one-quarter to one-half circle around the gestational sac. At first the nutrients reach it by diffusion, but in the surprisingly short time of about 13 days after commencement of implantation (20-day-old embryo or 34 days from LMP), a simple circulatory system is formed in the embryo, chorion, yolk sac, and connective stalk. This precocious development of the embryonic heart and blood vessels is correlated with the rapid enlargement of the chorionic vesicle.[4] By the twenty-first day postimplantation, 5 weeks of gestational age (1.5 mm embryo), circulation from the embryo through the blood vessels is established and the fetal heart is pulsating. This may be seen by the sixth week of gestation (from the LMP) only by transvaginal sonography. Thus the detection of fetal heartbeats by transvaginal sonography becomes possible within several days to a week of its chronological development.

First trimester detection of embryonic cardiac activity was published by Robinson in 1972.[8] In 1973 Robinson reported seeing the heart motion by transabdominal ultrasonographic method at 44 days postconception.[9] More than a decade later, using more sophisticated transabdominal scanning equipment, the earliest gestational age at which the heartbeats were seen was "pushed back" by Cadkin and McAlpin several days to an average mean gestational age of 42 days (with a range of ±4 days, 95% confidence limits).[10] The embryonic heart rate in this study was in the range of 96 to 120 beats/minute with a mean of 110 beats/minute. DuBoise studied the embryonic heart rate and compiled a graph displaying the heart rate changes as a function of early gestational ages.[11,12] Descriptive information regarding the imaging of the developing heart is forthcoming in this chapter.

THE MATERIAL

The authors reviewed material published in the literature[2,3,7,13–28] or accepted for publication[29–31,45] at the time of the printing of this book.

DATING THE GESTATION

Expressing the chronological age of any first trimester gestation has not only clinical significance but it is of utmost importance to arrive at a consensus in dating the pregnancy. There are three ways to express the age of the conceptus.

1. *Conceptual age.* This term is used mostly in embryology and relates to the true age of the gestation. It is counted in days beginning the day of the presumed conception, or the day of fertilization of ova if an in vitro fertilization was performed. Articles and information dealing with various external effects on the embryo usually express the exposure time in conceptual age to enable an accurate research of the possible teratological impact.
2. *Gestational age.* Gestational age is expressed in weeks from an arbitrary

date computed by the addition of 14 days to the conceptual age. This compensates for the 2 weeks of a normal menstrual cycle from the first day of the last menstrual period (LMP) and the day of ovulation/conception, enabling the "translation" of the conceptual age into a clinically agreed upon and used age of the pregnancy. Example: A 41-day embryo is consistent with a gestational age of 7 weeks (completed) and 6 days.

   3. *Menstrual age.* Expresses the time elapsed from the LMP in weeks, but does not take into consideration the actual day of ovulation/conception. The menstrual age is widely used by obstetricians/gynecologists. The crown-rump length (CRL) measurements are expressed in menstrual age.

   In the studies performed at the Sloane Hospital for Women (Columbia Presbyterian Medical Center), the gestational ages were expressed in *completed weeks* and days from the first day of a certain LMP, or the known day of ovulation induction, in vitro fertilization, to which 14 days were added. Example: 5 weeks and 3 days means five completed weeks and 3 days into the sixth week. In other words, *the sixth week* means 5 completed weeks and 1 day to 5 weeks and 6 days. Before any work in sonoembryology is evaluated, it is important to understand the way the gestational age is expressed since there is no international consensus to use for a standardized dating nomenclature.

   Another duty of the researcher studying sonoembryology is to study only those gestations dated with extreme accuracy. This enables the comparison and study of embryos of the same ages. Embryologic structures appear at predictable and well-timed conceptual ages. Streeter, a prominent researcher, wrote: "It is in embryos of the first seven weeks that the external form and structural organization are more informative as to age than its size alone."[33] In the material studied by our group,[2,7,19,21,27,29–31] the menstrual age and the gestational age computed from measurements of the crown–rump length were within ± 4 days of each other in *all* embryos studied. In about 75%, the difference was only ±3 days.

THE DISCRIMINATORY ZONE OF ßhCG FOR VAGINAL PROBES

Before proceeding to the ultrasonographic evaluation of embryonic structures, the concept of the discriminatory βhCG zone must be discussed.

   This concept was developed by Kadar[40] to answer a very simple question: At what serum βhCG level should a sac be seen on ultrasound examination? If serum βhCG level is above the discriminatory zone, an intrauterine gestational sac should be seen, and if it is not seen, the pregnancy is either abnormal, has aborted, or is in an ectopic location. This is an excellent clinical tool which can guide our approach to the early normal and abnormal pregnancy.

   The physiology behind the discriminatory zone is important. As pregnancy progresses, the volume of trophoblastic tissue increases, leading to an increase in the production of βhCG. At the same time, the sac and the embryo are growing in size. Once the sac becomes large enough, it will become visible during an ultrasound examination. If the sac diameter reaches a certain point, it will be consistently detected by an examiner. If the level of the serum βhCG corresponding to that particular sac size is determined, this is called the *discriminatory* zone value. Both the cells and the βhCG increase exponentially, and the doubling time of the cells is about 1.2 days, with βhCG doubling in about 2 days.[41] It is worth mentioning that the βhCG is measured in different units of measurement, ie, the First International Reference Preparation (IRP) and the Second International Standard. It is important to know that 2.2 mIU/mL Second Reference Standard = 1 mIU/ml of the First IRP.

Abdominal scanning detects a sac size that is usually close to 1 cm in diameter, or perhaps somewhat less with a higher resolution scanner. Transvaginal sonography allows the detection of a sac as small as 2 mm in diameter.[7]

There are many ways to calculate the value of the discriminatory zone. Kadar picked a value when the intrauterine sac was always seen.[40] Other investigators used the same concept.[14,42] They compared the presence or the absence of an intrauterine gestational sac to the value of the serum βhCG for a series of early pregnancies. Then they compared it to the βhCG value corresponding to the presence of the sac (Table 11.1). Peisner et al[16] chose another method of determining the discriminatory zone for the vaginal probe. The natural logarithm of the βhCG and sac values were taken using the following equation:

$$\log (\beta hCG) = 6.56 + 0.34 \times \log (\text{sac volume}) \ [R^2 = 49\%]. \ (\text{Table 11.2})$$

The βhCG that corresponds to a sac diameter of 1 mm is about 840 IRP in our institution. This calculation method is so simple that it can be calculated in a matter of minutes.

When using a 3.5 MHz abdominal scanning probe, the discriminatory zone was calculated to be between 6000 and 6500 mIU/ml.[40] However, the introduction of higher resolution (5 MHz) abdominal ultrasound equipment allowed the threshold to be dropped to 1800 mIU/mL.[42] With vaginal sonography, the boundary value of the discriminatory zone that is currently being reported ranges from 600 mIU/mL to 1025 mIU/mL.[14,15,18,28]

The derivation of the discriminatory zone varies with the type of scanning, equipment, and the nature of the βhCG determination. To derive a discriminatory zone for an institution does not require a large number of patients. *Because of its importance, it is imperative that the appropriate discriminatory zone for each equipment and laboratory employed be determined in each institution where transvaginal sonography is used.*

TABLE 11.1 Graphic Representation of hCG Levels (mIU/mL) as a Function of Maximal Gestational Sac Diameter in 20 Cases $\leq$1.0 cm (After Goldstein et al.[42])

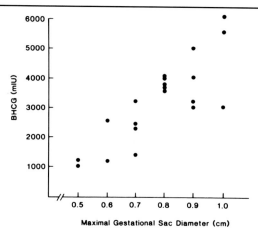

TABLE 11.2 Correlation of Sac Volume with Beta-hCG

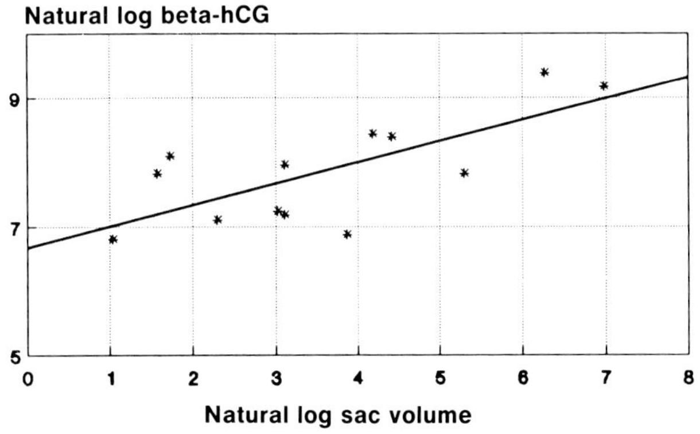

Natural log beta-hCG

Natural log sac volume

After Peisner et al.[28]

The βhCG discriminatory levels can be determined for other than the gestational sac. The first appearance of the yolk sac and the embryonic heartbeats can also be determined. Table 11.3 summarizes the findings reported by Bree et al[26] regarding the above issue.

THE TECHNIQUE

The scans are usually performed with a high-frequency transvaginal transducer probe. The higher the frequency, the higher the resolution. *The first prerequisite* of a detailed sonoembryologic study is a probe with a frequency of at least 6.5 MHz. *The second indispensable necessity* is the availability of equipment with "zooming" ability (or high-power magnification). As said in a previous chapter, because of the high resolution there is no loss of detail if high magnification is used. *The third requirement* is to "place" the embryo or the examined structure in the focus of the transducer crystal employed. If this is not known (from the specifications supplied by the manufacturer), the exact depth has to be determined by trial and error. The operator should push or pull the probe gently until the embryo appears absolutely clear and best "focused."

An *empty bladder* is a must if a very early pregnancy is scanned. A full bladder distorts the gestational sac and causes less-than-perfect imaging.

If an early gestation is scanned where the first appearance of embryonic heart-

TABLE 11.3 Discriminatory Zone for the Early Pregnancy

βhCG mIU/mL (IRP)	Chorionic Sac	Yolk Sac	Embryo and Heartbeat
<1000	±	0	0
1000–7200	+	±	±
7200–10,800	+	+	±
>10,800	+	+	+

After Bree et al.[26]

beats is the issue, a high scanning frame-rate mode should be selected. This may be an option on some ultrasound machines. The higher the scanning frame-rate, the easier it is to discern the tiny beating heart from the random flickering of echoes or the disturbing but obvious trophoblastic blood flow.

The use of high-quality *video recording equipment* with high-quality tapes played back on a high-definition TV screen not only enhances picture quality but decreases the scanning time. Structures or organs can be scrutinized off-line by the frame-by-frame feature of the equipment.

The chief disadvantage of the vaginal probe is caused by its lack of mobility in the vagina. It is not always possible to use all three conventional scanning planes to study all organs. Fortunately, the fetus changes its position within the amnion rapidly enough to "expose" all the desired positions to the examining probe. Patience is imperative; rescan after walking the patient for a short time; gentle attempts to use the abdominal hand to change the fetal position can help.

WHAT DOES TRANSVAGINAL SONOGRAPHY SEE IN EARLY PREGNANCY?

Fifth Week (4 weeks 0 days to 4 weeks 6 days)

The gestational or chorionic sac can usually be detected at 4 weeks 1–4 days from the LMP (or 15–18 days after ovulation). The average level of serum βhCG at this gestational age is 400–800 mIU/mL (IRP). At this time the gestational sac measures 4–5 mm and is usually detected within the "shining" endometrium, on one side or another of the cavity line. In one of these carefully dated pregnancies, the gestational sac was detected at 4 weeks 1 day and measured 4.2 mm. The serum β-hCG was found to be 820 mIU/mL (IRP) on the same day. The lowest serum βhCG level at which a gestational sac was detected was 420 mIU/mL (IRP); the gestational age was 4 weeks 1 day (Fig 11.6).

By the end of the fifth week, transvaginal sonography detected all intrauterine gestation in patients with well-documented dates. On the average, the transabdominal 3.5 MHz sector transducer probe detected the gestational sac for the first time about 1 week after the 6.5 MHz vaginal probe produced its first image of the same patient.

Sixth Week (5 weeks 0 days to 5 weeks 6 days)

Although diagnosis of pregnancy at this gestational age is possible, but difficult, by transabdominal ultrasound,[6] it becomes *feasible* and *relatively easy with transvaginal sonography* (Figs 11.1C and 11.6). An important characteristic of the early gestational sac is the double line, differentiating it from other intrauterine elements, such as uterine bleeding or the decidual reaction of a pseudogestational sac, described in ectopic pregnancies. These have a single echogenic rim and may suggest an erroneous diagnosis of intrauterine pregnancy.

The origin of the double contour or double ring at this gestational age may be attributed to the rapidly proliferating inner cytotrophoblast and outer syncytiotrophoblast. One or two weeks later, the hyperplastic endometrium is "invaded" by the trophoblast, thus creating the decidua basalis and chorion frondosum on one side and the decidua capsularis and parietalis (or vera) on the other side. All of these contribute to the later sonographic appearance of the previously described echo-dense ring around the true intrauterine gestational sac.

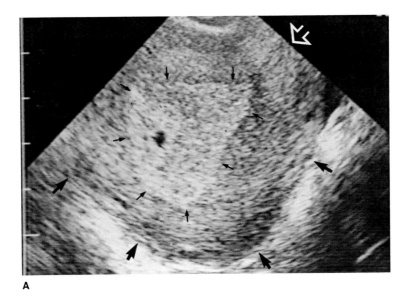

A

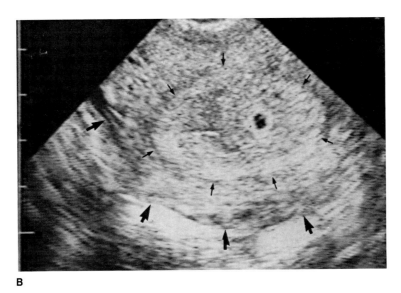

B

Figure 11.6 (**A**) Transvaginal sonographic picture of a 4-week 1-day intrauterine pregnancy. The serum βhCG level was 420 mIU/ml (IRP). In this longitudinal (vertical) section the cervix points to the right (open arrow). The endometrium is highlighted by small arrows, and the posterior aspect of the uterus, by large arrows. (**B**) Transverse section of the same uterus.

In contrast to this, Cadkin et al[34] propose that the decidua vera does not form part of the echo-dense ring immediately surrounding the true intrauterine gestational sac, because it is less echogenic than the chorionic villi, per se. Furthermore, in this eloquent article which is based on observations obtained by TAS, the authors feel that the inner ring is composed almost entirely of the hyperechoic sphere of chorionic villi surrounding the gestational sac fluid and that the surrounding, less echogenic area peripheral to this inner ring represents the surrounding decidual tissues. They feel that this is an important diagnostic point when trying to reliably diagnose an early intrauterine pregnancy.

The above theory seems to hold true even more if TVS is considered.

Indeed, the chorionic sac measuring 2–4 mm is embedded in the decidua on one side of the cavity line. This can easily be detected by "zooming in" on the chorionic sac on the image obtained by transabdominal scanning.

Two structures deserve to be mentioned:

1. The yolk sac becomes evident at 5 weeks 0 days and fills about one-third of the cross section of the gestational sac. At this time it measures 4 mm (Figs 11.1**D** and 11.1**E**). Its cross section in a normal pregnancy is always a circle because of its spherical shape. Transabdominal sonography will consistently detect the yolk sac from 6 weeks onward (Figs 11.5 and 11.7). The potential clinical importance of the yolk sac is discussed in Chapter 7 in conjunction with the missed abortion.
2. Lacunar structures of 2–3 mm are appreciated by transvaginal sonography on one side of the gestational sac (Fig 11.1**D**). They are located along a curved line forming about one-fourth of a circle. Flow was clearly seen in these structures when a high frame rate or color coded Doppler flow techniques are employed. The authors believe that these vascular elements are the forerunners of the maternal placental circulation. They are described in classic textbooks of embryology.[4,5]

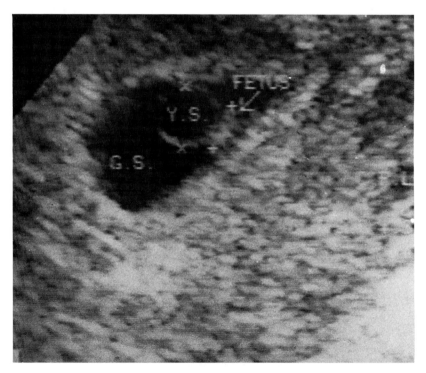

Figure 11.7 In this 7-week 2-day pregnancy, the gestational sac (G.S.), yolk sac (Y.S.), and fetal pole (fetus) are shown. The fetal pole measures 5 mm. Heartbeats are evident on real-time scanning.

As mentioned before briefly, embryonic heartbeats can be detected toward the end of the sixth week. They can be seen as early as 5 weeks and 5 to 6 days. If M-mode techniques are used, the heart rate and rhythm can be determined (Fig 11.5**B**). It should be stated that an experienced sonologist or sonographer using reliable equipment can detect embryonic heartbeats at 42 days.[10] However, the transvaginal route is less dependent on the thickness of the abdominal wall and experience of the operator.

Seventh Week (6 weeks 0 days to 6 weeks 6 days)

A 15 mm cystic structure representing the gestational sac (Fig 11.5) is outlined with great precision by transvaginal sonography. The main "landmark" now is an echogenic fetal pole consisting of the 2 to 4 mm embryo adjacent to a cystic yolk sac. One should remember that the yolk sac is an extraembryonic structure. The amniotic membrane is the partition between the two (see Figs 11.4**A** and 11.8). Fetal heartbeats are seen from 6 menstrual weeks onward in all well-dated pregnancies (Fig 11.5**B**). The double contour of the trophoblast (chorion) and the decidua are now much more evident. The thickness of the trophoblast should be one-fifth to one-third of the diameter of the gestational sac, and must be included in the measurement of the sac.[6] Throughout the sixth and seventh weeks, the fetal pole becomes more evident and measurements are now available for dating purposes.[31] It would appear that tables and graphs of crown-rump lengths compiled from data obtained by transabdominal sonography may not be as accurate as believed, because they were obtained by the transabdominal approach with a transducer of relatively low resolution; thus, part of the yolk sac may have been included in the measurements. This confusion, or rather imprecision, is reflected in the recent literature.[31]

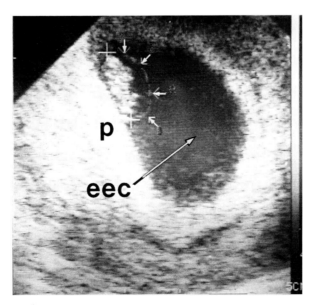

Figure 11.8 An 8-week 0-day pregnancy. CRL = 12 mm. Note the membranes (arrows), the placental site (p), and the large extraembryonic coelom (eec). The yolk sac is normal but visible in a different plane.

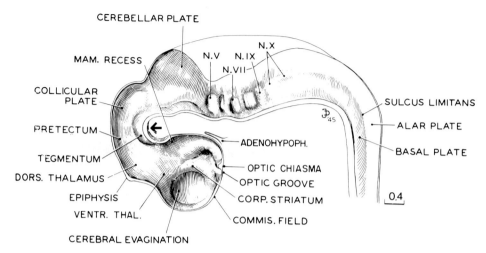

Figure 11.9 The line drawing represents the slightly convoluted arrangement of the ventricular system at 6 weeks and 5 days. The size of the embryo was 7–9 mm. Note: the only significant flexure is marked by the arrow. (Reprinted with permission O'Rahilly and Muller.)[47]

During the seventh week, the developing embryo measures 5–9 mm. Its central nervous system is a rather minimally convoluted system located in the sagittal midline (Fig 11.9). We tried to image the developing brain structures and its ventricular system. This is beyond the resolution of even the high-frequency probes at this gestational age (Fig 11.10**A**). However, in spite of the extremely curled up position of the embryo the coronal plane revealed for the first time the structure of the neural tube. This appeared as two parallel echo lines shown in Fig 11.10**B,C**.[30]

Eighth Week (7 weeks 0 days to 7 weeks 6 days)

The gestational sac has increased in size to 22 mm, and the embryo can be perceived clearly by the vaginal route. The trophoblastic rim is only one-fifth to one-fourth the thickness of the gestational sac. From the seventh week onward, measurements of the gestational sac are less informative but the crown-rump length measurements become meaningful. Because of the high resolution, a clear outline of the fetal pole enables a precise CRL measurement at this very early stage of the pregnancy. The membranes are starting to appear by TVS.

During the eighth week the anatomy of the embryo starts to "unfold," lending itself to the scrutiny of the high-resolution probes.

The Extraembryonic Coelom

This is still larger in volume than the amniotic sac. No matter what power/gain is used the extraembryonic space will always be somewhat more echogenic than the amniotic sac. The yolk sac is a prominent structure at this time.

Limbs

Mostly the lower limb buds can be seen. These are short but discernible. The upper limb buds usually blend into the echoes of the chest area since they are not

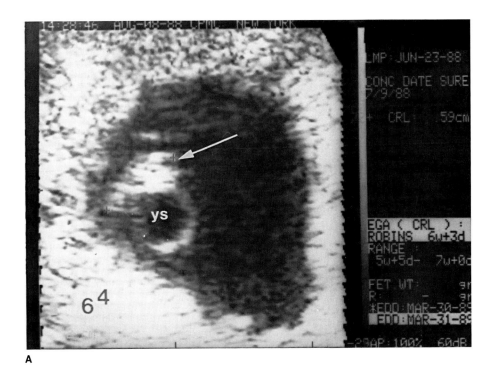

A

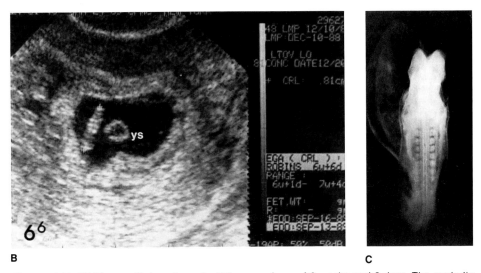

B   **C**

Figure 11.10 (**A**) The sagittal section of a 5.9 mm embryo of 6 weeks and 3 days. The cephalic pole is marked by an arrow. No brain structures were imaged. (**B**) A 6-week 6-day embryo is imaged. Its CRL is 8.1 mm. Note that on the coronal section the parallel lines of the neural tube are seen. (Reprinted with permission of C.V. Mosby Company. Mosby Year Book, Inc.)[27] (**C**) The neural tube of a 5-week 6-day specimen is shown for comparison. (Reprinted with permission O'Rahilly and Müller.)[46]

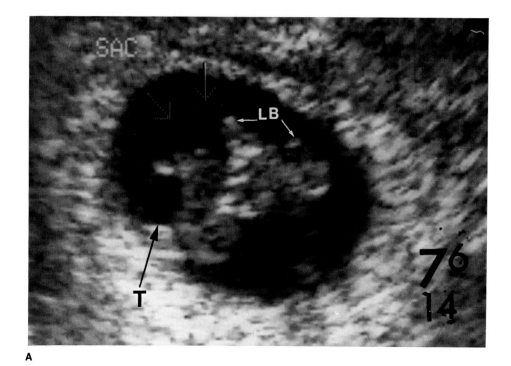

A

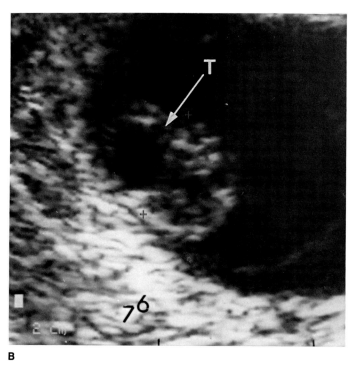

B

Figure 11.11 (**A**) A 7-week 6-day embryo is imaged in the coronal plane. Its CRL is 14 mm. Note the limb buds (LB) and the telencephalic vesicle (T). (**B**) On the axial image of the cephalic pole, the unpartitioned telencephalic vesicle is depicted.

yet prominent; however, toward the end of the eighth week their prominence is already evident (Fig 11.11**A**).[7]

The Heart

Its motion is clearly detectable within the central area of the curled up embryo. Using the M-mode, the heart rate and rhythm can be evaluated in addition to its small dimension. The heart rate at this time is between 112 and 136 beats/minute; the size is about 2 mm.[7]

The Posterior and Anterior Sagittal Contours

These cannot yet be evaluated.

The Central Nervous System (CNS)

The cerebellar plate develops a rostrally directed curve (pontine flexure) (Fig 11.12). It is still hard to depict structures by TVS. The unpartitioned telencephalic and mesencephalic vesicles can be seen (Fig 11.11). Close to the end of the eighth week, on a tangential (coronal) plane, the myelocele can be seen (Fig 11.13). For comparison, a line drawing of the ventricular system is presented (Fig 11.14).

The Genitalia

At the end of week 8 and on the coronal plane a small protrusion can be observed. This of course is the tail section of the spine which at this time is longer than the lower limb buds protruding caudally, creating the false impression of the genital tubercle which in reality is 1–2 mm above it on the ventral side.[35]

In Fig 11.15 a concise recapitulation of the more important structures is presented.

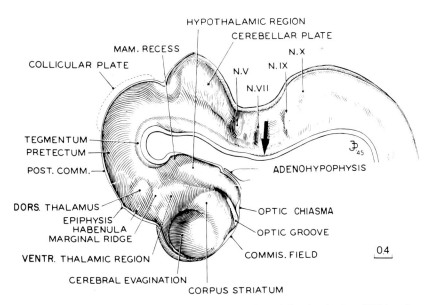

Figure 11.12 This drawing represents the sagittal section of the developing CNS in a 7-week 2-day, 11–14 mm embryo. Note that cerebellar plate develops a pontine flexure marked by the black arrow. (Reprinted by permission O'Rahilly and Muller.)

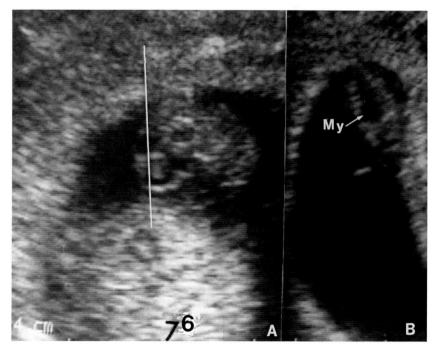

Figure 11.13 (A) Midsagittal section of a 7-week 6-day embryo. The white line depicts the coronal plane through which image **(B)** was obtained. The sagittal and the coronal plane of the ventricular system are clearly imaged. The funneling into the spinal cord of the myelocele is seen on the coronal plane. My = Myelocele.

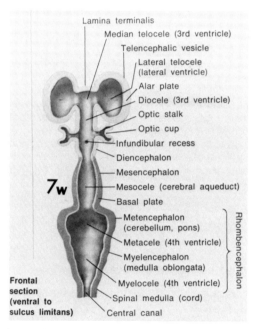

Figure 11.14 Frontal (coronal) section of the ventricular system at 7 completed menstrual weeks. The depicted anatomical structures follow a convoluted path which is evident only if it is looked at from the sagittal plane. This sagittal depiction is evident in Figure 11.25**A**. (Reprinted by permission from Clinical Symposia, Ciba. Illustration by F. Netter.)[47]

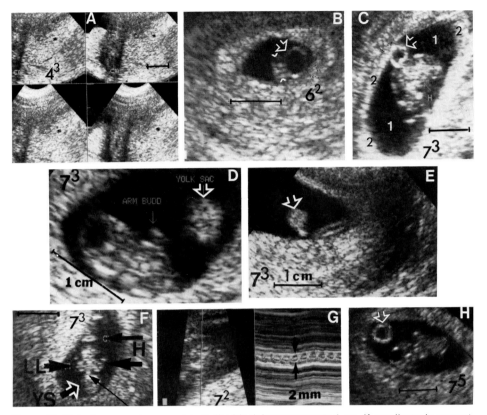

Figure 11.15 In the seven images shown, the black bar represents 1 cm. If a yolk sac is present, it is marked by an open arrow. Gestational ages are expressed in weeks and days and are indicated on each picture. (**A**) Gestational sac of 2 mm at 4 weeks and 3 days. (**B**) At 6 weeks and 2 days the fetal pole is seen to be attached tangentially to the lower left side of the yolk sac. Crown-rump length is 5 mm and is measured between the markers. (**C**) The embryo at 7 weeks and 3 days is curled up. The yolk sac is in the extraembryonic coelom (1) between the amnion closely surrounding the embryo and the chorion lining the uterine cavity (2). (**D**) A coronal section showing the still undivided ventricle in the head. (**E**) This coronal section passes through the spine represented by the parallel lines. (**F**) A coronal section through the lower body. LL = Lower limbs; H = part of the head; YS = yolk sac. The tail section is marked by a long, narrow arrow. The two limb buds protrude laterally and are marked by the two larger, symmetrically placed arrows. (**G**) The M-mode sweep clearly shows the heart size and rhythm. The rate can also be computed. (**H**) The still unpartitioned single ventricle in this embryo at 7 weeks and 5 days Crown-rump length is 15.3 mm; the yolk sac measures 4.8 mm. (Reprinted by permission of C.V. Mosby Company.)[17]

Ninth Week (8 weeks 0 days to 8 weeks 6 days)

The placenta becomes more demarcated and its relationship to the uterine cavity may be extrapolated (Fig 6.8). At this stage the embryonic structure is represented by distinct parts of the fetal body—the head, trunk, and limbs (Fig 11.16). The size of the fetal head surpasses the diameter of the yolk sac and it becomes a distinct anatomical structure. The amnion expands more and more at the expense of the extraembryonic coelom; flow is first seen in the tiny umbilical cord.

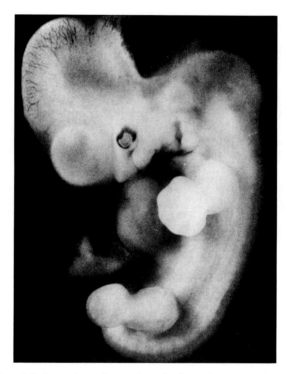

Figure 11.16 An 8-week 3-day embryonic specimen is shown (conceptual age 44 days). Note the appearance of the small cerebral hemispheres and the upper limb paddle, which is more developed than the lower limb bud. (Reprinted with permission O'Rahilly and Müller.)[46]

Limbs

At this stage, the upper limbs develop faster than the lower limbs (Fig 11.16).[35] The arms are seen on sonograms, not only as a result of their size and the position they assume at the side of the body, but due to their movements which start about the middle of the ninth week. Between days 36 and 44 (conceptual age) the ridges and grooves separating the fingers deepen, and toward the end of week 9 they are almost entirely formed. Their final form is reached only during the tenth week. In our material we were able to see clear upper and lower limbs and sometimes the cross-section of the hand.

The lower limb and its motion are seen but the neighboring cord interferes with a clear image.

The Heart

In addition to what was already described, there is no additional structural sonographic information available.

The Posterior and Anterior Sagittal Contours

As the embryo unfolds from its curled up position, the contour of the spine on the midsagittal picture becomes clearer (Figs 11.17, 11.18, and 11.19). This is significant because it enables diagnosing cystic nuchal structures or edematous changes of the neck and the entire silhouette of the back (see Chapter 13).

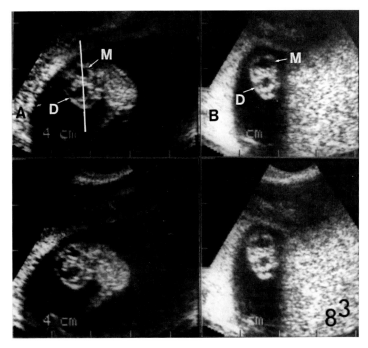

Figure 11.17 Two pairs of images show sagittal plane (**A**) and the axial plane (**B**). The diencephalon and metencephalon are marked by D and M respectively. The falx is not yet present.

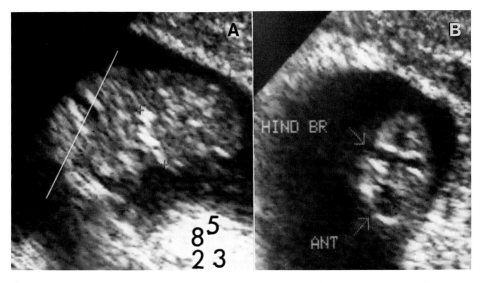

Figure 11.18 (**A**) An 8-week 5-day embryo is shown on the sagittal plane. The white line represents the section at which image **B** was obtained. (**B**) Semicoronal plane. Note the echogenic borders of the sulcus of the rhombencephalon (the hindbrain), as well as the sonolucent appearance of the diencephalon marked by ANT and an arrow.

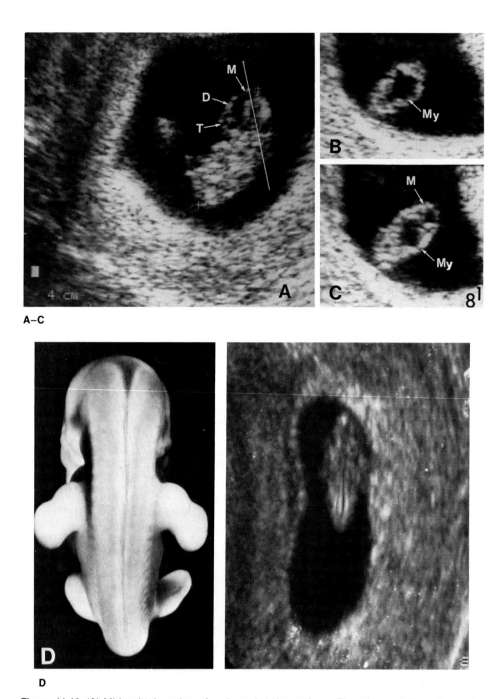

A–C

D

Figure 11.19 (**A**) Midsagittal section of an 8-week 1-day embryo. The telencephalon, diencephalon, and mesencephalon are marked by T, D, and M, respectively. The white line represents the planes at which section **B** showing the funneling of the myelencephalon (My) was obtained. Section **C** is slightly more anterior and shows a small portion of the mesencephalon. (**D**) The neural tube of a 7-week 5-day specimen (reprinted by permission from O'Rahilly and Müller[46]) and the coronal scan of an 8-week 0-day embryo are compared. Note the similar appearance of the spine.

The Physiologic Midgut Herniation

All the studied embryos demonstrated this structure,[21] which was first observed during this week.

The physiologic (ventral) midgut hernia is dealt with in textbooks of embryology.[4,5,35,36] It is a normal developmental finding between the eighth and twelfth weeks (gestational age). During this time the gut completes a 270° rotation "returning" into the abdominal cavity by the end of the twelfth week.

The sonographic description of this midgut herniation was performed by using transabdominal scanning.[38,39] The transvaginal sonographic image of the physiologic midgut herniation consists of a hyperechoic thickening of the cord just before its abdominal insertion (Fig 11.20).[7,19,21] The size of the cord insertion containing the midgut, in the study performed by us, was at least 1.5 times the size of the cord thickness.[21] This is, therefore, the suggested definition to diagnose the physiologic ventral hernia.

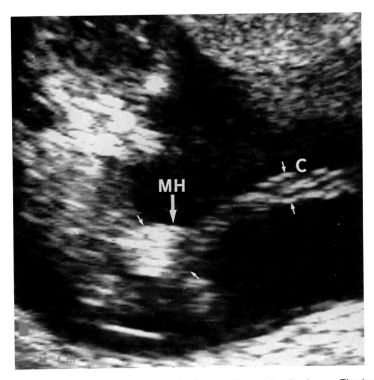

Figure 11.20 The anterior sagittal contour of a 9-week 6-day fetus is shown. The hyperechoic physiologic midgut hernia (MH) at the cord insertion is shown (C = cord). Note the larger size of the midgut hernia and then that of the cord (arrows). (By permission of C.V. Mosby Company.)[21]

Central Nervous System

The hallmark of the ninth week embryonic brain continues to be the lack of the falx cerebri which is reflected in the sonographic picture. (Fig 11.17**B**) The lack of the choroid plexus is also evident, at least in the first part of week 9.

The progressively convoluted arrangement of the brain ventricles—at this time still in the sagittal plane—without significant lateral protrusions is demonstrated on the line drawing 11.21. On the transvaginally obtained sagittal images, the forebrain vesicles (telencephalic, diencephalic, and metencephalic) were successfully imaged (Figs 11.17**A** and 11.19**A**). On the coronal plane the future aqueduct, fourth ventricle and its lower funneling into the spinal tract (mesocele, metacele, and myelocele, respectively) were imaged (Fig 11.19**C** and **D**).[30] The brain structures mentioned are part of larger sections, or cavities, called mesencephalon, metencephalon and myelencephalon.

Both on the sagittal and the axial planes the cavity of the future hind brain (rhombencephalon) can be imaged (Fig 11.18**A** and **B**).

Genitalia

The coccygeal region is still more prominent than the lower limb buds (Fig. 11.22**A** and **B**) and the genital tubercle. Therefore, imaging this relatively hidden area during the ninth week with current technology is presently impossible.

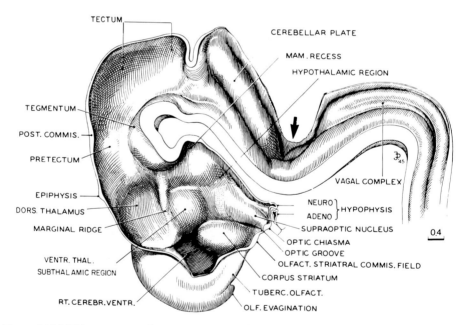

Figure 11.21 This represents the reconstruction of the right embryonal brain at 8 weeks and 3 days, at a CRL of 13–17 mm. Note the developing right cerebral ventricle, the tectum, which covers the mesencephalic vesicle, and the cerebellar plate, which is part of the metencephalon. The roof of the fourth ventricle is marked by a solid arrow, which also shows the direction of the pontine flexure. (Reprinted with permission O'Rahilly and Müller.)[46]

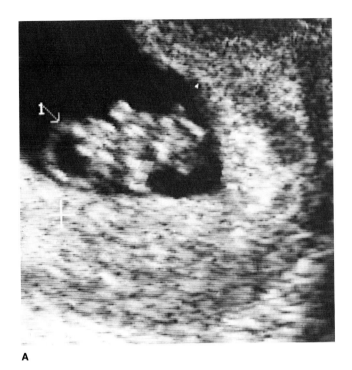

A

B

Figure 11.22 (**A**) At 8 weeks 2 days, one single ventricle is visible in the head (1). The limb buds are prominent. (**B**) The lower part of the same fetus is magnified. The lower limb buds are marked by open arrows. The sacrococcygeal region (white arrow) is still prominent at this gestational age.

Tenth Week (9 weeks 0 days to 9 weeks 6 days)

During this week the yolk sac is "pushed" aside by the continuously enlarging amniotic sac. This process involving the yolk sac continues into the twelfth and thirteenth weeks at which time it is almost absorbed and incorporated into the umbilical cord.

Imaging the fetus by TVS during this week becomes increasingly informative and clinically meaningful. The contours of the fetus created by the mounting amniotic fluid volume are clear. Early first trimester biometry is now feasible.[31] The biparietal diameter, and the head and abdominal circumferences can be measured.

From an anatomical standpoint, imaging by TVS in the tenth week is a turning point. A relative abundance of structures can be depicted by a higher frequency probe. Coincidentally, now the "embryo" suddenly changes its name to "fetus."

The Limbs

The upper and lower limbs have now undergone a 90° "torsion" around their longitudinal axes, but in opposite directions. The elbows point caudally and the knees cranially.[37] Almost the entire length of the upper and lower limbs can now be seen (Fig 11.23A).[2,7] The toes form during the eighth and ninth weeks and by ten weeks they are fully developed.[35,37] In fact, they can be detected consistently after this time.

Imaging the upper limbs is somewhat easier. The arms stand away from the body; therefore, their imaging is more successful. During the tenth week the forearm and fingers can be detected in more than 25% but not in all the fetuses studied[2,29] (Table 11.4; see further discussion on p. 304.) Sporadically (less than 25% of the cases), the hand can be imaged. The cross section of the fingers (or metacarpals) can be seen (Fig 11.23B).

The active movements of the limbs can easily be appreciated during this gestational week.

TABLE 11.4 Evaluation of Structures From 9–14 Weeks

Weeks	n	Ant. & Post. Contours	Long Bones	Fingers	Face Palate	Foot Toes	4 chamb. view
9	17	+	F&H ± / T&R −	±	−	−	−
10	16	+	F&H ± / T&R −	±	±	−	−
11	17	+	+	±	±	±	−
12	15	+	+	+	+	±	±
13	14	+	+	+	+	+	±
14	18	+	+	+	+	+	+

− = Seen 25% or less
± = Seen > 25% but not in all
+ = Seen in all cases
F = femur
H = humerus
T = tibia
R = radius

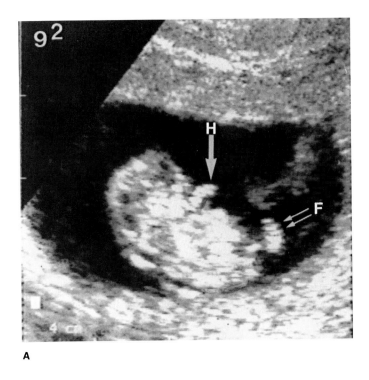

A

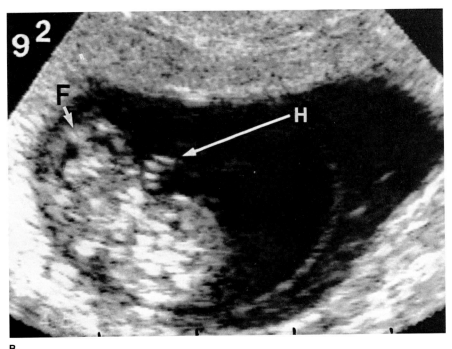

B

Figure 11.23 A 9-week 2-day fetus is depicted. (**A**) shows the hand (H) and feet; (**B**) shows the cross section of the hands marked by (H).

The Heart

At the end of the tenth week we believe the septum could be seen (Fig 11.37**F**).[2]

The Posterior and Anterior Sagittal Contours

The posterior contour (silhouette) becomes crisp and is easy to "interrogate" for irregularities. (Figs 11.24 and 11.25**C**) This is the first time cystic structures of this region can be observed. The abdominal wall displays the described physiologic midgut herniation (Fig 11.23).

The Central Nervous System

An abundance of structures can now be imaged. These crisp and clear images are the result of the developing fluid-filled quite tortuous ventricular system along a sagittal plane (Fig 11.25**A**, **B**, and **C**). However in the coronal planes, up to the tenth week, there are almost no bulging "side pouches" (the future lateral ventricles). During and after nine completed weeks the telencephalic vesicles (cerebral hemispheres) develop. Within these "hemispheres" the lateral ventricles occupy most of the space. During this week the falx develops alongside the choroid plexus.

The transvaginal sonographic "hallmark" of the tenth week is the falx and the echogenic choroid plexus. Their presence is obvious even with lower frequency or less than high-quality vaginal probes (Figs 11.26 and 11.27). If the falx and the choroid plexus are present, the pregnancy is at least 9 weeks.[19] Because of the increasing size of the fetus, beginning with the ninth week, more than one sagittal or coronal scanning plane can be obtained.

On the serial *coronal* sections, the structures to be mentioned are the *facial bones* (orbits, maxilla, and mandible) shown in Fig 11.28, the *falx,* and the *choroid plexus* (Figs 11.26 and 11.27**A**). The sonolucent ventricular system and the upper spinal canal are depicted as the coronal sections progress toward the back (Fig 11.27**B,C**).

Three *sagittal* sections are feasible. *The midsagittal* depicts the tortuous ventricular system. The rostral telencephalic vesicle leads into the wide diencephalon, then, turning almost 180° around, follows the cephalic flexure. The cephalic flexure is a prominent echogenic landmark structure that protrudes into the ventricular system as a peninsula between the dicencephalon and the metencephalon (Fig 11.25**A–C**). Caudally, the metencephalon bends posteriorly, forming the roof of the fourth ventricle and the rhombencephalon (hindbrain), leading into the last wide space, ie, the myelencephalon (the future medulla oblongata). From this point the ventricular system narrows and forms the spine (Figs 11.18, 11.25**A**, 11.26**C**, and 11.27).

At times, a true or partial axial section through the head is obtained (Fig 11.24**A,B**) enabling a more detailed scrutiny of the developing brain.

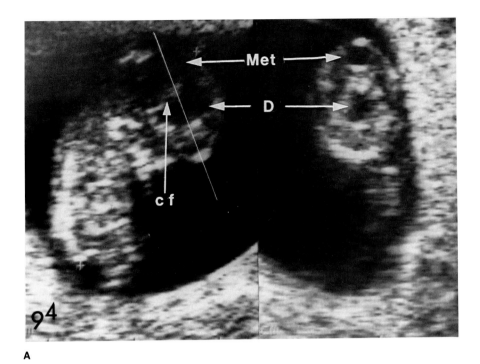

A

B

Figure 11.24 (**A**) Sagittal and axial section of the brain of a 9-week 4-day fetus. The metencephalon (Met), the diencephalon (D), and the cephalic flexure (cf), marked by arrow, are seen. (**B**) The sagittal section and a different, more coronal, section of the same embryo is shown.

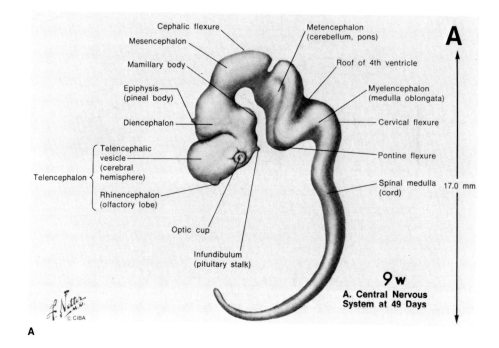

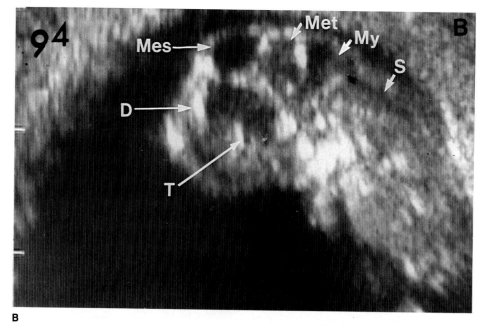

Figure 11.25 (A) Schematic presentation of the CNS at 9 weeks. (By permission Clinical Symposia, CIBA.) **(B)** The ventricular system of a 9-week 4-day fetus is shown through the midsagittal plane. **(C)** For easier identification, the ink drawing outlines the ventricular system. T = telencephalon; D = diencephalon; Mes = mesencephalon; Met = metencephalon; My = myelencephalon; S = spine.

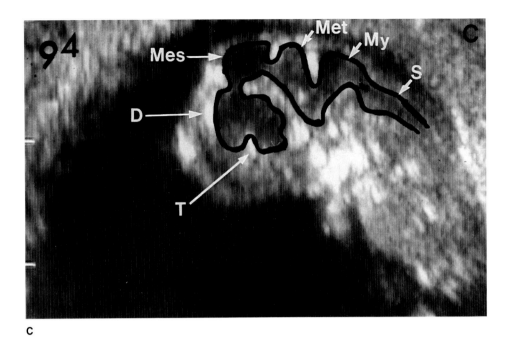

C

Figure 11.25 (*continued*)

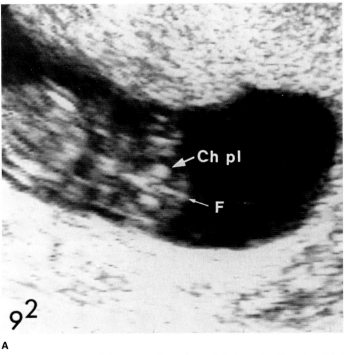

A

Figure 11.26 Coronal sections of fetuses at 9 weeks and 2 days. (**A**) The choroid plexus (Ch pl) and the falx (F) are shown. (*continued*)

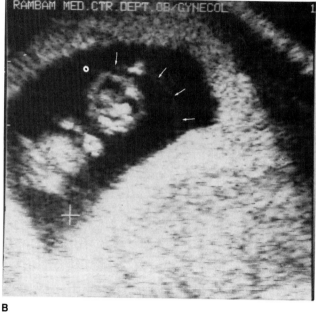

B

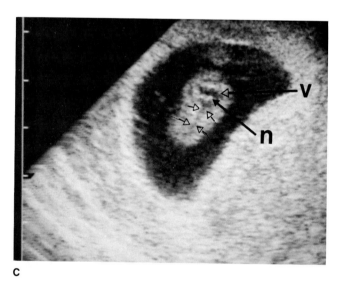

C

Figure 11.26 (*continued*) (**B**) The ventricles and the partition into two hemispheres are visible. The left and the right choroid plexus are well delineated in the ventricles. Above the head a small segment of the yolk sac and the thin amnion are imaged (small arrows). The extraembryonic coelom (eec) is still extant at this age. (**C**) This coronal section of the fetal body crosses the fetal head and the spinal canal (pairs of small arrows); n = two minute protuberances into the ventricle (v), which may represent some of the midbrain nuclei.

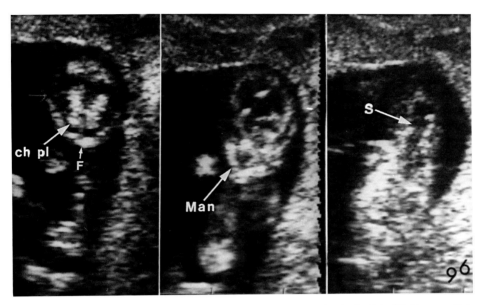

Figure 11.27 Serial coronal sections show the choroid plexus (ch pl), the falx (F), the mandible (Man), and the spine (S) in this 9-week 6-day fetus.

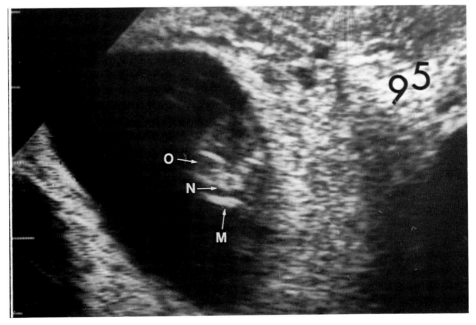

Figure 11.28 A 9-week 5-day fetus is shown. The facial structure of a 9-week 5-day fetus is shown. O = orbit, N = nasal bones, and M = the tip of the mandible.

Eleventh Week (10 Weeks 0 Days to 10 Weeks 6 Days)

The amniotic cavity increases in size pushing the yolk sac more and more to the side in the shrinking extraembryonic coelom (Fig 11.29).

Limbs

Upper and lower limbs can be scanned partially or throughout their entire length (Figs 11.29 and 11.30**A**,**B**). The number of fingers can be counted (Figs 11.29, 11.31, and 11.32) and a cross section shows their arrangement along a curve (grip) as well as the opposing thumb, now evident for the first time (Fig 11.32).

Heart

The four-chamber view has not yet been seen by us at this gestational age.

Posterior and Anterior Sagittal Contours

These can be seen crisply and are of diagnostic quality. The physiologic midgut herniation is of a size that may mislead the uninitiated observer to falsely imply pathology (Fig 11.33). Just above this midgut hernia a perfect cross section of the upper abdomen is evident; measuring the abdominal circumference is feasible (Fig 11.34).

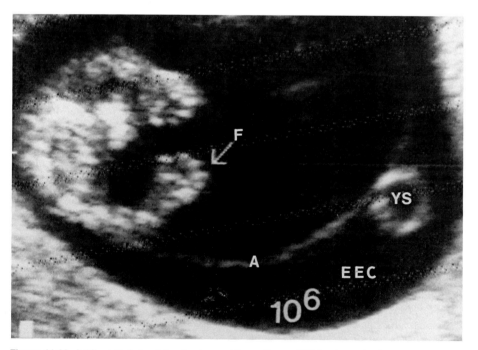

Figure 11.29 A 10-week 6-day fetus is shown. The yolk sac (YS) is shown in the extraembryonic coelom which is outside the amnion (A). Also represented is a cross-section of the fetal body at the level of the chest showing the entire length of the arms and the fingers (F).

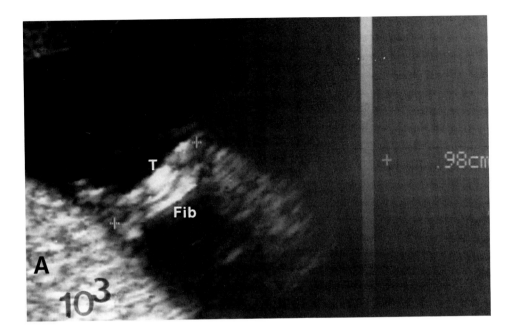

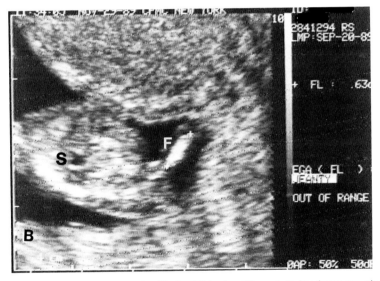

Figure 11.30 (**A**) The tibia (T) and the fibula (Fib) of a 10-week 3-day fetus are shown. The distance from the knee to the bottom of the foot is barely 1 cm. (**B**) The femur length of a 10-week 4-day embryo is 6.3 mm (F). The stomach (S) is also depicted.

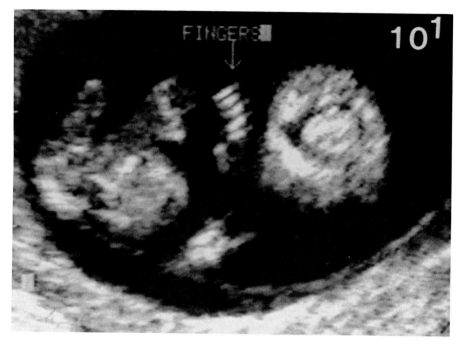

Figure 11.31 The fingers of a 10-week 1-day fetus are imaged. (Most probably a cross section.)

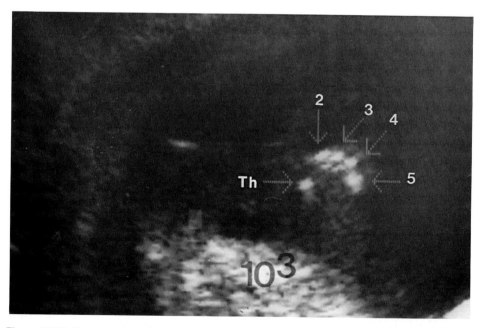

Figure 11.32 Cross section of the fingers at 10 weeks and 3 days. The opposing thumb (Th) is shown.

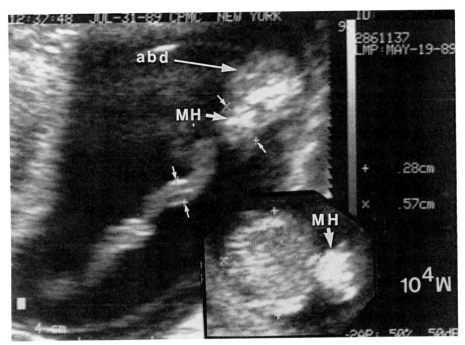

Figure 11.33 Both cross-sectional images of the fetal abdomen at 10 weeks and 4 days show the midgut herniation (MH). The approach of the cord (C) is also depicted. The measurement of the cord is 2.8 mm and the midgut hernia measures 5.7 mm.

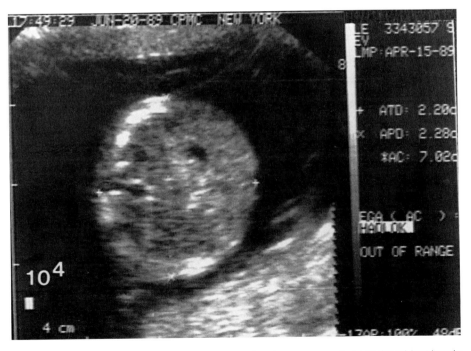

Figure 11.34 At 10 weeks and 4 days, the cross-sectional measurement above the midgut herniation of the fetal abdomen is visible. The abdominal circumference is 7 cm.

Central Nervous System

This can now be better defined. The ventricular system is outlined on almost all planes. The fourth ventricle and its funneling into the spine is shown in Fig 11.35. The third ventricle is still a sonolucent structure at this time.

The Face

Facial structures look appealing to the sonographer and the images can be used clinically. However, one must remember that the palate starts the process of fusion at 10–11 weeks and is completed at 13 weeks.[35]

This incomplete fusion accounts for the tiny midline gap of the palate on the coronal plane (Fig 11.36). The mandible is seen at this age.[7]

The Genitalia

The genitalia are not yet seen at this stage; the final phenotypic appearance is due only after the thirteenth week.[35]

A recapitulation of the major structural hallmarks of the tenth and eleventh weeks are shown in Fig 11.37.[7]

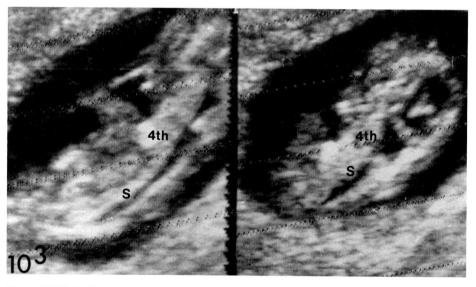

Figure 11.35 At 10 weeks and 3 days a semicoronal section shows the fourth ventricle and its funneling into the spine (S). (Reprinted with permission: Mosby Year Book, Inc.)[30]

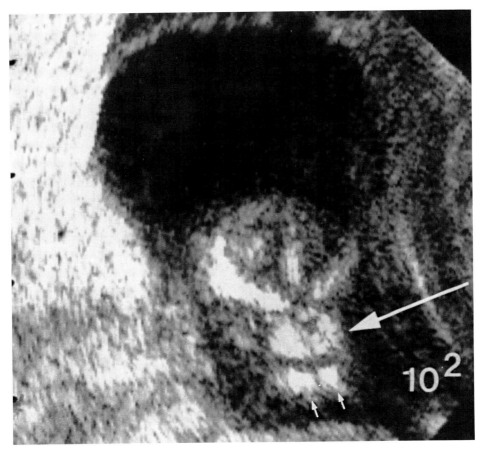

Figure 11.36 The coronal section of the face is shown. Two small arrows mark the cross sections of the mandible. The palate is marked by a larger arrow. Note that at this time, the midline is not yet completely closed. (With permission of C.V. Mosby Company. Mosby Year Book, Inc.)[27]

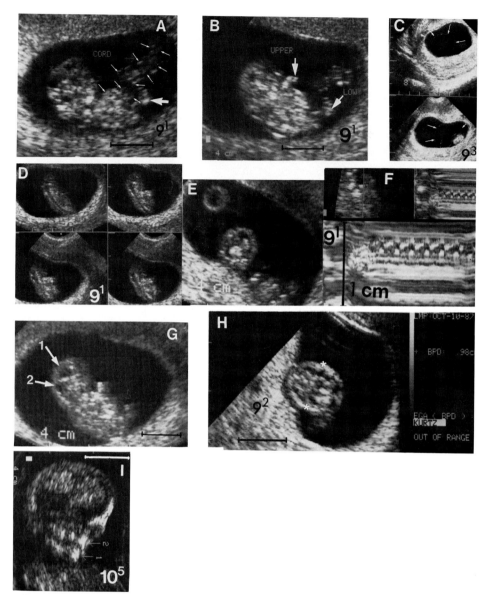

Figure 11.37 On these pictures the gestational ages are expressed in weeks and days; 1 cm is marked by a *solid bar* or the original grid. (**A**) The cord is outlined by *small arrows*. There is a change in the caliber of the cord before it reaches the abdomen. The foot is marked by a *larger arrow*. (**B**) The upper and lower limbs are seen sectioned by a parasagittal plane. (**C**) The extraembryonic coelom is still present between the amnion, marked by *small arrows*, and the chorion, lining the wall of the cavity. (**D**) Serial sections imaging the spine at 9 weeks and 1 day. (**E**) A coronal section through the head at 9 weeks and 1 day shows the complete partition of the ventricles and the echogenic choroid plexi. (**F**) At 9 weeks and 1 day the M-mode sweep reveals intracardiac echoes that may represent the septum. (**G**) On a sagittal plane through the head, two sonolucent structures are evident: the ventricle in the forebrain (1) and the hindbrain (2). (**H**) On a horizontal plane the biparietal dimension can be measured accurately. Conversion tables were not yet compiled for this range. (**I**) A sagittal plane through the forehead, orbita, and both the mandibula (1) and the maxilla (2). (Reprinted by permission of the C.V. Mosby Company).[7]

Twelfth Week (11 weeks 0 days to 11 weeks 6 days) and Thirteenth Week (12 weeks 0 days to 12 weeks 6 days)

The twelfth and thirteenth weeks will be considered together since there was no significant change from the twelfth to the thirteenth week in terms of structures seen.

The extraembryonic coelom becomes more and more obliterated. With some degree of patience during scanning the yolk sac can still be found.

Limbs

In spite of the fact that all long bones can be imaged and measured without difficulty, there are no standard tables available for their evaluation. Some of the examples for picturing the long bones are shown in Fig 11.38**A,B**.

The hands appear in their final development. The tiny metacarpal and phallangeal bones are sufficiently echogenic to enable their examination for clinical use since they are consistently scanned in these age groups (Fig 11.39). As to the feet, we *always* "invest" more time in obtaining a diagnostic quality image of the toes than we do for the fingers. The position of the foot in relationship to the tibia/fibula (to rule out clubfoot), and the shape of the plantar plane (to rule out rocker-bottom foot) are a realistic demand of TVS at this age. The imaging technique is similar to the one presented in Figure 11.30**A**.

The Heart

In a study performed at Columbia Presbyterian Medical Center, the four-chamber view was seen in more than 25%, but not in all, the examined fetuses (Table 11.4).[29] Its position, axis, and size in the fetal chest can be evaluated. Some of the larger fetal blood vessels can be imaged (Fig 11.52**B**).

The Anterior and Posterior Sagittal Contours

Studying the well-discerned *posterior contours,* the sonographer should always make sure the amnion is accurately and correctly identified not to create a false nuchal cyst by its close juxtaposition to the occipital area. If the posterior contour is scanned, a reverberation artifact should not appear as the amnion, implicating the real—but close by—amnion as a cystic hygroma (Fig 11.40). By enlarging the picture of the occipital and upper thoracic silhouette on the midsagittal image, the resolution permits a close scrutiny of the covering skin (Figs 11.41, 11.42). The posterior can conveniently be seen even if the back of the fetus is on the opposite side of the beam direction (Fig 11.43).

The anterior contour created by the chest and the abdominal wall undergoes a major change during these two weeks. The size of the physiologic midgut hernia diminishes, and by the end of the thirteenth week in well-dated fetuses it retracts into the abdominal cavity (Fig 11.43). Sometimes this retraction of the gut occurs somewhat earlier.

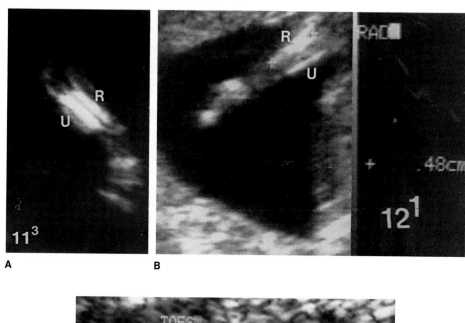

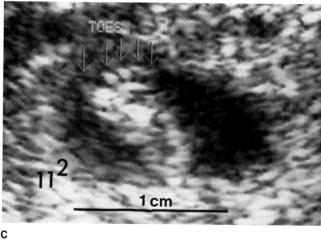

Figure 11.38 The radius (R) and ulna (U) of an 11-week 3-day (**A**) and a 12-week 1-day fetus (**B**) are shown. The latter measures 4.8 mm. (**C**) The foot and the toes of a 22-week 3-day fetus.

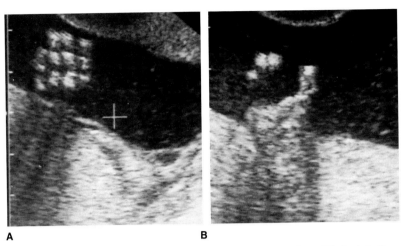

A   B

Figure 11.39 Hand of a 12-week 4-day fetus. The first scanning plane (**A**) depicts fingers 2–5; another plane (**B**) reveals the thumb.

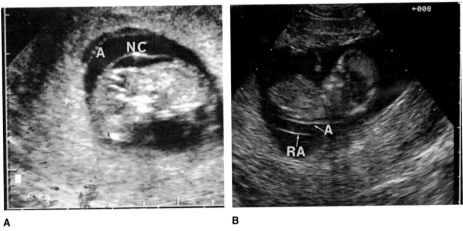

A   B

Figure 11.40 Pitfalls of studying the posterior sagittal contours are shown. (**A**) A true nuchal cyst (NC) is shown; however, the amnion (A) is clearly depicted separately. (**B**) If the fetus turns the back upside down, special care must be taken not to identify the amnion (A) or any artifacts such as reverberation artifacts (RA), as belonging to the fetal posterior contours.

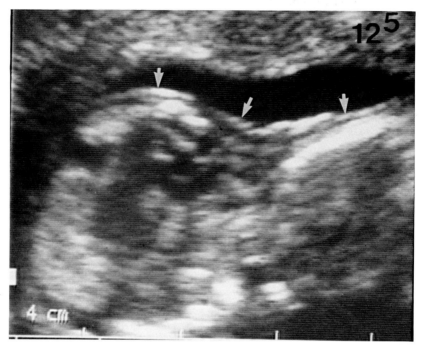

Figure 11.41 The nuchal area with the covering skin marked by arrows is shown in a 12-week 5-day fetus. Note the convulted sonolucent ventricular system.

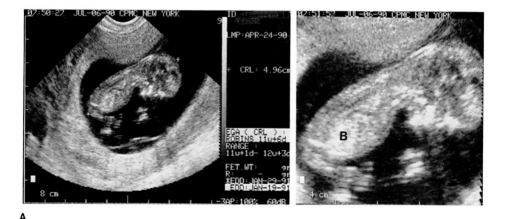

A

Figure 11.42 (**A**) The posterior and anterior sagittal contours of a fetus are imaged. Note that by enlarging the picture, no detail is lost. The fetal bowel (B) is clearly shown within the abdominal cavity. (**B**) Kidney (black arrows) with the renal pelvis (white arrow) at 11 weeks and 4 days.

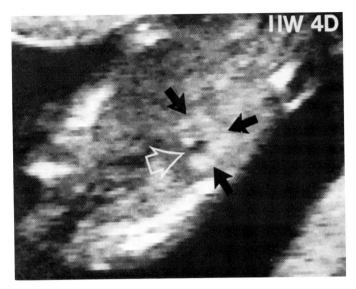

B

Figure 11.42 (*continued*)

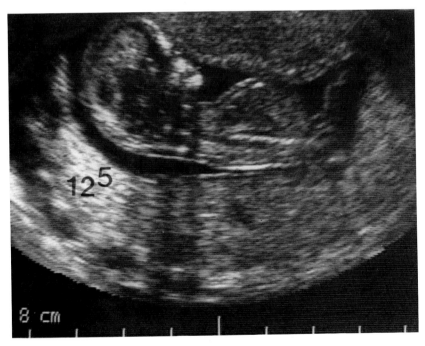

Figure 11.43 The posterior sagittal contour as well as the anterior chest wall contour are seen in this fetus. This image demonstrates that even a posterior location of the nuchal area can be evaluated with the transvaginal transducer. Fetal age was 12 weeks and 5 days.

The Central Nervous System

Scanning Planes.   During the twelfth and thirteenth weeks multiple sections can be achieved through each of the three planes: axial, coronal, and sagittal. However, one must remember that it is not always possible to obtain the classical and "pure" planes. In many instances the planes obtained may, for all practical reasons, be a combination of the conventional and classical planes.

The Sagittal Plane.   The "precise" *midsagittal plane* reveals the tortuous ventricular system (Fig 11.41). However, at this time we could not yet demonstrate the imaging of the corpus callosum. The parasagittal section reveals the lateral ventricle in which the hyperechoic choroid plexus is seen to fill the whole available space. The thalamus is also seen on this plane (Fig 11.44).

Figure 11.45 shows a slightly parasagittal section aimed at the longitudinal axis of the spinal canal. This structure seems to have an intact and normal appearance. The result of the combination of an axial and a semi-coronal plane (a backwards tilted axial section) is shown in Figure (11.46**A**). The latter combines the choroid plexus, usually seen on a "high" axial, and the cerebellum—fourth ventricle image of the posterior fossa seen on a "low" axial or a posterior-coronal plane.

The Axial Plane.   On a "high" axial plane (Fig 11.46**A**), the still large lateral ventricles can be seen portioned by the falx which sometimes appears multilayered. The hyperechoic choroid plexus fills the frontal horns almost completely. A "mid" axial section shows the thalami and the penduculi (Fig 11.46**B**). Sometimes the third ventricle may be seen. The "lower" axial section usually reveals the posterior fossa with the cerebellum, the cysterna magna, and, finally, the lowest plane reveals the foramen magnum (Fig 11.47). Several axial sections in the same fetus at 11 weeks and 3 days are presented in Fig 11.48.

One of our observations was that the actual brain tissue lining the ventricular system at these gestational ages is still extremely thin, almost impossible to detect, even with the high-resolution TVS.

The Coronal Plane.   Several coronal planes can be obtained. The most anterior one (Fig 11.49**B**) reveals the hyperechoic choroid plexus in the frontal horn, and the "steer head" appearance generated by the skull, orbits, and maxilla. This is the hallmark of an extremely rostral coronal section. The next section more occipitally "cuts" through the thalamus (Fig 11.49**A**). About midway to the occiput the main structure in the midline seems to be the still wide third ventricle depicted on Fig 11.50**C**. The cysterna magna (behind the cerebellum) is imaged on a still more occipital coronal section (Fig 11.50**B**). An almost tangentially apposed coronal section images the fine line of the spinal processes of the thoracic and cervical vertebral column (Fig 11.50**A**). This image is valuable to ascertain the integrity of the vertebral arch in the process of ruling out spina bifida or rachischisis.

The Genitalia

It is possible to image the perineal area of the fetus; however, the imaging of the external genitalia was not performed by us. This topic will be touched upon discussing the next gestational weeks.

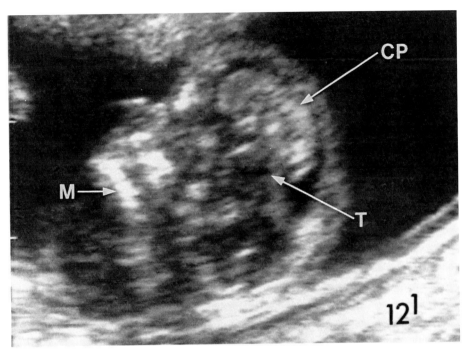

Figure 11.44 Note the mandible (M). The brain structures clearly seen here are the echogenic choroid plexus (CP) and the sonolucent appearance of the round thalamus (T). The facial contours can also be seen.

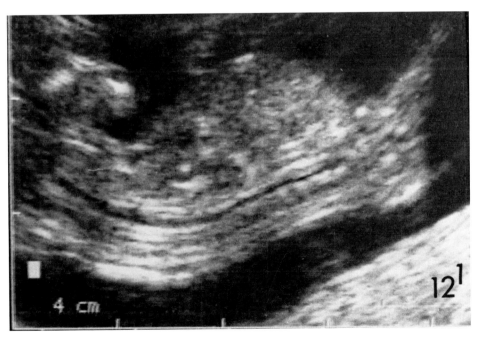

Figure 11.45 This is a slightly tilted parasagittal section along the longitudinal axis of the fetal spine in a 12-week 1-day fetus. Note the sonolucent normal-appearing spinal canal.

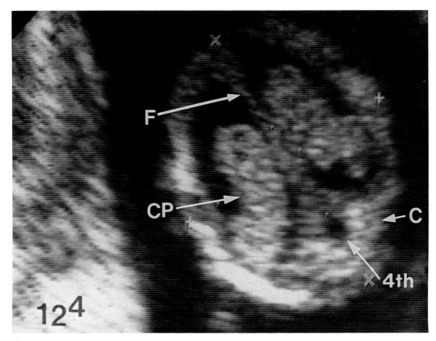

A

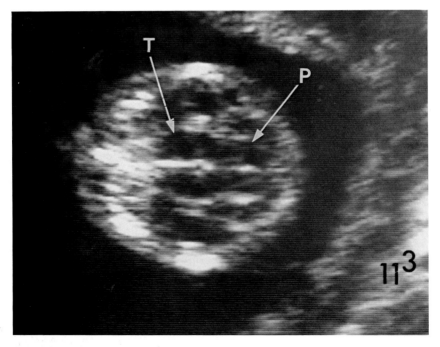

B

Figure 11.46 (**A**) The slightly backward tilted axial section of a 12-week 4-day fetus. Depicted are the falx (F), the choroid plexus which is typically hyperechoic (CP), and the structures of the posterior fossa, such as the cerebellum (C) and the fourth ventricle. (**B**) Mid-axial section at 11 weeks and 3 days. The thalami (T) and the pedunculi (P) are shown.

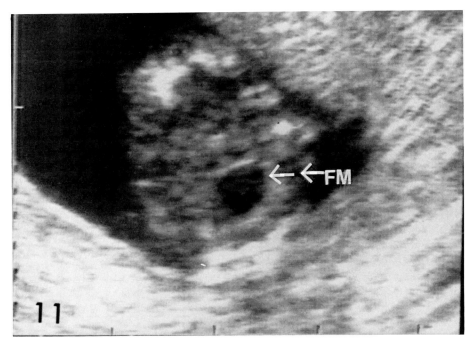

Figure 11.47 The lowest possible axial section showing the foramen magnum at 11 weeks.

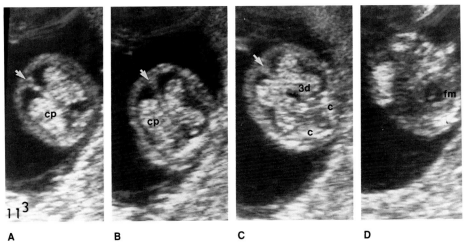

A   B   C   D

Figure 11.48 A complete series of axial sections are shown at 11 weeks and 3 days. (**A**) The highest and (**D**) the closest to the base of the skull. (**B**) and (**C**) in between. cp = choroid plexus, f = falx, c = cerebellum, fm = foramen magnum. (Reprinted with permission: Mosby Year Book Inc.)[30]

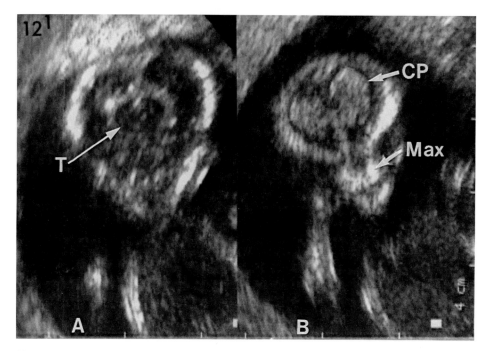

Figure 11.49 Serial coronal planes of the head and the body of an 11-week 5-day fetus. (**A**) The thalami (T). (**B**) The choroid plexus (CP), and the maxilla (M) (slightly more anterior section).

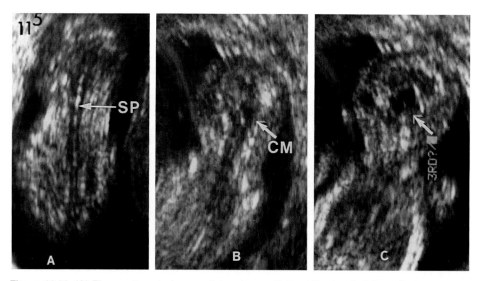

Figure 11.50 (**A**) The most posterior one, taken tangentially at the level of the spinal possesses (SP). (**B**) Depicts the cisterna magna (CM) and the upper portion of the neck. (**C**) Shows the third ventricle, which is still wide open at this gestational age.

TABLE 11.5 Evaluating Patients in Late First or Early Second Trimester Who Are at Risk for Fetal Kidney Abnormalities

	Weeks of Pregnancy		
	12 Weeks	13 Weeks	14 Weeks
Fetal Kidney	cm	cm	cm
Anteroposterior diameter			
Mean	0.40	0.53	0.56
SD	0.12	0.08	0.09
Transverse diameter			
Mean	0.40	0.52	0.59
SD	0.09	0.06	0.12
Longitudinal diameter			
Mean	0.61	0.83	0.92
SD	0.06	0.18	0.11
Other measurements			
Biparietal diameter			
Mean	1.89	2.27	1.65
SD	0.12	0.16	0.15
Crown-rump length			
Mean	5.35	6.30	7.12
SD	0.23	0.17	0.46

After Bronshtein et al.[45]

The Fetal Kidneys

The possibility of imaging the fetal kidneys and the urinary bladder was entertained by many. However, no published work was available until 1990.

The fetal kidneys reach their final position and form by 10–12 weeks (menstrual age). In the past it was possible to image the fetal kidney only later in pregnancy using the transabdominal route.[43,44] More recently, the renal size in the first trimester of pregnancy was evaluated in 50 low-risk pregnant patients resulting in normal deliveries.[45] Both kidneys were consistently identified at 12, 13, and 14 completed weeks. Table 11.5 illustrates the measurements of the kidneys and the corresponding BPD and CRL measurements. Figure 11.42**B** illustrates a very early detection of the fetal kidney and its renal pelvis at 11 weeks and 3 days.

Fourteenth Week (13 Weeks 0 Days to 13 Weeks 6 Days) and Fifteenth Week (14 Weeks 0 Days to 14 Weeks 6 Days)

As a rule, progressing along the gestation from the end of the first into the early second trimester, structures become successively larger; hence, the odds of their being imaged and the clarity of the image are improving.

The Extraembryonic Coelom

This is now almost completely obliterated by the adherence of the amnion to the chorion.

Limbs

Shape and measurements can be determined without significant obstacles. The fetal movements become so active that tape-recording the examination for slow playback and later scrutiny is imperative. The hand and the fingers can now be imaged only if multiple planes are used (Fig 11.51**A**). As opposed to the hand, the toes can be imaged on one plane since they are aligned in the same plane (Fig 11.51**B**).

The Heart

The four-chamber view is now of such quality as to enable conclusions that are clinically important (Fig 11.52). Normative evaluation of fetal heart measurements was attempted by Bronshtein et al. They tabulated measurements of the right and left heart chambers as well as the heart-to-chest size ratios from 11–17 weeks.[45] The heart-to-chest diameter ratio was almost constant from 11 to 17 weeks.

The Anterior and Posterior Contours

There is very little to add to the information already known regarding these contour projections. Their diagnostic value is highly reliable (Fig 11.53). The silhouette of the nuchal area, head, and face should be interrogated for their normal (Fig 11.54) or abnormal appearance.

The Face

The "workup" of the facial bones can be considered at the fourteenth and fifteenth weeks. The midsagittal contour is evident in Fig 11.54. The *orbits* and interorbital distances are depicted using several different scanning planes (Figs 11.55, 11.56, 11.57, and 11.59**A,B**). The ringlike structure of the *lens* becomes increasingly discrete. The *palate* can also be examined from different angles and at least two planes: the coronal and midsagittal (Figs 11.56 and 11.59**A,B**), but a slightly oblique plane—a combination of the above two—is also feasible (Fig 11.57). The *mandible* is visible on an axial scan (Fig 11.58).

The Central Nervous System

The increasing number of sections possible now, in almost all three conventional planes, makes the scanning of the brain plausible.

Coronal Planes.   Here all important brain structures such as the falx, eyes, thalami, cavum septi pellucidi, choroid plexi, superior sagittal sinus, cysterna magna, and cerebellum can be outlined (Figs 11.59**C,D** and 11.60).

Axial Planes.   These planes, particularly the highest one, show the trend of the relative regression of the choroid plexus into the antrum (of the lateral ventricle) from the rostral position it assumed in the frontal horn (Fig 11.61**A**). The thalamus and the peduncle of the brain stem, and the third ventricle (which is still present and visible at these ages) are imaged (Fig 11.61**B,C**). At the occipital pole of the axial image, the fourth ventricle and the cerebellum as well as the cysterna magna can be depicted (Fig 11.62).

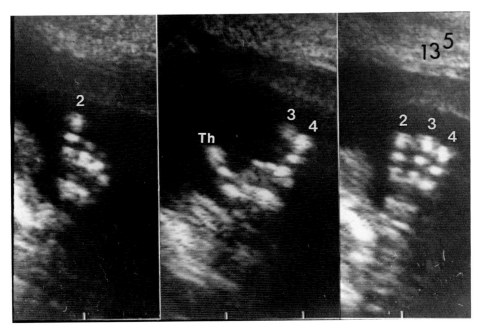

A

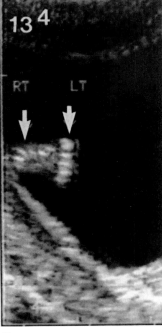

B

Figure 11.51 (**A**) The hand is imaged at 13 weeks and 5 days. Serial pictures and planes are necessary to depict all the bony structures of the hand. Because of the slightly semicircular grip-like position of the hand (Th = thumb), the fifth finger is not in the picture. (**B**) The toes are depicted on the cross section of both feet.

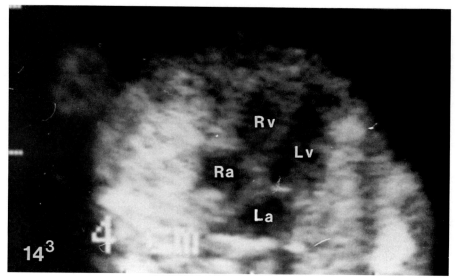

A

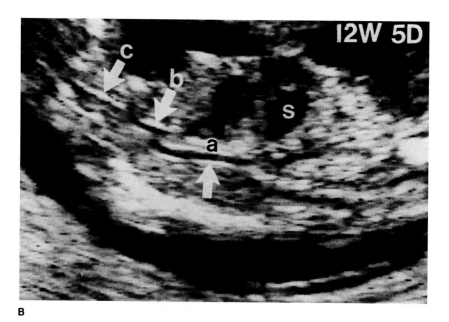

B

Figure 11.52 (A) The four-chamber view of the heart at 14 weeks and 3 days. The right and left atria and ventricles are marked respectively. **(B)** The larger blood vessels are imaged at 12 weeks and 5 days: the aorta (a), brachiocephalic artery (b), and the common carotid artery (c). S = stomach.

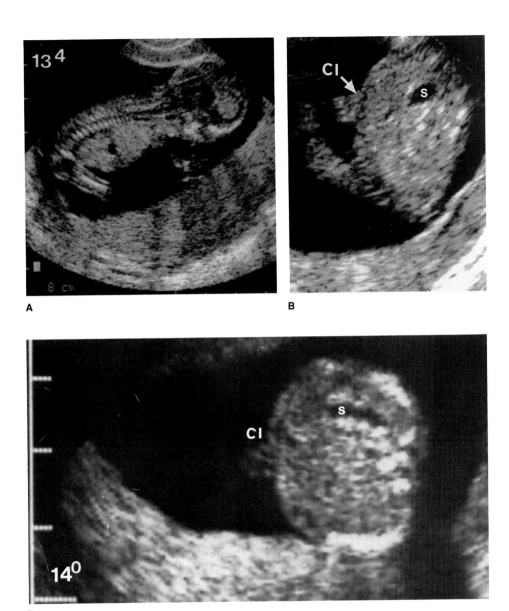

Figure 11.53 The posterior contours (**A**), and the anterior midsagittal contour (**B**) are shown, in a 13-week 4-day fetus. The cord insertion is marked (CI). The stomach (s) is also seen. A "perfect" abdominal cross section is shown in **C**.

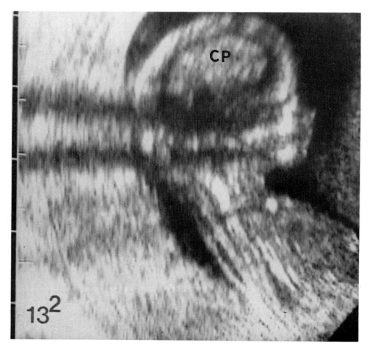

Figure 11.54 The contours of the upper part of the body are seen at 13 weeks and 2 days. CP = choroid plexus.

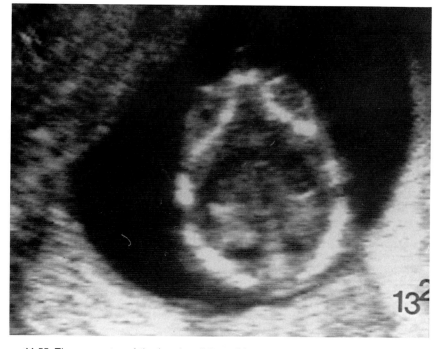

Figure 11.55 The symmetry of the head and the orbits are imaged on this picture at 13 weeks and 2 days.

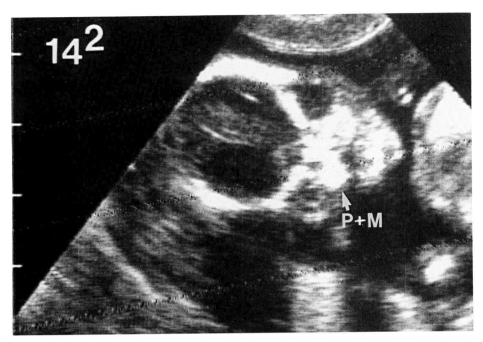

Figure 11.56 At 14 weeks and 2 days, the orbit, the arch of the palate, and the maxilla (P + M) and the tip of the mandible are shown on this coronal section.

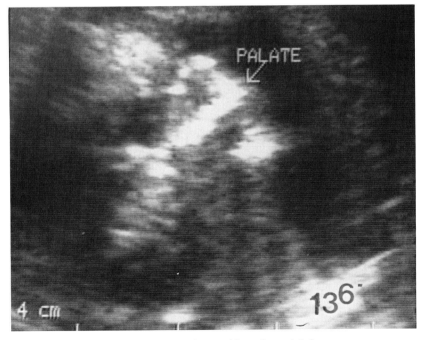

Figure 11.57 Parasagittal section of the palate at 13 weeks and 6 days.

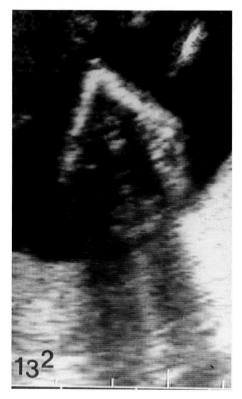

Figure 11.58 Horizontal section showing the mandible, throughout its lower branch, at 13 weeks and 2 days.

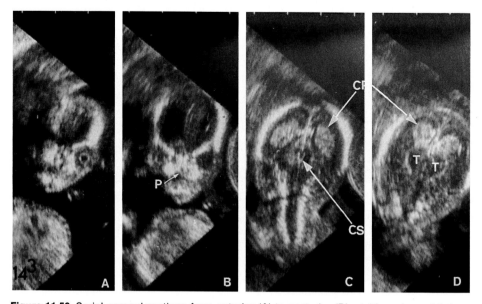

Figure 11.59 Serial coronal sections from anterior (**A**) to posterior (**D**), at 14 weeks and 3 days. (**B**) The palate is shown (P). (**C**) The choroid plexus (CP) and the cavum septi pellucidi (CSP) are evident. (**D**) The choroid plexus is shown to ride on top of the thalami (T).

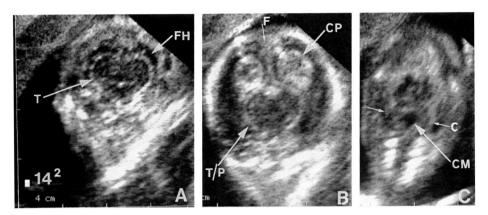

Figure 11.60 At 14 weeks and 2 days, serial coronal sections show the clear outline of the thalami (T) and the sonolucent frontal horn (FH), as well as the falx (F) and the choroid plexus (CP), and the thalami and pedunculi complex (T/P). The most posterior scanning plane (**C**) shows the cisterna magna (CM) and the cerebellum marked by two small arrows (C).

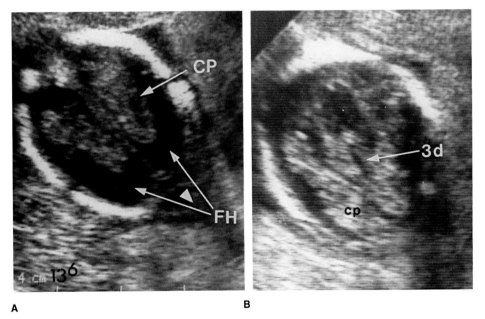

A   B

Figure 11.61 Three axial sections at 13 weeks and 6 days. (**A**) Shows a high section with the hyperechoic choroid plexus (CP) and the relatively free frontal horns (FH). The frontal direction is marked by an arrowhead. (**B**) Slightly below the previous one, showing the third ventricle and the hyperechogenic choroid plexus (cp).

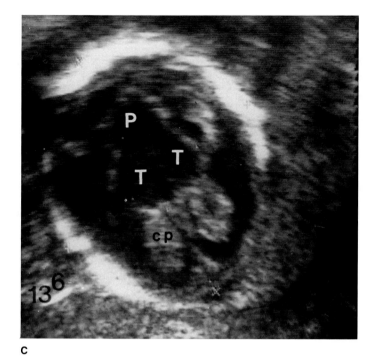

C

Figure 11.61 (*continued*). (**C**) A lower axial section, showing the choroid plexus (cp), the thalami (T), and the pedunculi (P).

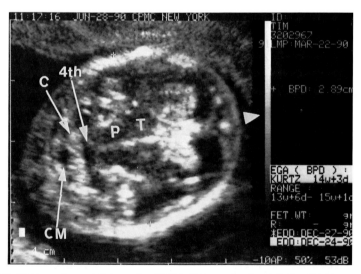

Figure 11.62 At 14 weeks and 2 days, the BPD is 2.9 cm, the frontal direction is marked by an arrowhead. In the posterior part of the axial section: the fourth ventricle, the cerebellum (C), and the cisterna magna (CM).

The Genitalia

During the fourteenth and fifteenth weeks the genitalia assume their final pheno-typic appearance.[35] Their transvaginal sonographic imaging can now be reliably used (Fig 11.63). In a recent study the clinical importance of imaging the fetal gender by TVS was discussed.[46] The prediction rate of fetal sex at 15 and 16 weeks by this group (n = 968) was 99.7% for males and 100% for females. A learning curve was evident: in the second year of the study (n = 781) the accuracy was 100% for both genders. This rate of accuracy is not paralleled by any of the previously published material.[47,48]

Other Organs

The identification of the normal lungs, stomach, bowel, liver, and kidneys presents no real challenge for the experienced sonographer or sonologist.

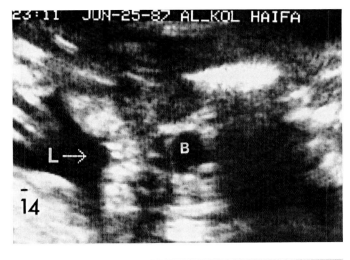

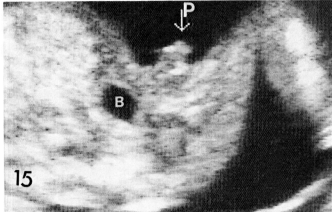

Figure 11.63 The upper image shows the labia majora (L) at 14 weeks; whereas the lower picture shows the phallus (P), and the bladder (B) at 15 weeks. (Courtesy of Dr. M. Bronshtein, Haifa, Israel.)

Sixteenth Week (15 Weeks 0 Days to 15 Weeks 6 Days)

This may be another turning point in sonoembryology. The reasons for this are: (1) By the sixteenth week, almost all organs usually interrogated by ultrasonography can *consistently* be imaged for malformation workup (see Table 11.4). (2) The size of the entire fetus is still within the reach of a 5.0 MHz transvaginal probe. (3) It is the last opportunity to effectively use the higher frequency (6.5 to 7.5 MHz) probes for those organs which at any given time are within the short focal range of these probes.

For the above-mentioned reasons week sixteen should be considered an ideal time to perform a detailed malformation workup of the fetus.

The question of malformation workup is addressed in a separate chapter (Chapter 13). However, before a detailed malformation workup is undertaken, one basic question has to be answered: What is the gestational age at which all, or the overwhelming majority of organs, systems, and structures can be consistently imaged?

To answer this practical question we undertook a study to look at selected structures from the ninth week to the fifteenth week of gestation.[29] Ninety-seven low-risk patients were scanned once each. The structures scanned were the posterior and anterior midsagittal body contours, long bones (femur, humerus, tibia/ fibula, radius/ulna), hand and fingers, face and palate, feet and toes, and the four-chamber view of the heart. The structures were evaluated as to the percentage of their detection within the peer group of the same gestational age.

Successful imaging of the structures during each gestational age was evaluated by labeling the structure as: (1) *negative detection,* if it was detected in 25% or less of the fetuses; (2) *occasional detection,* if it was detected in more than 25% but not in all; and (3) *consistent detection,* if it was in all examined fetuses of the same menstrual age.

The *contours* could be seen at 9 weeks (completed) and above, *long bones* at 10–11 weeks, *fingers* at 11 weeks, *face and palate* at 12 weeks, *feet and toes* at 13 weeks, and, finally, the *four-chamber view* at 14 completed weeks. Table 11.4 illustrates the results.

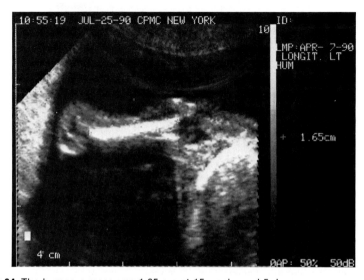

Figure 11.64 The humerus measures 1.65 cm at 15 weeks and 5 days.

The results of this study indicate that: (1) a *comprehensive malformation workup* of the fetus, looking at the studied structures, can be undertaken from week 15 and on; (2) one can look at *selected structures* at different but earlier gestational ages; and (3) if a *routine malformation workup* is planned, using only one scan at the earliest possible gestational age, this should not be offered before the fifteenth week.

A similar study was conducted to establish the evaluation of the developing a central nervous system.[30] Since the gestational ages at which brain structures could be imaged are different, the study concluded that a central nervous system malformation workup should be done at a time at which landmark structures can consistently be imaged. This gestational age is probably at or shortly after the sixteenth menstrual week. It should be emphasized that many major brain structures can be reliably imaged earlier; therefore, in experienced hands the brain can be scanned at even younger ages.

Following this, a series of images are presented to illustrate the performance of TVS in imaging the fetus during the sixteenth week. The humerus is depicted in Fig 11.64, the posterior and the anterior contours, the lung, the diaphragm, and liver are seen in Figs 11.65, 11.66, and 11.67. Figure 11.68 is a sonogram of the

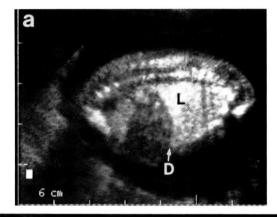

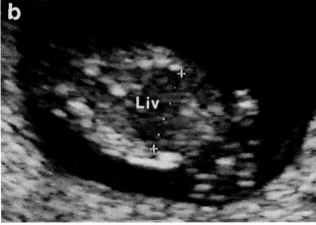

Figure 11.65 (A) The slightly echogenic lung (L) is shown. The outline of the diaphragm is clear (D). **(B)** Coronal plane. The semicircular diaphragm is above (left side of picture) the liver (Liv).

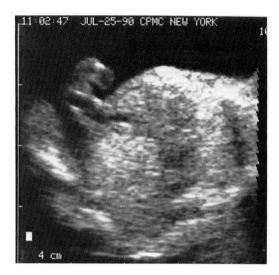

Figure 11.66 At 15 weeks and 5 days, the insertion of the cord into the anterior abdominal wall is shown.

four-chamber view and the three vessel *cord*. The examination of the *palate* in three successive coronal planes is seen in Fig 11.69**A–C**. The *lips* and the *nostrils* are evident in Fig 11.69**D,E**. A series of *axial* sections of the *brain* demonstrate the major structures imaged across multiple successive parallel planes (Figs 11.70**A–F** and 11.71). *Coronal* sections and a *parasagittal* section of the same fetal head are captured in Figs 11.72 and 11.73.

Sagittal and coronal sections of the entire spine are demonstrated in Fig 11.74. A meticulous, cross-sectional scanning of the spine (vertebra-after-vertebra) should also be performed. The bladder and bowel are shown in Fig 11.75.

Other organs (not illustrated here) to include in the scanning routine at this gestational age are the stomach, gall bladder, kidneys, and, if needed, the genitalia.

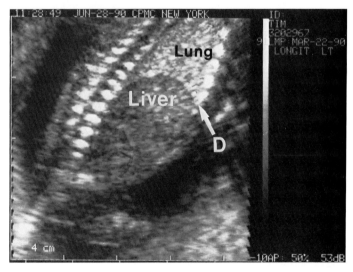

Figure 11.67 At 14.5 weeks, the lung–liver interface is depicted. D = diaphragm.

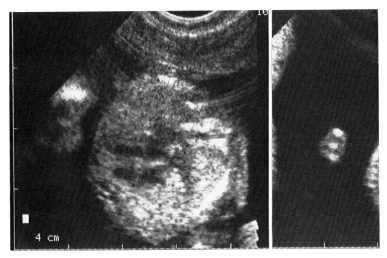

Figure 11.68 The four-chamber view is imaged on the left; the thre vessel cord on the right.

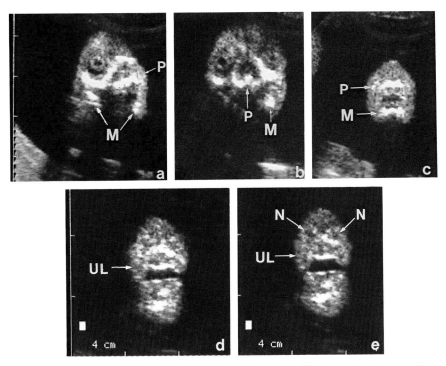

Figure 11.69 15 weeks and 5 days. (**A–C**) Workup of the palate (P). The rami of the mandible are also shown (M). On panel (**C**) the tip of the mandible is imaged. (**D–E**) The workup of nostrils and the upper and lower lips. N = nostrils, UL = upper lips.

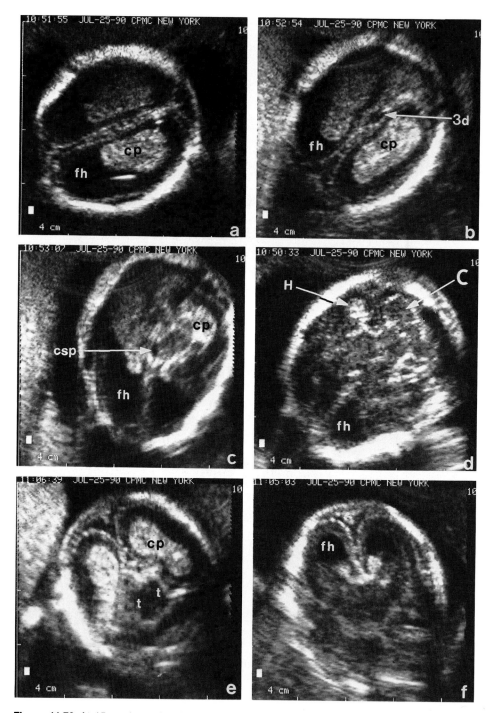

Figure 11.70 At 15 weeks and 5 days, six axial sections are shown. Of these, (**E**) and (**F**) are slightly posteriorly tilted axial planes. Structures seen here among others are multilayered falx (F), the frontal horns (fh), the third ventricle, the cavum septi delucidi (csd), the choroid plexus (cp), the cerebellum (C), the hippocampus (H), and the thalami (t).

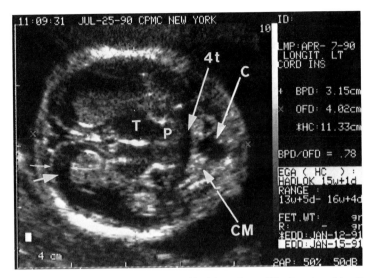

Figure 11.71 At 15 weeks and 5 days, horizontal/axial section of the head enables the measurement of the head circumference, as well as imaging of various brain structures, such as the thalami (T), fourth ventricle, the cerebellum (C), and the cisterna magna (CM). The thickness of the brain is also evident at the frontal horn, marked by a white arrow.

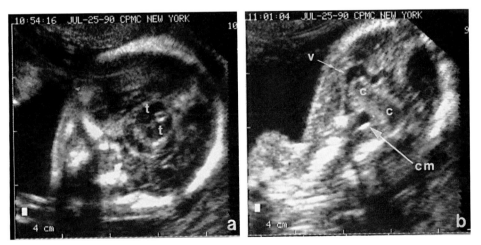

Figure 11.72 Two coronal sections are shown on the fetus imaged in Fig 11.70. (**A**) Depicts the section crossing the thalami (t). (**B**) Is a slightly more posterior section, clearly showing the cerebellum (c) below which the cisterna magna (cm) is seen. The sonolucent structure that demarcates the upper pole of the cerebellum is thought to be a venous structure (v).

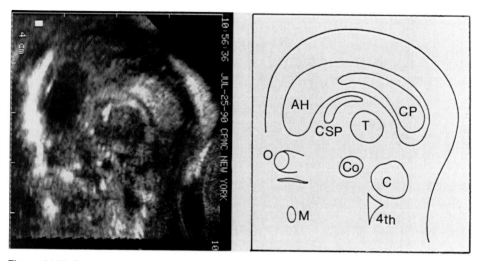

Figure 11.73 Parasagittal section of the fetus imaged in Figs 11.70 and 11.72. The ink drawing outlines the main structures: AH = anterior horn, CP = choroid plexus, CSP = cavum septi pellucidi, T = thalamus, Co = cochlea, C = cerebellum, M = mandible, O = orbits, 4th = ventricle.

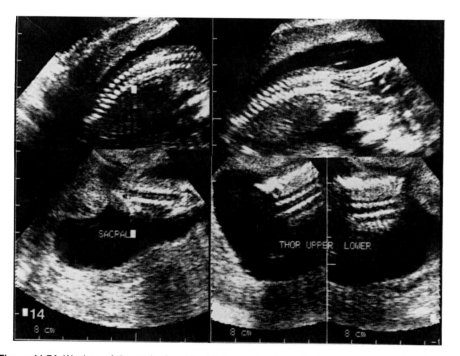

Figure 11.74 Workup of the entire length of the spinal column is shown. The upper two images show the sagittal, and the lower three images, the cross-sectional imaging of its integrity.

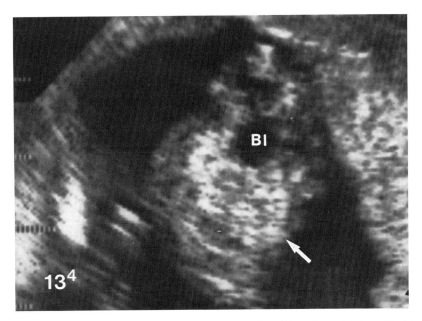

Figure 11.75 Coronal section of the lower part of the trunk at 13 weeks and 4 days. The bladder (Bl) and the hyperechoic bowel (arrow) are imaged.

Careful documentation and labeling of the depicted and studied organs or structures cannot be overemphasized.

COMMENTS

The high resolution of the 6.5 MHz probe makes possible a closer look at the early pregnancy through more detailed imaging of different embryonic structures. This property of the higher frequency transducer can be compared to the use of a high-power microscope to increase picture resolution. An important observation was made: almost every anatomical structure of early pregnancy was detected earlier by transvaginal than by transabdominal sonography. A closer look was taken at a selected group of 15 patients with well-documented and dated pregnancies. The performance of the generally used 3.5 MHz linear or sector scanner and the time of first detection of certain embryonic structures, as opposed to those of the 6.5 MHz transvaginal probe, were reviewed. The transvaginal probe detects the same embryological structures up to 3 weeks earlier, on the average, than the generally used, customary transabdominal probe.

Knowledge of the transvaginal sonographic appearance of embryonic and fetal structural anatomy enables us to determine the appearance of the normal embryo/fetus. In the embryonic period, ie, until the eighth week, this used to be important in determining whether a pregnancy is developing in the expected normal fashion. Recognizing the embryonic and extraembryonic structures, such as the gestational or chorionic sac, the yolk sac, the fetal pole with heart motion, the presence or absence of the single unpartitioned front brain, the falx, and finally the appearance and the disappearance of the midgut herniation, enables a "Gestalt" dating of the early pregnancy. This may be performed even before the conventional and

TABLE 11.6 Percent of Embryonic Structures Present or Absent (19)

Weeks of Gestation	4	5	6	7	8	9	10	11	12
Gestational sac only	100	→							
Yolk sac	0	91	100	→					
Fetal pole with heart motion	0	0	86	100	→				
Single ventricle	0	0	6	82	70	25	0	0	0
Falx	0	0	0	0	30	75	100	100	100
Midgut herniation	0	0	0	0	100	100	100	50	0
Total cases	6	11	15	17	10	13	15	11	6

☐ Structure present, ■ Structure absent

classical CRL measurements for dating are feasible. Table 11.6 depicts our experience in trying to determine the dating of the pregnancy just by observing the above-mentioned structures.[19]

Transvaginal sonography has certain limitations in scanning late second-trimester as well as third-trimester fetuses. One limitation, obviously, is the advancing gestational age leading to a rapidly increasing volume of amniotic fluid and a fast-growing fetus. Starting from the first days of the second trimester, the fetus literally outgrows the 2–7 cm "effective" focal zone of the 6.5 MHz transducer probe. A 5.0 MHz transvaginal probe can extend the focal range to about 10 cm at the expense of its resolution. However, in the second trimester, because of an increase in amniotic fluid production, fetal presentation and position change more often. Thus, there is good reason to believe that the body part, or organ of interest, will potentially come within reach of the vaginal probe. If the resolution of a 5.0 to 6.5 MHz probe is needed to image a second-trimester or early third-trimester fetus, one or several attempts should be made with a reasonable expectation of success. The benefits of external maneuvering of the fetus into the desired position can also be considered against the low risk of this procedure.

From the ninth and the tenth weeks onward, there is a possibility to scan and scrutinize fetal anatomy in a meaningful way and determine the presence or the absence of certain structural anomalies. As the pregnancy progresses, an increasing number of organs and body parts become visible using the high-frequency transvaginal probes. By determining the sequential appearance of structures that consistently lend themselves to sonographic examination, the groundwork is laid for possible selective or perhaps even routine anatomical workup of the first- or early second-trimester fetus.

Sonoembryology, or sonofetology, will definitely push back the frontiers of the classical fetal testing into the first half of the pregnancy.

In conclusion, transvaginal sonography detects various anatomical structures of the early pregnancy approximately 1 to 4 weeks earlier than the widely employed transabdominal scanning. We predict that this new method will be useful in the diagnosis of early and possibly second-trimester gestation as well as in learning more about early fetal anatomy and physiology. Its value in the indicated use for malformation workup should not be doubted anymore. We should now plan for its *routine* use in the near future.

REFERENCES

1. Popp LW, Lueken RP, Muller-Holne W, et al: Gynecologishe Endosonographie, Erste Erfahrungen. Ultraschall Med 1983;4:92.
2. Timor-Tritsch IE, Peisner DB, Raju S: Sonoembryology: an organ-oriented approach using a high frequency vaginal probe. J Clin Ultrasound 1990;18:286–298.
3. Neiman HL: Transvaginal ultrasound embryography, Seminars in Ultrasound, CT and MR, 1990;11:22–23.
4. Hamilton WJ, Boyd JD, Mossman HW: The implantation of the blastocyst and the development of the fetal membranes, placenta and decidua, in Human Embryology. Cambridge, W Heffer & Sons Ltd, 1945, pp 49–76.
5. Rock J, Hertig AT: Some aspects of early human development. Am J Obstet Gynecol 1942;44:973–983.
6. Jeanty P, Romero R: What does early gestation look like? in Jeanty P, Romero R (eds): Obstetrical Ultrasound. New York, McGraw-Hill, 1984, pp 34–40.
7. Timor-Tritsch IE, Farine D, Rosen MG: A close look at early embryonic development with the high frequency transvaginal transducer. Am J Obstet Gynecol 1988;159:676–681.
8. Robinson HP: Detection of fetal heart movement in first trimester of pregnancy using pulsed ultrasound. B Med J, 1972;4:466.
9. Robinson HP, Shaw-Dunn J: Fetal heart rates as determined by sonar in early pregnancy. J Obstet Gynaecology Br Commonw 1973;80:805.
10. Cadkin AV, McAlpin J: Detection of fetal cardiac activity between 41 and 43 days of gestation. J Ultrasound Med 1984;3:499–503.
11. Shenker L, Astle C, Reed K, et al: Embryonic heart beat before the seventh week. J Reprod Med 1986;31:333–335.
12. DuBose TJ, Cunyus JA, Johnson LF: Embryonic heart rate and age. J Diag Med Sonographers 1990;6:151–157.
13. Goldstein S: Early pregnancy scanning with the endovaginal probe. Contemporary Ob/Gyn, 1988;31:54–64.
14. Goldstein S: Very early pregnancy detection with endovaginal ultrasound. Obstet Gynecol 1988;72:200–204.
15. Timor-Tritsch IE, Rottem S, Thaler I: Review of transvaginal ultrasonography: a description with clinical application. Ultrasound Quart 1988;6:1–32.
16. Peisner DB, Timor-Tritsch IE, Margulis E, et al: Analysis of beta-hCG and sac size in early pregnancy. J Ultrasound Med 1988;7(suppl):5106.
17. Fossum GT, Dvajan V, Kletzky DA: Early detection of pregnancy with transvaginal ultrasound. Fertil Steril 1988;49:788–791.
18. Bernaschek G, Ruaelstorfer R, Csaicsich P: Vaginal sonography versus serum human chorionic gonadotropin in early detection of pregnancy. Am J Obstet Gynecol 1988;158:608–612.
19. Warren WB, Timor-Tritsch IE, Peisner DB, Raju S, Rosen MG: Dating the early pregnancy by sequential appearance of embryonic structures. Am J Obstet Gynecol 1989;161:747–753.
20. Cullen MT, Green JJ, Reece EA, Hobbins JG: A comparison of transvaginal and abdominal ultrasound in visualizing the first trimester conceptus. J Ultrasound Med 1989;8:565–569.
21. Timor-Tritsch IE, Warren WB, Peisner DB, Pirrone E: First trimester midgut herniation: a high frequency transvaginal sonographic study. Am J Obstet Gynecol 1989;161:831–833.
22. Bree RL, Edward M, Bohm-Velez M, et al: Transvaginal sonography in the evaluation of normal early pregnancy: correlation with HCG level. Am J Radiol 1989;153:75–79.
23. Kushnir O, Shalev J, Bronshtein M, Ben-Rafael Z, Mashiach S: Fetal intracranial anatomy in the first trimester of pregnancy: evaluation by transvaginal sonography. Neuroradiol 1989;31:222–225.
24. Bronshtein M, Kushnir O, Ben-Rafael Z, Shalev E, Webel L, Mashiach S, Shalev J: Transvaginal sonographic measurement of fetal kidneys in the first trimester of pregnancy. J Clin Ultrasound 1990;18:299–301.
25. Bronshtein M, Rottem S, Yoffe N, Blumenfeld Z, Brandes JM: Early determination of fetal sex using transvaginal sonography: technique and pitfalls. J Clin Ultrasound 1990;18:302–306.
26. Bree RL, Marn CS: Transvaginal sonography in the first trimester: embryology anatomy and hCG correlation. Seminars in Ultrasound, CT and MR 1990;11:12–21.
27. Timor-Tritsch IE, Montegudo A: Transvaginal ultrasonography in obstetrical care: a new frontier. Obstet Gynecol Reports 1990;2:210–220.
28. Peisner DB, Timor-Tritsch IE: The discriminatory zone of βhCG for vaginal probes. J Clin Ultrasound 1990;18:280–285.
29. Timor-Tritsch IE, Montegudo A, Peisner DB: High frequency transvaginal sonographic examina-

tion for the potential malformation workup of the 9–14 week fetus. Am J Obstet Gynecol (submitted).

30. Timor-Tritsch IE, Monteagudo A, Warren WB: Transvaginal sonographic definition of the central nervous system in the first and early second trimester. Am J Obstet Gynecol 1991;164:497–503.

31. Lasser D, Vollebergh J, Peisner DB, Timor-Tritsch IE: First trimester biometry using high frequency transvaginal ultrasound. Obstet Gynecol (submitted).

32. Rottem S: Targeted scanning of fetal organs in the first trimester. Doctoral thesis 1989, Technion Institute for Technology, Haifa, Israel.

33. Streeter GL: Developmental horizons in the human embryo. Contrib Embryol Carnegie Inst. 1942;30:211.

34. Yeh HC, Goodman JD, Carr L, Rabinovitz JG: Intradecidual sign: a US criterion of early intrauterine pregnancy. Radiology 1986;161:463–467.

35. England AM: Color Atlas of Life Before Birth: Normal Fetal Development. Chicago Year Book Medical, 1983.

36. Moore KL: The Developing Human. Philadelphia, W.B. Saunders, 1988.

37. Crelin ES: Development of the musculo skeletal system. Clin Symp 1981;33:1.

38. Cyr DR, Mack LA, Schoenecker SA, et al: Bowel migration in the normal fetus. Radiology 1986;161:119–121.

39. Schmidt W, Yarkoni S, Crelin ES, Hobbins JC: Sonographic visualization of physiologic anterior abdominal wall hernia in the first trimester. Obstet Gynecol 1987;69:911–915.

40. Kadar N, DeVore G, Romero R: Discriminatory hCG zone: its use in the sonographic evaluation for ectopic pregnancy. Obstet Gynecol 1981;58:156.

41. Braustein GD, Grodin JM, Vaitukastus J, Ross GT: Secretory rates of human chorionic gonadotropin by normal throphoblast. Am J Obstet Gynecol 1973;115:445.

41. Nyberg DA, Filly RA, Mahoney BS, et al: Early gestation: correlation of hCG levels and sonographic identification. Am J Radiol 1985;144:951.

42. Grannum P, Bracken M, Silverman R, et al: Assessment of fetal kidney size in normal gestation by comparison of ratio of kidneys circumference to abdominal circumference. Am J Obstet Gynecol 1981;136:249.

43. Sagi J, Vagman I, David MP, et al: Fetal kidney size related to gestational age. Gynecol Obstet Invest 1987;23:1.

44. Bronshtein M, Kushnir O, Ben-Rafael Z, Shalev E, et al: Transvaginal sonographic measurement of fetal kidneys in the first trimester of pregnancy. J Clin Ultrasound 1990;18:299–301.

45. Bronshtein M, Siegler E, Eshcoli Z, Zimmer EZ: Transvaginal ultrasound measurements of the fetal heart at 11 to 17 weeks of gestation. Accepted for publication.

46. O'Rahilly R, Müller F: Developmental stages in human embryos. Carnegie Institution of Washington. Publication 637. Washington, D.C. 1987.

47. Crelin ES: Development of the nervous system. Clin Symp 1974;26(2):1.

CHAPTER 12

Pathology of the Early Intrauterine Pregnancy

Ilan E. Timor-Tritsch, MD
Shraga Rottem, MD, DSc

INTRODUCTION

Abortion is the termination of pregnancy by any means before the conceptus is developed sufficiently to survive. If it occurs spontaneously, the term used is *miscarriage*, a term that has been applied by lay persons.

In the United States the *definition of miscarriage* or *abortion* is confined to termination of pregnancy before 20 weeks gestation based on the date of the first day of the last menstrual period. Another commonly used definition is: the delivery of a conceptus weighing less than 500 gm. In some European countries, the weight even for this definition is less than 1000 gm.[1]

In the previous chapter, the role of transvaginal sonography in diagnosing the normal intrauterine pregnancy was described. While this chapter bears many similarities to the previous one, this chapter, Chapter 12, will deal with the various features of TVS as far as the workup of a patient suspected of an abnormal gestation is concerned.

Categories of Spontaneous Abortion: In classical textbooks the categories of spontaneous abortion usually belong in the following 5 subgroups: *threatened, inevitable, incomplete, missed,* and *recurrent.*

None of these diagnoses was based on ultrasonography. It is probably a good idea to revise the above-cited terms in the light of the viability of the conceptus. Symptoms and signs such as slight vaginal bleeding, cramping, and lower abdominal pain in a patient having a short or more prolonged amenorrhea bring far more patients to the emergency room or the office than any other gynecological or obstetrical complaint. Combining the signs and symptoms with the findings of the bimanual examination, revealing a closed or a lightly opened cervix, results in the diagnosis of threatened abortion.[1] The term *threatened abortion* is applied to all slightly bleeding, early pregnancies which, at the time of the office or emergency room visit, do not have a specific, more accurate diagnosis. Usually these patients are referred for ultrasonography, a serum βhCG test, or simply left alone to be reexamined after a period of time. A vaginal probe in the office or the emergency suite would shorten the time to a more accurate diagnosis and would in most cases render the hormonal pregnancy test superfluous. We sincerely hope that the term "threatened abortion" will soon be abandoned in favor of a more precise nomenclature describing the underlying picture of the pregnancy abnormality.

The most confusing term in the category is *missed abortion*, which refers to the

299

prolonged retention of a fetus during the first half of the pregnancy. The dead products of conception have to have been in utero for 4 to 8 weeks or more in order to comply with this definition. The rationale for the aforementioned period for the diagnosis of missed abortion is of no useful clinical purpose. The definition was "inherited" from times when it was almost impossible to determine the viability of a first- or second-trimester gestation. The term "missed abortion" implies that the diagnosis of fetal demise was missed at the time it occurred. Most clinicians agree that once the death of a conceptus is established, the uterus has to be emptied. The use of transabdominal or transvaginal sonography enables us to establish an accurate diagnosis as soon as these modalities are used. The term that probably will gain acceptance in time will be "early fetal demise" or simply "fetal demise." Therefore, the term "missed" should be dropped.

The incidence of *spontaneous abortion* has been estimated to be 10 to 15% of all pregnancies.[2,3] Two areas of imprecision are attributed to these figures, namely, lack of inclusion of very early unrecognized abortions, and inclusion of illegally performed abortions claimed to be spontaneous. Since as many as 30% of abortions go unrecognized, this means they occur very early. Demographically, fetuses that were confirmed to be alive at 8 weeks of gestation abort only at a rate of 3.2%.[4] Stabile et al[5] demonstrated that the spontaneous abortion rate after fetal heart beats were seen was 5 to 6%. An abortion rate of 16.4% has been reported in patients bleeding during the first trimester.[6] In short, roughly 25% of pregnant women have uterine bleeding during the first trimester. It is widely accepted that more than 50% of these abort spontaneously.[7]

Despite the fact that nonviable gestations ultimately undergo abortion, the uterus may not expel the products of conception for weeks. Thus, it is of some importance to correctly identify those gestations that are nonviable before complications occur. Among the complications may be prolonged uterine bleeding, septic abortion, and, of equal importance, psychological upset of the patient and her family. The information has equally high clinical importance when recurrent abortions or the complications of chorionic villus sampling are considered. Genetic abnormalities of the conceptus are considered to be the major causes of early pregnancy loss.

Two main tools are known to evaluate the early pregnancy: the first is *hormonal assays*, but these lack the ability to correctly determine all potentially nonviable gestations. The second is *ultrasonography* which was and is extensively used. The gestational sac and its contents were considered to be reliable evidence of abnormal gestation.[8,9] In this chapter we will expand on the use of ultrasonography in the workup of a patient suspected of pregnancy abnormalities. First, the classical transabdominal approach will be mentioned, then the better and more accurate transvaginal scanning route will be widely discussed.

TRANSABDOMINAL SONOGRAPHY

Transabdominal sonography can correctly identify 53% of abnormal gestational sacs,[8] and transabdominal ultrasound, in conjunction with radioimmunoassay of human chorionic gonadotropin, beta subunits (βhCG), was found by Nyberg et al[9] to be useful in the diagnosis of early intrauterine pregnancy. The same author extended these studies to the pathological early pregnancy and reported on the successful use of simultaneous βhCG-level measurements and gestational sac size in the identification of abnormal gestation.[10] Previous studies reported that a gestational sac should be detected by transabdominal sonography when the βhCG level is ≥6500 mIU/mL (IRP). This level of βhCG was called the "discriminatory zone."[11] This "discriminatory zone" was updated by Nyberg et al[12] after consistently demonstrating a normal gestational sac when the βhCG level was greater than 1800 mIU/mL (Second Reference Preparate). As they applied this cutoff level of βhCG to ultrasound findings, a discrepancy was discovered between the sonographic finding and the expected βhCG level: only 36% of abnormal pregnancies were detected by the hormonal ascites. When gestational sac size was used in comparison with the βhCG level, 65% of the abnormal gestations were detected.[10] To consider transabdominal ultrasound a reliable method of gestational sac assessment an experienced sonographer for correct interpretation is required.

The following are some of the morphological characteristics of abnormal gestation detected by the *transabdominal method:*

1. *A small-for-date gestational sac.* This diagnosis is based on the knowledge of accurate menstrual dates which are often unknown.[13]
2. *The presence or absence of fetal heart motion* by the end of the seventh menstrual week. Good dating of the pregnancy is crucial for this.[13-15]
3. The appearance of the gestational sac of *irregular* or even *bizarre shape,* an *unnaturally large sac* that lacks an embryo, *and the absence of the double decidual reaction* ("double sac sign").[8,15,16]
4. An anembryonic pregnancy, which may result from an embryo that never developed.[8,15,16]

Nyberg et al[9] further refined the morphological description of a normal gestational sac using transabdominal sonography, which is considered as such if the following conditions apply:

1. It is larger than 24 mm without an embryo.
2. It has a distorted shape.
3. It has a thin choriodecidual reaction that measures 2 mm.
4. The choriodecidual echoes are of low amplitude.
5. An irregular contour is seen.
6. The typical double gestational sac is lacking and the sac is greater than 10 mm.
7. The sac is in a very low position within the uterine segment.

Detection of the first 3 criteria by transabdominal sonography was associated with 100% specificity as well as a positive predictive value in diagnosing an abnormal pregnancy. Because of the ability of these sonographic signs to define missed abortion, they are considered "major criteria."

The remaining criteria are considered "minor criteria" because they are more subjective in their interpretation as well as somewhat less specific in diagnosing an abnormal gestation. Several of these "minor criteria" can be combined to raise the positive predictive accuracy to 100%. This high level of accuracy is needed when the decision is made to evacuate the uterus in the case of an abnormal gestation.

Following the first reports of sonographic detection and description of the yolk sac,[17] several communications have pointed out its potential value in the diagnosis of normal or abnormal gestation.[18-20] By transabdominal sonography the human yolk sac is viewed from the seventh week on. At 10 weeks of menstrual age it starts to shrink, and by the eleventh week on it is gradually incorporated into the umbilical cord[17,20] (see Chapter 11). It should also be remembered that the yolk sac and the yolk stalk are extraembryonic structures. If the yolk sac is seen and no fetal pole is evident, the diagnosis of missed abortion should be made.[19] These criteria as well as a small-to-date and free-floating yolk sac were suggested by Hurwitz to be the "yolk sac sign."[20]

One should always emphasize that at times an abnormal-appearing gestation may develop normally. This seems to be a generally accepted clinical observation. Therefore, caution must be exercised, and it is advisable to give the patient with suspected threatened abortion the benefit of the doubt when sonographically there is normal-appearing or mildly atypical gestation. The patient should be re-examined in 1 week.[9]

The aim of sonography in the diagnosis of possible pathology during early pregnancy is twofold: *First* is the reliable, early, and expeditious detection of a pregnancy failure to enable emptying the uterus. This will shorten uterine bleeding and psychological upset of the patient. As mentioned before, at this time we should think of changing the term "missed abortion" to "early fetal demise". Similarly, making the diagnosis will reduce the rate of first-trimester complications. *Second,* if the pregnancy is normal, it will reassure both the patient and her obstetrician simultaneously.

THE USE OF TRANSVAGINAL SONOGRAPHY IN ABNORMAL GESTATION

Because of its *high resolution,* transvaginal sonography (TVS) generates clear, crisp pictures, and because of its *unobstructed view* in obese patients, TVS presents clear advantages in the diagnostic algorithm of pathology in early pregnancy. Experience gained throughout the world in the use of TVS in the workup of suspected pathological pregnancy has proven that this scanning route should be *the first choice* in the laboratory workup of the above-mentioned patients. From the data presented in Chapter 11, it is clear that the basic embryological structures of the early gestation are seen about 1–3 weeks earlier with TVS than with transabdominal scanning. *The prerequisite of accurate pregnancy dating and the knowledge of normal sonoembryology must once again be stressed.*

The discriminatory βhCG zone has to be reassessed if TVS is considered. Different levels of discriminatory zone have been proposed by several authors.[21–26] A detailed discussion of the discriminatory zone for vaginal probes is found in Chapter 11.

Discriminatory zones were also proposed for the identification of a yolk sac and embryonic cardiac activity. Bree et al[27] set the level for identifying a yolk sac at 7200 mIU/mL and for the detection of embryonic heart beats at 10,800 mIU/mL.[27]

Since the discriminatory βhCG zone is a function of equipment, the sonographer's experience, and the laboratory for βhCG determinations used, it is of utmost importance that an appropriate βhCG value for the equipment and method of assay in each institution be developed and available.[25]

Transvaginal Sonographic Morphology of the Abnormal Gestation

One way of describing the normal gestation would be to follow the classical classification appearing in textbooks such as threatened, inevitable, incomplete, and missed abortions, and describe the transvaginal sonographic features of each of them.

In this chapter, however, a different approach will be adopted. Sonomorphologic description of the major uterine and gestational structures making the diagnosis of an abnormal pregnancy will be looked at in a systematic way. First- and early second-trimester pregnancy abnormalities could be classified by transvaginal sonographic findings. However, experience shows that there is quite a large overlap in their sonographic appearances. Therefore, definitions may be adversely affected by new and more artificial classifications.

The sonographic pathology of the normal gestation involving the different structures may appear alone or in any combination, and may involve (1) the *uterus* with its *decidual reaction*; (2) the *gestational sac* and its *membranes;* (3) the *fetal pole itself;* and, finally, (4) the *placenta.*

Uterus and the Decidua

The following are the sonographic signs of abnormal gestation:

1. *Irregular appearance* of the normal echogenic decidual double ring with unclear lacunar structures (Fig 12.1**A,B**). Decidua/chorion complex seems to become significantly thicker and edematous, with numerous foci of hyperechoic and hypoechoic areas. The hypoechoic areas demonstrate blood flow. This blood flow is turbulent and becomes even more evident if the scanning frame-rate is increased. If the time lag between the actual fetal death and its detection by TVS increases, this irregularity of the decidua/chorion unit will become increasingly evident (Fig 12.2). The fetal pole will shrink accordingly and disappear, probably as a result of reabsorption. This late shape of fetal demise was called "missed abortion."

2. *Partial or complete disappearance* of the echoic double ring, the echogenicity of which approaches that of uterine muscles (Figs 12.3 and 12.4).

3. *Partial or complete detachment of the decidua* by fluid-filled spaces (Figs 12.2 and 12.5). These subdecidual sonolucencies consist of hemorrhages which, if their number and size increase, finally detach products of conception in order to expel from the uterus. The sonolucencies of this sort should not be confused with the subchorionic hemorrhage in very early pregnancies which will be discussed later.

4. *Complete disappearance of the products of conception* following spontaneous expulsion. Diagnosis of complete abortion or diappearance of the products of conception is a relatively difficult diagnosis to make. This is usually confirmed by a previous positive test and/or a previous ultrasound examination showing the clear sonographic features of pregnancy. The uterus may contain a larger blood clot (Fig 12.3) or just a hyperechogenic structure continuing into the area of the cervical canal and consisting of a firm blood clot (Fig 12.4). The "empty sac" will be discussed later.

5. *Subchorionic or subdecidual hematoma.* This entity was described previously by transabdominal sonography.[28] Sonographers and sonologists suspected for a long time that sonolucent crescent- or wedge-shaped structures between the uterine wall and the chorion may be a subchorionic hemorrhage (Figs 12.5, 12.6, and 12.7). Only recently, after chorionic villus sampling and multifetal reductions resulted in similar structures in patients with normal appearance of the pregnancies prior to the procedure, did origin of this structure become established without any doubt (Fig 12.8 and Fig 16.7 from Chapter 16).

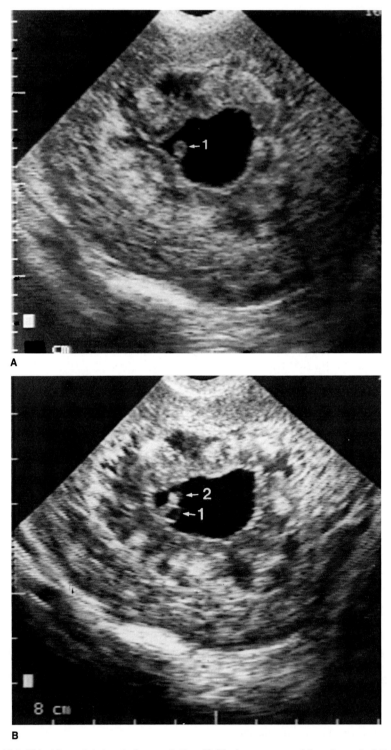

Figure 12.1 This 10-week intrauterine gestation (**A,B**) shows some of the characteristics of an abnormal pregnancy: the sac itself is small (23 × 16 × 15 mm) and irregular; a small yolk sac (1), an irregularly echogenic decidual ring, unclear lacunar structures, and a small, amorphous fetal pole (2) are also observed.

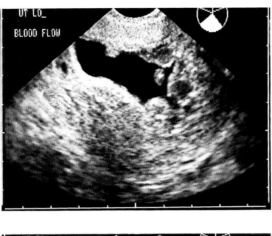

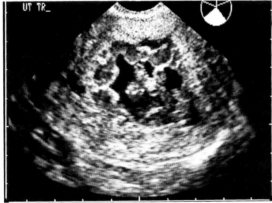

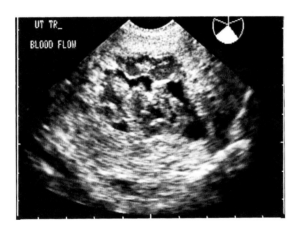

Figure 12.2 The larger the time lag between actual fetal demise and the detection/expulsion, the more accenuated the irregularity of the chorion/decidual and the surrounding blood flow will become. Depicted are serial images of a 20 week gestation. Sac and wall size is $6 \times 5 \times 4\frac{1}{2}$ cm. The fetal pole was smaller than $1 \times \frac{1}{2} \times \frac{1}{2}$ cm (not shown here). The structures seen within the sac are protrusions of the wall irregularities.

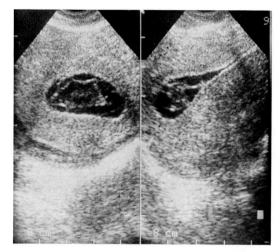

Figure 12.3 A 9-week abnormal pregnancy showing a blurred decidual ring and a clot within the uterine cavity. The left side is a cross section; the right side, a longitudinal section.

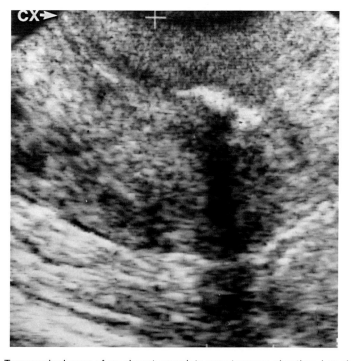

Figure 12.4 Transvaginal scan of an almost complete spontaneous abortion. Longitudinal section of the uterus showing the echogenic structures (blood clots?) along the cavity line. The cervix faces the upper left corner. Several days before, fetal heart beats had been observed in a normal-appearing gestational sac.

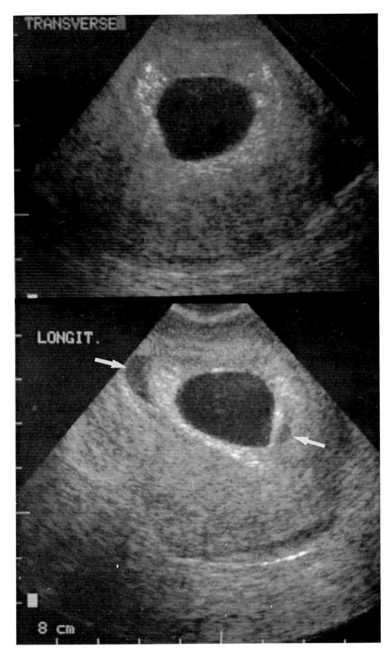

Figure 12.5 A blighted 8-week 5-day ovum is clearly seen in the uterine cavity. The sac is empty and measures 22 × 18 × 23 mm on the longitudinal section. Note the partial detachment of the decidual ring (arrows). The meaning of the strongly echogenic areas in the decidual ring is unknown.

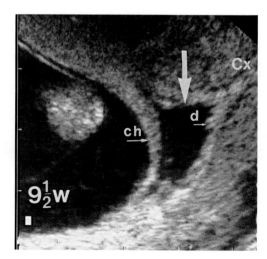

Figure 12.6 Subchorionic hemorrhage. Longitudinal sagittal section of the uterus at 9 weeks and 3 days. The arrow points to a small 1.5 × 1.0 cm sonolucent area at the internal os of the cervix (Cx). Its position between the chorion (ch) and decidua (d) is evident.

An office patient in whom the subchorionic hematoma is observed close to the internal os (Figs 12.6 and 12.7) may be reassured of good outcome after the bleeding has cleared. In contrast, a patient in which the chorionic hematoma is seen undermining the placental site may not have a particularly good outcome. The details observed on TVS regarding the position and place of subchorionic bleeding may enable introduction of definitions such as early placental separation. These extensive placental separations may explain some of the early fetal demises occurring from 9–12 or 13 weeks. Transvaginal sonography enables the diagnosis of small subchorionic hemorrhages such as those shown in Fig 12.7. The definition of *threatened abortion,* which is a *clinical diagnosis,* may have to be changed according to the transvaginal sonographic picture. The TVS image can more accurately describe the existence or nonexistence of fetal heartbeats and possible bleeding which does not involve the placental site and clears out through the cervix. This results in the clinical site of vaginal bleeding or a more complicated clinical picture which would indicate that some of the placenta was separated, endangering embryonic or fetal life.

At the time of chorionic villus sampling (CVS), in a small number of cases, we observed a separation of the chorion from the decidua along the path of the sampling catheter (Fig 12.8). If this separation did not involve the placental site, the outcome was good. The hematoma reabsorbed in a couple of weeks. The same traumatic hemorrhage around the chorion was observed after needle penetration at multifetal reductions (Fig 16.7).

It seems clear to us that a more meaningful clinical evaluation of a bleeding early pregnancy is feasible using TVS.

Gestational Sac and Membranes

Discrepancy Between the Sac Size and Dates

In reviewing the literature it is evident that only a few articles exist to evaluate the measurements of the gestational sac.[29–34] Some of them use linear measurements,

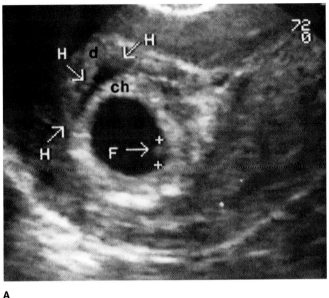

A

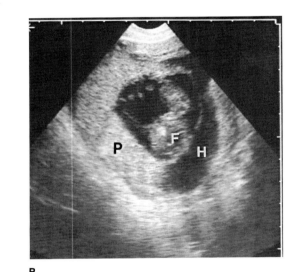

B

Figure 12.7 (**A**) Subchorionic hemorrhage. A longitudinal (sagittal) section of a 6-week 2-day gestation. A sonolucent, crescent-shaped structure marked by arrows and the letter "H" is evident between the decidua (d) and the chorion (ch). The fetal pole (F) had a heartbeat. Three days later the hematoma increased in size and the patient started bleeding from the cervix. Early fetal demise was diagnosed several days later. (**B**) Traumatic subchorionic hemorrhage (H) resulting from chorionic villus sampling. The patient bled; however, the tiny placenta (P) was not separated and the pregnancy progressed normally (F = fetus).

other graphs. From the articles it is not always evident whether the measurements were made from the sonolucent border of the gestational sac, or whether they included its solid wall component. It is equally unclear whether the measurement is an average diameter, since were that not the case, it would be very hard to compensate for the pressing full urinary bladder distorting the shape of the gestational sac.

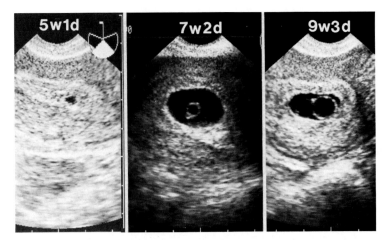

Figure 12.8 Serial images of an intrauterine pregnancy at 5 weeks and 1 day, 7 weeks and 2 days, and 9 weeks and 3 days. The chorionic sac does not grow, the fetal pole is not evident, and at 9 weeks and 3 days it is hard to distinguish which is the pathological amnion and which is the yolk sac. (The more hyperechogenic structure is probably the yolk sac.)

The most practical graph is the one suggested by Hellman et al.[29] However, it is not widely used by ultrasonography laboratories.

The use of transvaginal sonography makes the measurement of the gestational sac practical if only in one single instance, and this is determining the diagnosis of the empty gestational sac or, as it was called for years, "blighted ovum." It is very simple to remember that by using the average measurements of the sac, at 5 weeks the gestational sac measures 1 cm, a 2 cm sac is usually measured at about 6 weeks, and a 2.5 cm sac is seen around 7 weeks. At 8 weeks the sac should measure 3 cm.

Only in the very rare case would the diagnosis be made solely by the size of the gestational sac. In most instances, other parameters will attest to the abnormality of the gestation. Fig 12.8 shows serial images of the same early gestation. At 5 weeks and 1 day, the chorionic sac is seen amidst the hyperechoic endometrium on one side of the cavity line and appears to be normal. However, at 7 weeks and 2 days, and at 9 weeks and 3 days, the sac sizes were 2 cm and 1.5 cm, respectively. It is not only the sac size that is abnormal in this pregnancy; the fetal pole as well as the yolk sac are also pathological. No fetal heartbeats were seen at 7 weeks and 2 days, nor were they appreciated later on.

A note of warning should be inserted here: If any doubt exists as to the correct dating of the pregnancy and a smaller-than-expected gestation is observed, with or without fetal pole or heartbeat, the patient should be rescanned within 3 to 7 days in order to observe the expected growth in the gestational sac or fetal pole. Bear in mind that even if these patients start to bleed, the size of the pregnancy is so small that no significant blood loss should be feared.

An Empty Sac

As mentioned before, a gestational sac 24 mm and larger should be considered an anembryonic or empty sac, otherwise termed a blighted ovum.[9] However, after the more accurate TVS was developed and widely used, the term "empty sac" was redefined. Researchers agree that for purposes of definition the size has to be reduced to enable better imaging of the contents of the gestational sac. However, agreement on the exact size is not yet available. It was believed that a 16 mm gestational sac without fetal pole or any contents should be termed an empty sac.[35]

A significant amount of confusion exists around the term *blighted ovum*. Abdominal sonographic studies do not solve the problem.

With the introduction of TVS, those who acquired the experience have long suspected that the term *blighted ovum* must be reassessed. Pirrone et al[37] compared the transabdominal images of empty gestational sacs with transvaginal findings. Patients between the menstrual ages of 6 and 18 weeks were scanned first abdominally, with a full bladder, using a 3.5 MHz transducer, and afterward, TVS was performed, with an empty bladder, using a 5 or 6.5 MHz transvaginal transducer probe. The study was prompted by 2 observations:

1. The discrepancy observed between transvaginal and transabdominal sonography in cases where transabdominal sonography showed an empty sac
2. Several weeks after fetal reduction, the gradual and, finally, total disappearance of the fetal pole, leaving behind an empty gestational sac

The results showed that from the 21 empty gestational sacs followed, only 5 were actually empty. Nine contained embryonic or fetal structures and 7 had embryonic and extraembryonic structures. Four of these demonstrated a faint but positive fetal cardiac activity by transvaginal sonography.

At the conclusion of this study there was clear indication that most ''empty sacs'' imaged by transabdominal sonography and pronounced to be empty, actually contained embryonic/fetal or extraembryonic structures Fig 12.9. Therefore it was postulated that the *blighted ovum* should be changed to *early embryonic or fetal demise*.

Supporting data were found in the study performed by Stabile et al, who looked at maternal serum alpha-fetoprotein levels in 21 women with threatened miscarriage, and an ultrasound diagnosis of anembryonic pregnancy was confirmed. Fourteen of the 21 patients had normal alpha-fetoprotein levels: the remaining 7 had levels above 95% of the reference range. This is in contrast to earlier findings

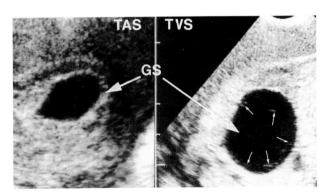

Figure 12.9 Transabdominal and transvaginal images of early embyonic demise at 8 weeks. Only the transvaginal image (on the right) shows embryonic structures.

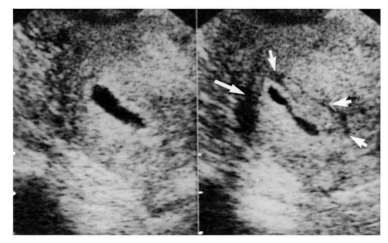

Figure 12.10 This flat gestational sac was found in a 7-week pregnancy. The "double-ring" sign can hardly be recognized, the sac is empty, and there is some detachment of the decidua (arrows).

of an association between low levels of alpha-fetoprotein in anembryonic pregnancy. It was concluded by that study that *most anembryonic pregnancies are in fact pregnancies in which the fetus has been lost rather than pregnancies in which the fetus was never present.* The authors concluded: "thus, the so called anembryonic pregnancy may prove to be a myth."[38]

Irregularly Shaped Sacs

These gestational sacs are usually flat (Fig 12.10) or polygonal in shape (Figs 12.11, 12.12, and 12.15). However, one should be extremely careful since sometimes an irregularly shaped sac may sometimes contain a normal pregnancy. Such a case is presented in Fig 12.13. In this case, the irregularity was caused by an incompletely removed intracavitory adhesion (Asherman's syndrome) which,

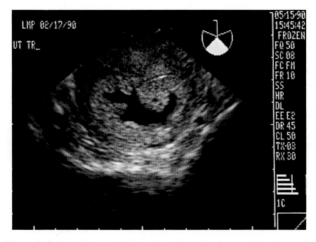

Figure 12.11 A 12-week 3-day abnormal gestation showing irregularly shaped sac, hypoechoic decidua/chorion, and fetal pole.

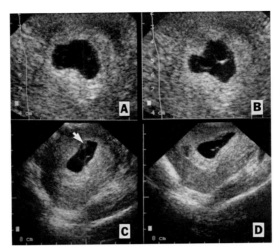

Figure 12.12 Four serial sections (**A–D**) of an 8-week abnormal pregnancy. (**A,B**) Cross sections showing fragments of membranes and the fetal pole. (**C,D**) Flat gestational sac; detached and shrunken membranes; small ill-defined, fragmented yolk sac (arrow); and poorly defined decidual ring.

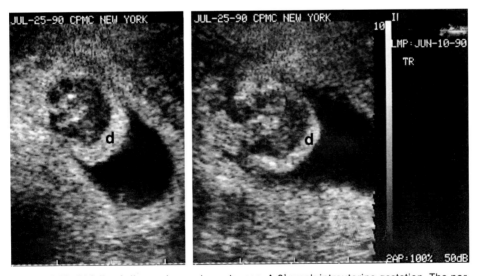

Figure 12.13 *Pitfalls of diagnosing an irregular sac.* A 6½-week intrauterine gestation. The normal decidua/chorion (d) covers a previously hysteroscopically treated intracavitary adhesion (Asherman's syndrome). The fetal pole with active heartbeats found is not in the plane of this image.

bulging into the normal cavity and covered by chorion, rendered this sac an irregular shape. A 6-week embryo with fetal heartbeats was found in the chorionic sac.

Irregular and Shrunken Amniotic Membranes

We speculate that together with the shrinking of the amniotic membranes they would be completely detached from any supporting decidual tissue in an advanced state of a long-standing fetal demise, previously called a "missed abortion" (Fig 12.12).

Fetal Pole and Yolk Sac

No Visible Fetal Heartbeats After 6.5 Weeks Menstrual Age

This has to be supported by accurate dating of the pregnancy or by previous, documented heart motion. Most significant changes in normal pregnancies really start within the fetal pole. The first and most important feature is that there are no visible fetal heartbeats. It is true that to reach the diagnosis of early pregnancy one has only to look at the presence or absence of the fetal heartbeats. However, we described in this chapter all the changes we were aware of which were observed by us and others that accompany at an earlier or later stage the cessation of the fetal heartbeats. If the sonographer or sonologist is unsure of the dates and there are no fetal heartbeats in a small fetal pole, one should scan the patient within 3 or 4 days to follow up on this observation.

Fetal Pole

The fetal pole usually grows at a rate of 0.8 mm per day CRL. This can be computed from the charts available. There is no indication to date in the literature as to the normal rate of growth of a fetal pole. It is important to know the normal or expected *rate of growth* since rescanning a patient after 3 or 4 days should enable observing normal or abnormal growth in the embryonic or fetal pole. An additional indication to inadequate growth is that the fetus itself may undergo *degenerative changes*. The transvaginal sonographic signs of these degenerative changes are an amorphous, irregularly echogenic, irregularly shaped tissue mass with no fetal heartbeats (Figs 12.1, 12.8, 12.9, 12.12, 12.14, and 12.15). The fetal pole may undergo cystic degenerative changes (Fig 12.16).

The Pathology of the Yolk Sac

1. *Nonexistent yolk sac.* This is usually diagnosed along with an anembryonic gestation. As said before, this is just probably the end result of a long-standing abnormal gestation in which significant reabsorption of the products of conception already was started (Figs 12.5, 12.9, and 12.15).
2. *Smaller than 4 mm yolk sac* (Figs 12.1A,B, 12.8, 12.12, and 12.14). The irregularly shaped and irregularly echogenic yolk sac (Figs 12.8 and 12.14).
3. *Pitfalls in imaging the yolk sac.* At times, during the ultrasonographic workup of a suspected abnormal gestation, it is hard to decide which one of two cystic structures, about 2–8 mm in size, is the actual yolk sac (Fig 12.8). At 5–6 weeks one may see 2 yolk sacs in one chorionic sac (Fig

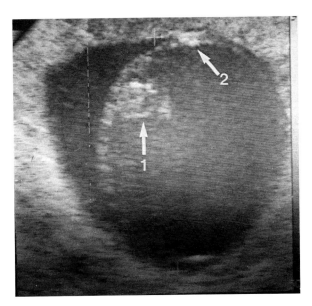

Figure 12.14 Completely detached spherical gestational sac in an 11-week 2-day pregnancy. No fetal heartbeats were detected during previous scans. Prominent signs of an abnormal gestation in this image are amorphous fetal pole (1) and small highly echogenic remnant of the yolk sac (2).

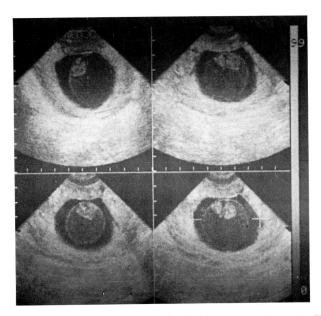

Figure 12.15 Four serial sections of the pathological pregnancy shown in Figure 12.14 are presented to demonstrate complete detachment of the amniotic sac floating freely in the gestational sac (measuring 5 cm). The amorphous irregularly echogenic fetal pole is obvious.

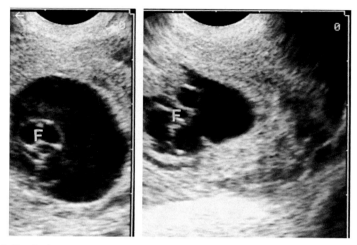

Figure 12.16 Cystic degeneration of the fetal pole (F) at 19 weeks in case of early fetal demise "(missed abortion)."

12.17**A**) which later on will give rise to a mono- or diamniotic twin with 2 yolk sacs (Fig 12.17**B**). Later, in the first trimester, cysts of the umbilical cord can be misdiagnosed as yolk sacs. The cysts of the umbilical cord raise several questions (see Chapter 13), and their correct diagnosis is important (Fig 12.18).

Studies on the normal and abnormal yolk sac and its potential clinical usefulness in diagnosing an abnormal pregnancy were performed and published only by using transabdominal transducers.[39-44] However, its size or its appearance seemed to be of little importance to predict the embryonic or fetal status and its potential clinical outcome. After reviewing the literature, the authors feel that unless the yolk sac shows markedly distorted shape or its size is far below or above the normally reported size throughout 8–12 weeks, it adds very little to the clinical management of the patient.

The Placenta

Cystic Changes

Abnormalities of the placenta such as significant thickening of cystic changes may be due to chromosomal abnormalities. Jouppila et al observed cystic areas of the placenta in 5 of 11 fetuses with trisomy 18 and 1 fetus with trisomy 13.[45] Triploidy in cases with multiple placental cysts was found by Rubenstein et al[46] and Lockwood et al.[47] These placental changes were described using transabdominal sonography. No such description of multiple cystic areas in the placenta was observed in the *very early pregnancy* by TVS. Therefore, if in the future multiple cystic areas are seen in the placenta, chromosomal workup of a first- or very early second-trimester fetus should be considered. Of particular advantage at this time would be the use of CVS.

A *solitary cyst* was seen by us in a placenta at 10 weeks and 2 days. This small cystic area did not show blood flow and disappeared completely after 6 weeks (Fig 12.19). The karyotype of the placenta was 46XY.

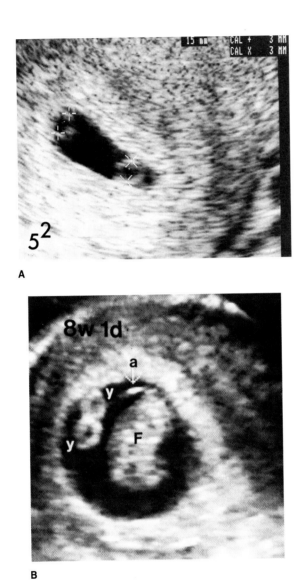

Figure 12.17 The yolk sac. (**A**) Two yolk sacs in a single chorionic sac at 5 weeks and 2 days. A normal twin gestation (monochorionic diamniotic) developed. (**B**) At 8 weeks and 1 day a normal monochorionic diamniotic twin pregnancy showing one of the fetuses and the two extraamniotic yolk sacs on the same image (a = amnion).

Hydatiform Mole

The sonographic picture of the hydatiform mole is typical and easily diagnosed even by the transabdominal approach. The transvaginal approach should be preferred in all patients, but its use is essential in obese patients or in patients in which the image obtained by transabdominal sonography is inconclusive. The sonographic picture of pain by TVS shows a multitude of different-sized sonolucent structures with high fidelity (Fig 12.20); thus, a reliable diagnosis of hydatiform mole or molar degeneration can be made. The earlier the diagnosis is made

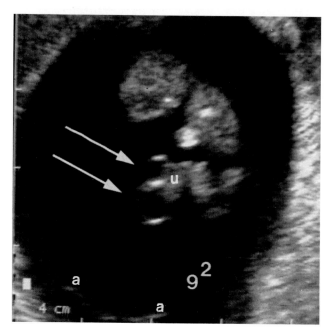

Figure 12.18 Cysts of the umbilical cord (arrows) mimicking yolk sacs. Note that they are close to the umbilical cord and inside the amnion.

cent "grape-like" configurations, and the more hyperechogenic placental echo-density will be evident.

The concomitant development of a live fetus with a partial hydatiform mole can also be observed at times (Fig 12.21). This diagnosis should be made early enough since the partial or incomplete hydatiform mole may represent triploidy 69 XXY or 69 XYY.[48] The typical fetus also has the stigmata of triploidy with multiple malformations and growth retardation. The risk of choriocarcinoma rising from a partial hydatiform mole is slight. There is no uniform approach to the management of a partial mole coexisting with a live fetus. There are reports of a successful pregnancy outcome with a healthy infant and mother in such cases.[49,50]

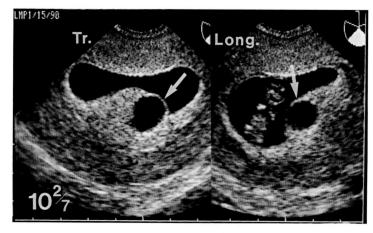

Figure 12.19 Placental cyst (arrows) at 10 weeks and 2 days.

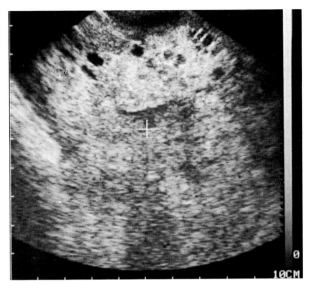

Figure 12.20 Hydatiform mole. The transvaginal image is typical, showing a large number of sonolucent round structures of various sizes.

Examination of the Cervix

The clue to an abnormal pregnancy or to the development of pathology of the first- and early second-trimester of pregnancy may lie in the cervix itself. Examining the cervix is an integral part of examining the entire pregnancy.

If the uterus is anteverted and the scanning is done in the transverse plane, the first structure to appear on the screen is the cervix. If a retroverted uterus is present, the transducer will first reveal the fundus of the uterus which, in this case, is close to the sacrum. Scanning in the longitudinal plane will easily reveal the exact position of the uterus and the cervix in the pelvis. The cervix is usually studied in the sagittal, longitudinal plane. On this longitudinal plane, the endocervical canal will become the most prominent structure on the screen. Sometimes, cystic formations of various sizes (0.5–1 cm) may appear along the endocervical

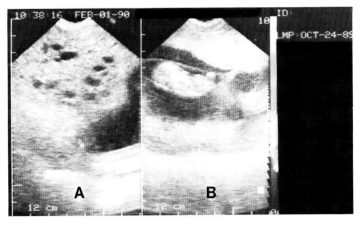

Figure 12.21 Concomitant molar placenta (**A**), and live 14-week 1-day fetus (**B**).

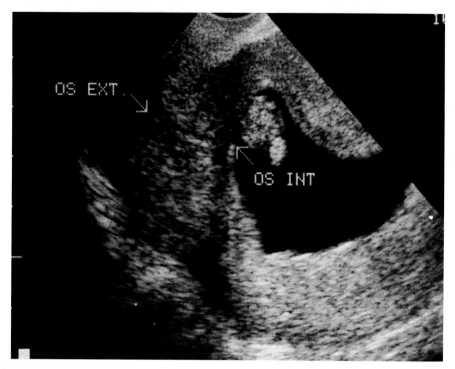

Figure 12.22 The normal uterine cervix of a 14-week-pregnant patient.

canal. These probably represent dilated endocervical glands termed nabothian cysts. The internal cervical os is more distinct in the pregnant than the non-pregnant uterus (Figs 12.22 and 12.23).

In cases of spontaneous abortion in progress, the images will show cervical dilatation of various degrees and the products of conception at different places within the gestational sac on their way to expulsion (Fig 12.24**A,B,C**).

Recently, Kushnir et al reported on measurements of the cervix performed by TVS.[51] For the first time we may have the right tools and the opportunity to make direct observations and study the entity called *cervical incompetence*. It is premature to draw clinical conclusions based on this new route of cervical scanning before more extensive descriptions of the normal and abnormal cervix, with or without the presence of an intrauterine pregnancy, are available.

Using TVS it is easy to follow up the patient with cerclage. In addition, the accuracy in placing the suture can be evaluated (Fig 12.25). If, in spite of the suture in place, the cervix is in the process of dilating, TVS is the right tool to follow up and report possible funneling and progressive dilatation of the cervix.

SUMMARY

We do understand that the basic fact in the ultimate diagnosis of early fetal demise is easy and is made if no embryonic/fetal heart activity is seen past 6 weeks gestational age. However, the high-resolution equipment enables the user to tell much more about the pathology involved.

In spite the fact that the old, classic terms and definitions of early pregnancy abnormalities still prevail, it is clear to all TVS operators that these diagnoses are

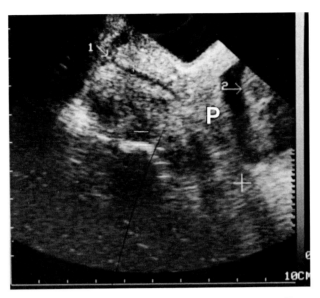

Figure 12.23 The placenta previa (p) overlying the internal cervical os. The external os (1) is visible. Part of the fetus (2) is also shown in this section.

continuously challenged and changed. The changes are mandated by the observations of detailed and clear images revealing information heretofore not seen.

In this chapter the basic building blocks of pathological pregnancies, as seen by TVS, were discussed. By looking at the transvaginal sonographic findings and by trying to understand the dynamic changes involved one can reach an unavoidable, but natural conclusion. The images are clear! This conclusion calls for the need to change some of the definitions, such as "threatened abortion," "missed abortion," "blighted ovum," and "anembryonic gestation." This need for the new and more specific and targeted diagnostic definition of the abnormal gestation became evident in the recent literature. This necessity is also prompted through the observations made by the individual sonographers and sonologists—at least of those who care to go one step beyond the customary phrase in the classical report on a pregnancy failure: ... "no fetal heart activity was seen."

The sonographic examination is the most appropriate laboratory tool in the diagnosis of any first- and early second-trimester pregnancy disturbance. If a definite answer as to the life of the embryo or the placenta is needed in the office or in the emergency department, without much ado (and many times without a lengthy hCG testing!) one should use TVS.

One should never forget that the diagnostic process of pregnancy anomalies is closely linked to a precise dating of the gestation. In the first trimester, the exact dating is even more important, since fundamental structural changes occur throughout each week. Knowledge of accurate dates will enable the clinician to determine the normal or abnormal progress of a very early pregnancy, based on the serial follow-up of the sonographic findings. The reverse is also true: In a normally progressing gestation, the age of the embryo/fetus can be determined according to the presence of the chronological appearance of the embryonic and extraembryonic structures.[56]

In conclusion, the use of the high-resolution TVS will leave very few questions unanswered in the case of a suspected pregnancy abnormality.

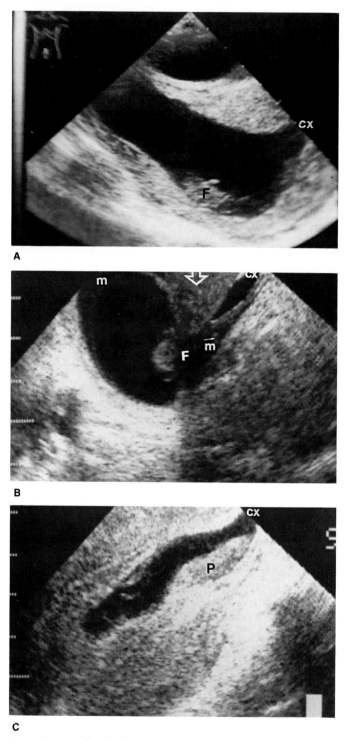

Figure 12.24 A spontaneous abortion in progress. (**A**) The cervix (Cx) is dilated. The fetal pole (F) has no heartbeats. (**B**) The membranes are still intact (M), the cervix (Cx) is in the process of dilatation. A contraction sweeps through the uterus (open arrow). This was clearly seen during the real-time examination of the patient. (**C**) The membranes ruptured suddenly, and the fetus was passed. The placenta (P) is in the process of being passed through the cervix.

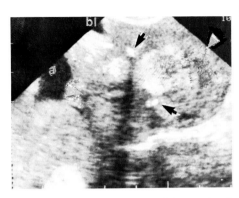 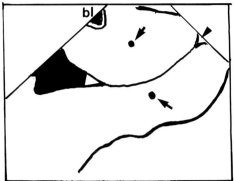

Figure 12.25 Sagittal section of the cervix after cerclage. Arrowheads point to the external and internal os. The bladder (bl) appears on the upper left side of the image. The arrows point to the cross-section of the sutures. The ink drawing on the right facilitates the understanding of the scan on the left side.

REFERENCES

1. Cunningham, MacDonald, Gant (eds): Williams Obstetrics, 18th ed. Norwalk, Conn., Appleton & Lange, 1989, pp 489–509.
2. Tietze C: Introduction to the statistics of abortion, in Engle ET (ed): Pregnancy Wastage. Springfield, IL, Thomas, 1953, p 135.
3. United Nations, Department of Social Affairs: Foetal, Infant, Early Childhood Mortality: I. The Statistics. New York, United Nations, 1954.
4. Simpson JL, Mills JL, Holmes LB, Ober CL, Aarons J, Jovanovic L, Knopp RH: Low fetal loss rates after ultrasound-proved viability in early pregnancy. JAMA 1987;258:2555.
5. Stabile I, Campbell S, Grudzinkas JG: Ultrasonic assessment of complications during first trimester of pregnancy. Lancet 1987;2:1237–1240.
6. Siddiqi TA, Caligaris JT, Miodovnik M, et al: Rate of spontaneous abortion after first trimester sonographic demonstration of fetal cardiac activity. Am J Perinatology 1988;5:1–4.
7. Fantel AG, Shepard TH: Basic aspects of early (first trimester) abortion, in Iffy L, Kaminetzky HA (eds): Principles and Practice of Obstetrics and Perinatology. New York, John Wiley & Sons, 1981, vol 1, pp 553–563.
8. Donald I, Morley P, Barnette E: The diagnosis of blighted ovum by sonar. Br J Obstet Gynecol 1972;79:304–310.
9. Nyberg DA, Filly RA: Threatened abortion: sonographic distinction of normal and abnormal gestational sacs. Radiology 1986;158:397–400.
10. Nyberg DA, Filly RA, Duarte-Filho DL, et al: Abnormal pregnancy: early diagnosis by US and serum chorionic gonadotropin levels. Radiology 1986;158:393–396.
11. Kadar N, DeVore G, Romero R: Discriminatory HCG zone: its use in sonographic evaluation for ectopic pregnancy. Obstet Gynecol 1981;58:156–161.
12. Nyberg DA, Filly RA, Mahoney BS, et al: Early gestation: correlation of HCG levels and sonographic identification. AJR 1985;144:951–954.
13. Anderson SG: Management of threatened abortion with real-time sonography. Obstet Gynecol 1980;55:259–264.
14. Hertz JB: Diagnostic procedures in threatened abortion. Obstet Gynecol 1984;64:223–229.
15. Robinson HP: The diagnosis of early pregnancy failure by sonar. Br J Obstet Gynecol 1975;82:849–857.
16. Jouppila P, Herva T: Study of blighted ovum by ultrasonic and histopathologic methods. Obstet Gynecol 1985;55:574–578.
17. Mationi M, Pedersen JF: Ultrasound visualization of the human yolk sac. J Clin Ultrasound 1979;7:759–762.
18. Sauerbrei E, Cooperberg PL, Poland BF: Ultrasound demonstration of the normal fetal yolk sac. J Clin Ultrasound 1980;8:217–220.
19. Bernard KG, Cooperberg PL: Sonographic differentiation between blighted ovum and early viable pregnancy. AJR 1985;144:597–601.

20. Hurwitz RS: Yolk sac sign: sonographic appearance of the fetal yolk sac in missed abortion. J Ultrasound Methods 1986;5:435–438.
21. Timor-Tritsch IE, Rottem S: Review of transvaginal ultrasonography: a description with clinical application. Ultrasound Quarterly 1988;6:1.
22. Timor-Tritsch IE, Farine D, Rosen MG: A close at early embryonic development with the high-frequency transvaginal transducer. Am J Obstet Gynecol 1988;159:676–681.
23. Bernashek G, Ruaelstorfer R, Csaicsich P: Vaginal sonography versus serum human chorionic gonadotropin in early detection of pregnancy. Am J Obstet Gynecol 1988;156:608–612.
24. Peisner DB, Timor-Tritsch IE, Margulis E, et al: Analysis of β-HCG and sac size in early pregnancy. J Ultrasound Med 1988; S106.
25. Peisner DB, Timor-Tritsch IE: The discriminatory zone of β-HCG for vaginal problems. J Clin Ultrasound 1990;18:280–285.
26. Goldstein SR, Snyder JR, Watson C, et al: Very early pregnancy detection with endovaginal ultrasound. Obstet Gynecol 1988;72:200.
27. Bree RL, Edwards M, Bohm-Velez M, et al: Transvaginal sonography in the evaluation of normal early pregnancy: correlation with HCG level. AJR 1989;153:75–79.
28. Goldstein SR, et al: Subchorionic bleeding in threatened abortion. Sonographic findings and significance. AJR 1983;141:975–978.
29. Hellman LF, Kobayashi M, Fillisti L, et al: Growth and development of the human fetus prior to the 20th week of gestation. Am J Obstet Gynecol 1969;103:784–800.
30. Hoffbauer H: The importance of ultrasonic diagnosis in early pregnancy. Electromedia 1970;3:227–230.
31. Piiroinen O: Studies in diagnostic ultrasound. Acta Obstet Gynecol Scand 1975;55:1–60.
32. Jouppila PC: Length and depth of the uterus and the diameter of the gestation sac in normal gravidas during early pregnancy. Acta Obstet Gynecol Scand 1971;50(suppl 15):29–31.
33. Kossoff G, Garrett WJ, Radovanoich G: Grey scale echography in obstetrics and gynaecology. Austr Radiol 1974;18:63–111.
34. Robinson HP: "Gestational sac" volumes as determined by sonar in the first trimester of pregnancy. Br J Obstet Gynecol 1975;82:100–107.
35. Lyons E: Personal communication.
36. Bernard KG, Cooperberg PL: Sonographic differentiation between blighted ovum and early viable pregnancy. AJR 1985;144:597–601.
37. Pirrone EC, Monteagudo A, and Timor-Tritsch IE: Does "Blighted ovum" really exist? Presented at the 34th Annual Meeting of the Aium. New Orleans, 1990.
38. Stabile I, Olajide F, Chard T, Grudzinkas JG: Maternal serum alfa-fetoprotein levels in anembryonic pregnancy. Human Reproduction 1989;4:204–205.
39. Crooij MJ, Westhuis M, Shoemaker J, et al: Ultrasonographic measurement of the yolk sac. Br J Obstet Gynaecol 1982;89:931.
40. Reece EA, Pinter E, Leranth CZ, et al: Ultrastructural analysis of malformations of the embryonic neural axis induced by in vitro hyperglycemic conditions. Teratology 1985;3:363–373.
41. Sauerbrei E, Cooperberg PL, Plland BF: Ultrasound demonstration of the normal fetal yolk sac. J Clin Ultrasound 1980;8:217–229.
42. Bernard KG, Cooperberg PL: Sonographic differentiation between blighted ovum and early viable pregnancy. AJR 1985;144:597–601.
43. Hurwitz RS: Yolk sac sign: sonographic appearance of the fetal yolk sac in missed abortion. J Ultrasound Med 1986;5:435–438.
44. Reece E, Scioscia AL, Pinter E, Hobbins C, Green J, Mahoney MJ, and Naftolin F: Prognostic significance of the human yolk sac assessed by ultrasonography. Obstet Gynecol 1988;159:1191–1194.
45. Jouppila P, Kirkinen P, Kahkonen M, et al: Ultrasonic abnormalities associated with the pathology fetal karyotype results during the early second trimester of pregnancy. Official Proceedings of the 1988 World Federation for Ultrasound in Medicine and Biology Meeting. J Ultrasound Med 1988;7:218.
46. Rubenstein JB, Swayne LC, Dise CA, et al: Placental changes in fetal triploidy syndrome. J Ultrasound Med 1986;4:545–550.
47. Lockwood C, Scioscia A, Stiller R, et al: Sonographic features of the triploid fetus. Am J Obstet Gynecol 1987;157:285–287.
48. Berkowitz RS, Goldstein DP, Bernstein MR: Management of partial molar pregnancy. Contemp Ob/Gyn 1986;27:77.

49. Berkowitz RS, Goldstein DP, Bernstein MR, Sablinska B: Subsequent pregnancy outcome in patients with molar pregnancy and gestational trophoblastic tumors. J Reprod Med 1987;32:680.

50. Suzuki M, Matsunobu A, Watita K, Osanai K: Hydatidiform mole with a surviving coexisting fetus. Obstet Gynecol 1980;56:384.

51. Kushnir O, Vigie D, Izquierdo L, Schiff M, Curet L: Vaginal ultrasound assessment of cervical length changes during normal pregnancy. Am J Obstet Gynecol 1990;162:991–1000.

52. Grischke EM, Dietz HP, Schmidt W: Die Zervixlage im zweiten und dritten Trimenon: Vaginale Untersuchung versus Messung mittels Perinatal Scan—Verbesserte Indikationsstellung zur Cerclage? Geburtshilfe-Frauenheilkd 1988;48:364–368.

53. Ayers J, De Grood R, Compton A, Barclay M, Ansbacher R: Sonographic evaluation of cervical length in pregnancy: Diagnosis and management of preterm cervical effacement in patients at risk for premature delivery. Obstet Gynecol 1988;71:939–944.

54. Balde MD, Stolz W, Unteregger B, Bastert G: L'echographie transvaginale. Un apport dans le diagnostic de la beance du col uterine. J Gynecol Obstet Biol Reprod 1988;17:627–633.

55. Bohmer S, Dagenhardt F, Gerlach C, Jagala K, Schneider J: Vaginalsonographie versus vaginale Tastbefund: Erste Erfahrungen bei 120 schwangeren Frauen mit Verdacht auf Zervixinsuffizienz. Z Geburtshilfe Perinatol 1989;193:115–123.

56. Warren WB, Timor-Tritsch IE, Peisner DB, Raju S, Rosen MG: Dating the very early pregnancy by sequential appearance of embryonic structures. Am J Obstet Gynec 1989;161:749–753.

CHAPTER 13

Early Detection of Fetal Anomalies

Moshe Bronshtein, MD
Ilan E. Timor-Tritsch, MD
Shraga Rottem, MD, DSc

INTRODUCTION

The incidence of fetal anomalies warrants an extensive discussion of malformation detection by ultrasonography. It is estimated that about 3–5% of all newborns have congenital anomalies.[1] This figure does not take into consideration the anomalies for which detection occurred and pregnancy was terminated at an early stage.

The etiology of the congenital malformations is difficult to establish. In 1986, Beckman and Brent suggested the following breakdown of etiologies or the detected anomalies: genetic, chromosomal defects (20–25%); fetal infections (3–5%); maternal diseases (about 4%); drugs and medications (less than 1%); and unknown origin or multifactorial (65–75%).[2]

It is important to emphasize that birth defects are at the top of the list of causes for infant death before the age of one.

It is clear, therefore, that the detection of congenital anomalies is an important task of perinatal management. But more specifically, their early detection seems to be of utmost importance for taking the necessary steps in the management of patients demonstrating these anomalies. It has always been, and continues to be, the goal of perinatal medicine to detect malformations as early as possible. The reasons for this are multiple: to further test for chromosomal abnormalities; for early diagnosis to enable the termination of the pregnancy as early as possible; for planning the best way to follow up development of the fetus; for planning for delivery; and for planning for postnatal surgical intervention.

One example illustrating the yearning for early prenatal diagnosis is the evolution of the amniotic fluid testing for chromosomal anomalies.

Fetal karyotyping was initially based on amniocentesis performed at 16–18 weeks. Later, the possibility of an earlier amniocentesis was considered. With the development of transvaginally directed puncture procedures, the frontiers of the amniocentesis were pushed back further to 9–10 weeks of gestation. Performing chorionic villus sampling at 9 weeks is also aimed at early prenatal diagnosis.

Furthermore, the assessment of the fetal karyotype by examining fetal lymphocytes from maternal circulation was attempted in the late sixties, and is now reintroduced using the new technology. Recent experience from animal research showed that the karyotype may be obtained from in vitro embryos at the four-cell stage. However, testing for chromosomal abnormalities does not always lead to the detection of fetal anomalies, since a large number of structural anomalies do not carry chromosomal stigmata. Therefore, obstetrical ultrasound, more than any other technique, has complemented the prenatal diagnosis by permitting the detection of *structural anomalies*. The indications of prenatal ultrasonography have broadened dramatically over the past few years.

Among the major factors of importance that have to be considered in the management of a patient with a malformed fetus, the most important one seems to be *the gestational age at detection*. The options available for the patient are: (1) no intervention and follow-up scans, with a relatively insignificant malformation or the patient's desire for nonintervention; (2) future postnatal correction or selection of the best delivery route with a malformation amenable to surgical treatment (antepartum puncture or surgical treatment has been recently proposed and carried out in a selected number of specific anomalies); and (3) elective termination of the pregnancy or selective multifetal reduction of an affected twin or triplet.

All of the above-mentioned options take into consideration the gestational age at which the diagnosis can reliably be made. The earlier the diagnosis, the wider the management possibilities.

Ultrasonography is one of the important and probably most used laboratory modality for detecting fetal anomalies. This became evident after Campbell reported for the first time in 1972 the imaging of a fetal malformation by means of ultrasound technology.[4]

Two scanning routes are available at this time for sonographically imaging the fetus.

The Transabdominal Route

The contribution of TAS to detection of fetal malformations is uncontested. However, due to the resolution and other physical properties, the currently used transabdominal probes do not permit a *detailed* fetal structural evaluation prior to 16 weeks. Several very experienced centers have reported good results in relatively early detection of fetal structures. However, their accomplishment is due in great part to high skill. It is unreasonable to expect similar results of the larger body of operators. On the other hand, after 24 weeks, when imaging of anomalies becomes progressively easier, the legal aspects of a potential pregnancy termination may become an overwhelming factor.

The use of TAS in detection of fetal malformations and anomalies resulted in the compilation of extensive and detailed textbooks.[5,6]

It is undeniable that an early gestational age is of the essence in the detection of fetal abnormalities. Because of the small size of the first- and early second-trimester fetus and its close proximity to the vaginal vault, a new option is available in addition to the traditional transabdominal sonographic technique: high-resolution transvaginal sonography (TVS).

The Transvaginal Route

This route circumvents almost all physical obstacles of the transabdominal transducer probes and, as discussed in previous chapters (1, 3, and 11), allows for the use of high-frequency sound waves to create a clear, high-resolution image on the screen. The crisp, well-defined anatomy or pathology, therefore, becomes evident at an earlier gestational age. Even if better definition of an organ at a somewhat later gestational age is needed, this can be done with the vaginal probe provided the organ is within its focal range.

Since the introduction of high-frequency sonography, the list of malformations detected is continuously growing. The discovery of anomalies in the first or early second trimester has to be considered incidental since no widely applied screening programs have yet been launched. Only a few centers experiment with a centralized referral network; however, these scan a selected population, usually one at high risk for malformations. Not surprisingly, the time window, which until now was considered appropriate for the sonographic diagnosis of structural anomalies, slowly shifts from 16–24 weeks to 9–16 weeks. In Chapter 11 it was stated that a progressively increasing number of anatomic structures and organs can be imaged by transducer probes operating at 5–7.5 MHz.[7,8] The organ and structure detection rate and range is not only dependent on instrument quality but also on the sequential development of the targeted organs and structures.

This chapter, rather than pretending to be a systematic textbook of malformations, presents the updated literature and the experience of the authors in detecting early fetal structural anomalies. We thank those who have agreed to let their findings be included in this work.

A limited number of anomalies are included here simply because only a part of the potentially recognizable anomalies have been seen by the attentive eyes of a few who adopted this technique. As emphasized before, the list is not complete and new detections at surprisingly early gestational ages are continuously encountered.

Nevertheless, the malformations are discussed adhering to a systematic approach and discussion (organs and systems) where possible.

Guidelines for malformation workup using the vaginal probe. For technical information regarding the large variety of transvaginal probes and their use, the reader is referred to Chapters 1, 2, and 3. Some of the important work on which this chapter is based is discussed in Chapter 11.

The operator who is accustomed to the transabdominal route in malformation workup will immediately be aware of the similarities between TAS and TVS. However, there are important differences between the two ultrasonographic methods employed in scanning for abnormalities in the embryonic or early fetal period.

First, a good *knowledge of basic embryology* is required because the subsequently discovered structures can only be understood in light of their embryonic and fetal development. It is important, for example, to know that at 8–9 weeks of gestation there are ample sonolucent structures in the head which are not only normal, but cluster in a well-defined pattern (Figs 11.24 and 11.25). Furthermore, at 10–11 weeks the herniation of the midgut into the umbilical cord is normal. However, if the liver is herniated with the midgut into the cord this can be called omphalocele even before 11–12 weeks, based on the knowledge of embryology, reiterating the fact that the liver does not migrate throughout development as does the bowel. Finally, knowledge of physiologic brain development is essential to realize that around 14 weeks the choroid plexus "retracts" from the anterior horns of the lateral ventricles. Since the growth of the brain seems to lag behind in filling the space, an anterior cross section may falsely appear to the uninitiated as a ventricular enlargement (Fig 11.60).

Therefore, we not only emphasize the importance of the new imaging technique but also the importance of a thorough knowledge of embryology.

The *second* notable aspect differentiating TVS from TAS is *the use of scanning planes*. Scanning through the vagina allows only a certain restricted maneuverability of the probe. Therefore, the "scan-all-you-can-get" approach has to be adopted, rather than a more methodical and organized scanning routine searching for planes and sections as is usually done in abdominal scanning.

To improve the yield of scanning with TVS, listed below are several useful hints:

1. Record the scan by means of a high-definition VCR (the playback should be displayed on a high-definition TV screen). The structure in question may appear only for a short time on the screen. Therefore, playing back the tape using the frame-by-frame feature of the VCR enables scrutiny of the structure.

2. Be patient. Frequent and random fetal motion will eventually enable imaging of all or most structures.

3. If necessary, move the fetus gently by the abdominal hand while searching for anatomy or pathology.

4. If all fails, reschedule the patient for a rescan at a different time, hoping for a change in the fetal position.

5. Try to vary between the use of several available transducer frequencies. The 11–12 week fetus may "slip out" of the focal zone of a 7.5 MHz probe but can still be imaged using a 6.5 or a 5.0 MHz probe. Scanning a 14–15 week fetus may begin by using a higher frequency probe for the nearest fetal pole, but must be completed by using a lower frequency probe for the more remote pole of the fetus.

After this short technical consideration, several organs and organ systems will be reviewed as to their anomalies detected and defined by the transvaginal transducer probe.

EARLY SONOGRAPHIC FINDINGS OF MALFORMATIONS

The Central Nervous System (CNS)

For a broader list of brain malformations, see Chapter 15. Only a few CNS malformations detected by early TVS were reported.

Disorders of the Neural Tube Closure

The malformations belonging to this subcategory are: (1) anencephaly; (2) exencephaly; (3) anencephaly; and (4) meningoencephalocele, which include the spina bifida. The anencephaly and exencephaly will be discussed together.

Anencephaly. This disorder typically presents with the absence of cranial vault and brain tissue (Fig 13.1). The first report of an anencephaly at 11 weeks, and at the same time the first report of any anomaly diagnosed by TVS, was published in 1989 by one of the authors.[8]

The diagnosis of anencephaly can potentially be made starting from the tenth gestational week, since at this time, the shape of the normal head with the cranial

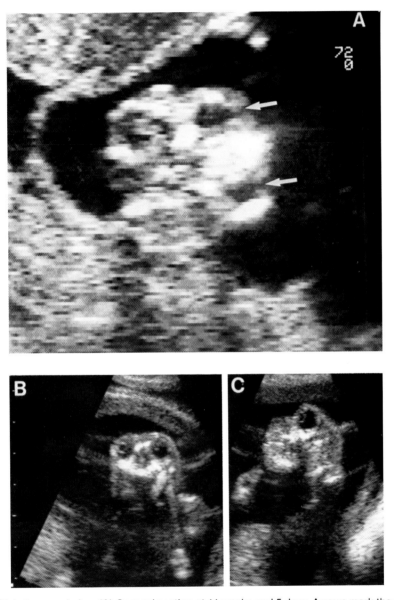

Figure 13.1 Anencephalus. (**A**) Coronal section at 11 weeks and 5 days. Arrows mark the orbits. (Rottem et al: Lancet, 1989;1:844. Used by permission.) (**B**) Typical coronal section through the orbits of an anencephalus at 14 weeks. (**C**) Sagittal images of the same fetus. Note the lens within the eye. (Courtesy of Dr. Israel Meizner. Soroka Medical Center, Beer Sheba, Israel.)

vault is final. However, it seems that there is some concern about *ruling out* the diagnosis of anencephaly until several weeks later. The reason for this may be its later development.

There is a significant controversy in the literature concerning the pathogenesis of this entity. Textbooks present anencephaly, exencephaly, and acrania as separate entities with scarce explanation as to their development. They merely reflect the pathological description of fetuses born with these anomalies. Transvaginal sonography may shed some light on the dynamic picture of the formation of this neural tube defect. Exencephaly was mentioned as the primary defect which may or may not progress to an anencephaly. It is not unreasonable to support a different theory: *acrania* may be the primary pathology that develops as a result of the absence of bony coverage of the brain (Figs 13.2 and 13.3). The soft brain tissue is left without adequate shielding, and is exposed to mechanical or chemical trauma.[9] Such an abrasion of the hemispheres may lead to their *partial destruction* resulting in *exencephaly*. If *extensive destruction* of the tissue occurs, the resulting and final pathological picture is the *anencephalic* fetus. In a small number of fetuses, for unknown reasons, the acrania is maintained without any apparent damage to the unshielded brain. However, as mentioned, this is a rare occurrence. This possible and local pathogenesis of the anencephalic fetus by means of abrasion and sloughing of the brain tissue to change the appearance of a fetus with acrania into an anencephalic is supported by an observation made by the author. In three out of five fetuses with acrania at 12 weeks, the "clear" sonolucent amniotic fluid which was present in a previous scan turned into one debris-containing and low-level echogenicity (Fig 13.4). This may have resulted from disintegration of brain tissue that took place in the time span between the scans. The final sonographic picture is that of a classical anencephalus. It is therefore important not to establish the final diagnosis of exencephaly, acrania, and anencephaly *before* the more extensive unification of the fetal cranium, ie, after 12 weeks of menstrual age.

Iniencephaly.   This is a complex neural tube defect involving the occiput (inion), foramen magnum, cervical and thoracic spine with exaggerated lordosis of the spine, as well as rachischisis. It is associated with omphalocele, gastroschisis, polycystic kidneys, and various limb deformities. It is easily diagnosed because of its typical appearance: a hyperextended head, no neck, and splaying of the spinal

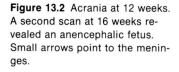

Figure 13.2 Acrania at 12 weeks. A second scan at 16 weeks revealed an anencephalic fetus. Small arrows point to the meninges.

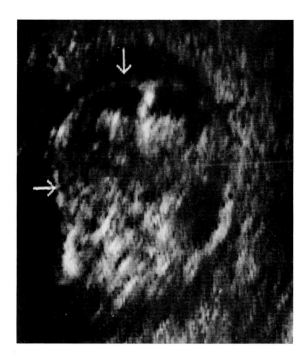

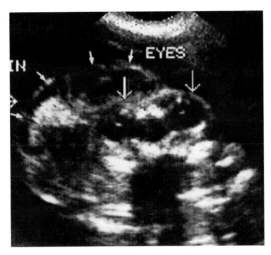

Figure 13.3 Acrania at 16 weeks. At 17 weeks an anencephalic fetus was diagnosed. Arrows point at the meninges.

column of various degrees. Its earliest diagnosis has been done at 9 weeks.[10] It seems that the first sign of this anomaly may be a lag in the expected measurement of the crown–rump length, due to the shortened section of the neck (Fig 13.5).

Meningoencephalocele.   This condition is diagnosed by the bulging of the meninges or the meninges-containing brain tissue through a bone deficiency in the

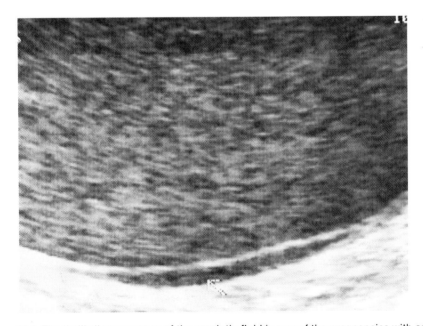

Figure 13.4 The "milky" appearance of the amniotic fluid in one of the pregnancies with anencephalus.

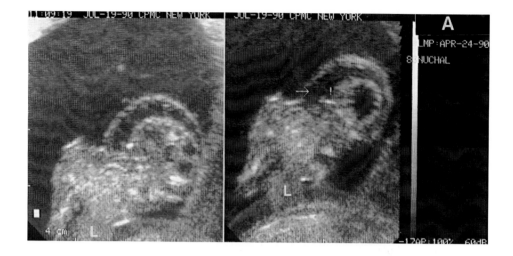

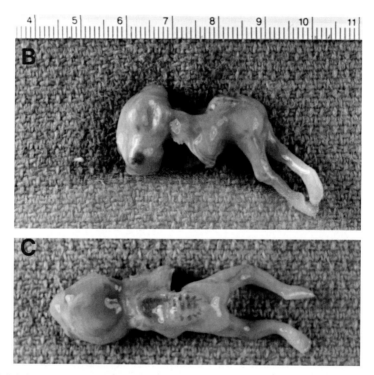

Figure 13.5 Iniencephalus. (**A**) Sonographic appearance: the sagittal plane at $12\frac{1}{2}$ weeks. Note the edematous appearance of the head, the brain anomaly, and the short trunk as well as the omphalocele, which contains the liver (L). (**B**) and (**C**) show the specimen with the shortened neck, the deformity of the spine, and the dorsal rachyschisis (the liver cannot be seen since it was disrupted as a result of termination of the pregnancy).

skull. The first time TVS was used in the diagnosis of an encephalocele, it was not in the first, but in the late second trimester.[11] This anomaly was diagnosed at the end of the first trimester by high-frequency TVS (Fig 13.6). The diagnostic features were: normal appearing face, small cranial vault, and brain tissue protruding posteriorly at the occipital area.

Spina Bifida.   Evaluation of the spine can be undertaken as soon as this structure can consistently be seen.[7,8] If only the contours are targeted and examined, this can be done as early as 9 weeks gestational age. At 12–14 weeks the individual vertebrae can be scrutinized, and a small spina bifida can be detected (Fig 13.7).

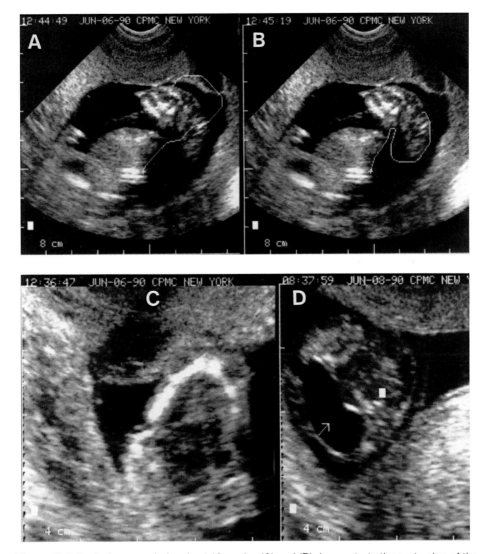

Figure 13.6 Posterior encephalocele at 12 weeks. (**A**) and (**B**) demonstrate the protrusion of the brain posteriorly (arrows). An outline of the imaginary normal skull as it would appear was drawn on the screen to demonstrate the pathology. (**C**) and (**D**) show axial sections of the head. (**C**) shows the brain within the sac of the encephalocele. (**D**) depicts the same section two days later. Note the empty structure representing the remnant of the previously seen image.

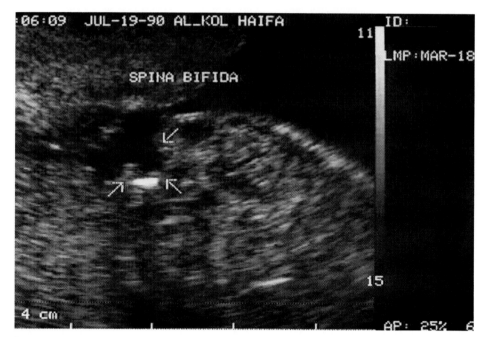

Figure 13.7 Spina bifida. Cross section of the fetal trunk at 14 weeks. Arrows point to the open spina bifida.

At this writing no reports are yet available in the literature of an early detection of small *occult spinal defects* or those involving one or two vertebrae. A more extensive involvement spanning across several vertebrae can be imaged as early as 11–12 weeks (Fig 13.8).[8]

Disorders of Ventral Induction

These malformations develop at 5 to 6 weeks of gestation. The representative lesion of this group is the holoprosencephaly. Depending upon the anatomic expression of the anomaly, one can distinguish between *alobar, lobar,* or *semilobar holoprosencephaly.* Figure 13.9 demonstrates some of the features of a monoventricular cavity lacking temporal and frontal horns.

Disorders of Agenesis and Disgenesis

These develop over a wide time span (8–24 weeks). For sonographic detection of the first subgroup of anomalies—*the cerebral abnormalities*—the role of TVS is rather limited. *Microcephaly*, for example, develops in the second trimester. Therefore, all TVS can offer, if used at all, is accurate biometry to lay the groundwork for a reliable comparative measurement in case the skull growth becomes stunted. *Hydranencephaly*, another anomaly of this group, is characterized by an "empty skull," postulated to be the result of occlusion of a major brain vessel. Figure 13.10 shows what was considered to be an "empty skull" at 11 weeks, but pathological confirmation in this case was not possible. Performing the termination of a pregnancy without obtaining the intact specimen usually leaves the question of morphological examination unanswered, because of its destructive nature.

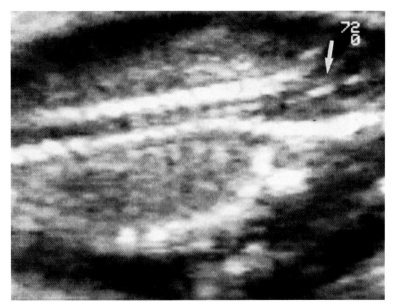

Figure 13.8 Spina bifida. Longitudinal scan of the fetal spine at 11 weeks and 5 days. The cervical spinal bifida is marked by the arrow. (From Rottem et al: First trimester transvaginal sonographic diagnosis of fetal anomalies. Lancet 1989;1:844. Used by permission.)

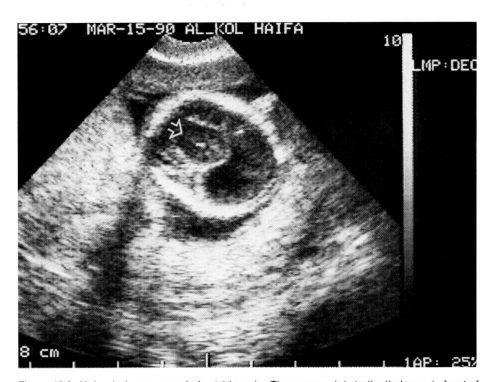

Figure 13.9 Alobar holoprosencephaly at 14 weeks. The arrow points to the thalamus in front of which the fluid-filled ventricle is seen.

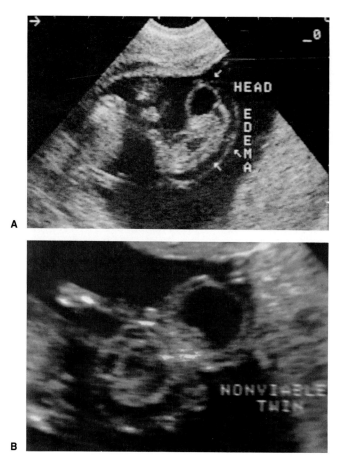

Figure 13.10 An empty skull at 10 weeks. This may be consistent with an early alobar holopro-sencephaly or a hydranencephaly. (**A**) The sagittal image showing the empty skull as well as some posterior contour edema. (**B**) A coronal section showing the fluid-filled skull. (Courtesy of Vickie Mahoney, Sonography Specialists, Virginia Beach, Virginia.)

The second group of abnormalities consists of *commissural anomalies* of which the agenesis of corpus callosum and septal agenesis were not yet described by early vaginal sonographic diagnosis.

Disorders of the Cortex

These cannot yet be addressed by TVS in the first and early second trimester since the surface of the brain is flat. The surface of the brain acquires gyri and sulci only in the latter half of the gestation.[12]

Disorders of Size

These are anomalies incorporating the *congenital hydrocephali* of various origins. Most experienced sonologists believe it is extremely difficult or virtually impossible to diagnose hydrocephalus in the first trimester. The same holds true for detection during the second trimester with one exception: a dilated ventricle can now be seen and imaged. The relative size of the lateral ventricle and the free-floating choroid plexus ("dangling choroid plexus") may be the only clues to the pathology. Unfortunately, in spite of some available measurements of the ventricles in early gestation,[12a] the diagnosis of ventricule megaly is still inconclusive due to their large standard deviations. Until more information is available, one should be cautious about diagnosing hydrocephalus in the first half of the pregnancy unless this is marked. Until then, it seems reasonable to use the word "ventriculomegaly" in order to express our gestalt diagnosis of a ventricle that appears larger than we would anticipate. The distancing of the choroid plexus from the midline and the "dangling choroid plexus" should represent serious warning signs as to the possibility of a developing ventriculomegaly. A series of axial images are presented here (Figs 13.11 and 13.12). These represent serial observations of patients with follow-up scans.

Dandy-Walker Malformation.   This consists of a posterior fossa-triangular-cyst, hypoplastic cerebellum, and partial or complete absence of the vermis, through which a communication with the dilated fourth ventricle exists. Sometimes agenesis of the corpus callosum as well as occasional chromosomal anomalies such as trisomy 18 and 13 can be associated.[13-17] There is some of the unknown in the structural pathogenesis of this disease.

Early diagnosis of Dandy-Walker malformation can potentially be done at or around 14 to 16 weeks, when the posterior fossa can reliably be scanned. Transvaginal sonographic examination of the posterior fossa can shed some light on the development of this disease. There are at least two yet unpublished cases of Dandy-Walker cysts which were diagnosed at 16 and 16½ weeks.[18] Figure 13.13 represents the cystic lesion as well as the absence of the vermis in a case of Dandy-Walker malformation detected at 17½ weeks in the posterior fossa.

Unclassified Anomalies

This is the last category of unclassified anomalies including the choroid plexus cysts and intracranial tumors as well as arachnoid cysts.

Choroid Plexus Cysts (Fig 13.14).   These are common findings and may be seen as early as 11 to 12 weeks, the time we can image the well-developed choroid plexi. They are found in about 50% of autopsied material.[19] Cundleish first described their sonographic appearance,[20] and there is controversy regarding their significance. The question remains: Are choroid plexus cysts a valid indication for chromosomal workup? A significant number of reports discuss the association or the lack of association of the choroid plexus cysts with trisomy 18.[21-32] Choroid plexus cysts can be seen early in pregnancy, about the time the choroid plexus can be imaged. By evaluating the data presented in the literature, it becomes clear that (1) a high-frequency probe results in a higher percentage of their detection;[31] (2) if a choroid plexus cyst is detected before the twentieth week, a sonographic malformation workup should be performed for aneuploidy-related malformations. The trisomy 18–related abnormalities include: neural tube defects, heart defects, cystic hygroma colli, diaphragmatic hernia, omphalocele, limb abnormalities, hydrocephalus, and micrognathia.[33-36] If such an anomaly is found, an amniocentesis or fetal blood sampling is warranted. (3) If no anatomic malformations are found in the presence of the choroid plexus cysts, a chromosomal mapping is probably not indicated, or the decision for its performance should be left to the provider. (4) Choroid plexus cyst size, number, and bilateralness may have a positive correlation with chromosomal abnormality and/or other malformations.[23,30]

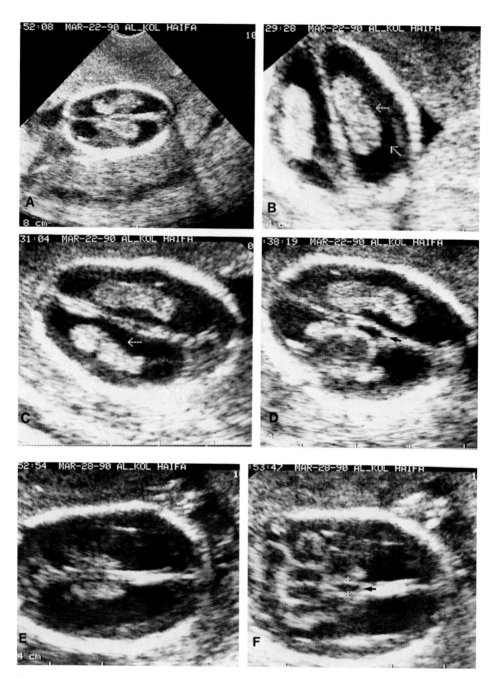

Figure 13.11 Ventriculomegaly at 14 and 15 weeks. Four axial sections at the level of the choroid plexus and the third ventricle. (**A–D**) demonstrate the relationship between the choroid plexus and the lateral ventricle at 14 weeks. The arrows mark the larger than usual gap between the inner lateral wall and the choroid plexus. (**C**) shows an unusually large distance between the midline and the choroid plexus (marked by an arrow). (**D**) reveals the third ventricle suspected to be slightly dilated (black arrow). (**E**) and (**F**) are follow-up scans one week later at 15 weeks, (**E**) showing widened lateral ventricle and relatively small choroid plexus, and (**F**) demonstrating, in addition to enlarged frontal horns, the continuing suspicion of widened third ventricle (black arrow).

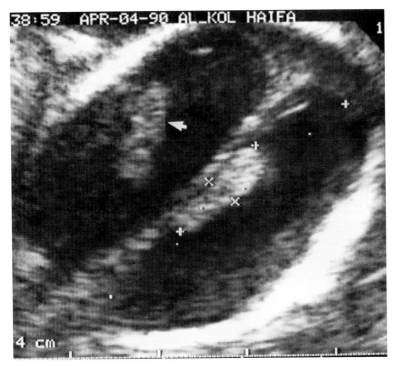

Figure 13.12 Ventriculomegaly at 16 weeks. Note the enlarged ventricles and the relatively small choroid plexus. The arrow points to the choroid plexus, which is freely moving within the lateral ventricle.

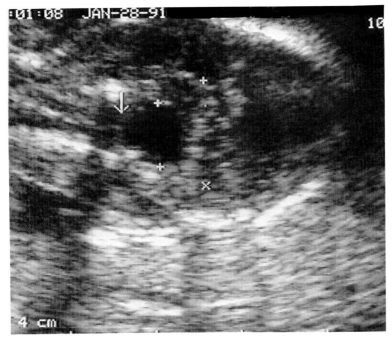

Figure 13.13 Coronal section of the posterior fossa. This 15-week fetus had holoprosencephaly and the dilatation of the posterior fossa is seen on this picture. This cystic dilatation is consistent with a Dandy-Walker cyst (arrow).

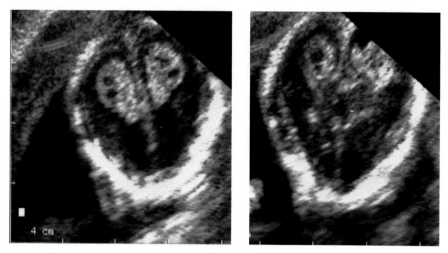

Figure 13.14 Choroid plexus cysts. Axial section at 14 weeks. The neonate appeared normal at birth. Neonatal brain scan was normal.

The question of management in the case of detection of choroid plexus cysts by high-resolution TVS still remains. Until more information on their transient nature or persistence, size and number, as well as uni- or bilateralness is available, it seems reasonable to adhere to the management guidelines emerging from the information available in the literature.

At times early TVS detects a fetus with obvious structural deformity of the head, brain, and spinal column (Fig 13.15). However, no positive identification of a specific anomaly or syndrome is evident. In these cases we believed the extent of the abnormality to be so extensive that termination of the pregnancy was undertaken. As mentioned before, because of tissue destruction inherent to some pregnancy termination techniques the specimen cannot be properly inspected and the anomaly diagnosed.

ANOMALIES OF THE GENITOURINARY TRACT

The fetal kidneys were sonographically imaged as early as $9\frac{1}{2}$ weeks;[37] however, detailed evaluation of their internal architecture using transabdominal sonography is possible at approximately 16–18 weeks.[38] Several excellent compilations of genitourinary anomalies based on transabdominal scanning are available.[5,6] Chapter 11 provides basic information about imaging the fetal kidneys and the urinary bladder by TVS. Early diagnosis of urinary tract anomalies is possible by TVS.

Ectopic kidney was diagnosed in the pelvis by imaging it at a close proximity to the iliac bone (Fig 13.16). Obstructive disorders of the urinary tract were imaged as early as 12 weeks (Fig 13.17**A,B**) and followed until 16 weeks by TVS to enable an accurate diagnosis (Fig 13.17**C–E**).

The multicystic dysplastic kidney or multicystic kidney diseases (MKD) were the earliest renal anomalies detected by TVS at 12 weeks.[39]

The affected kidney characteristically has no normal renal parenchyma.

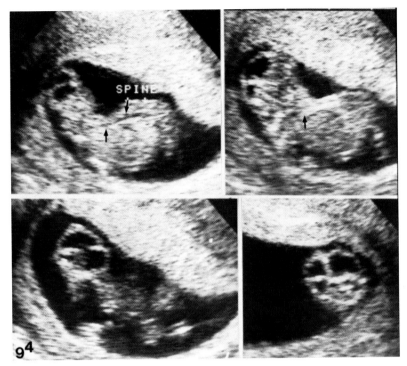

Figure 13.15 A fetus at 9 weeks and 4 days shows extensive anomalies. The spine is deformed and has kyphoscoliosis at around the thoracic area (arrow). The brain shows larger than usual and irregular sonolucent cystic areas. The final diagnosis of this anomaly was not made since termination of pregnancy resulted in destruction of the anatomy. (Courtesy of Vickie Mahoney, Sonography Specialists, Virginia Beach, Virginia.)

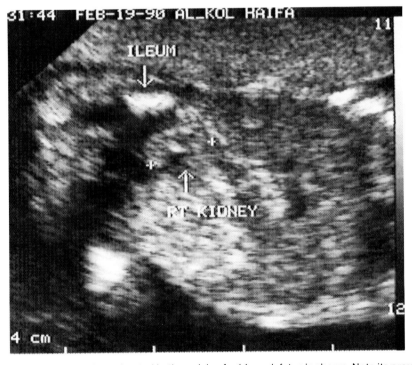

Figure 13.16 Ectopic kidney situated in the pelvis of a 14-week fetus is shown. Note its proximity to the iliac bone.

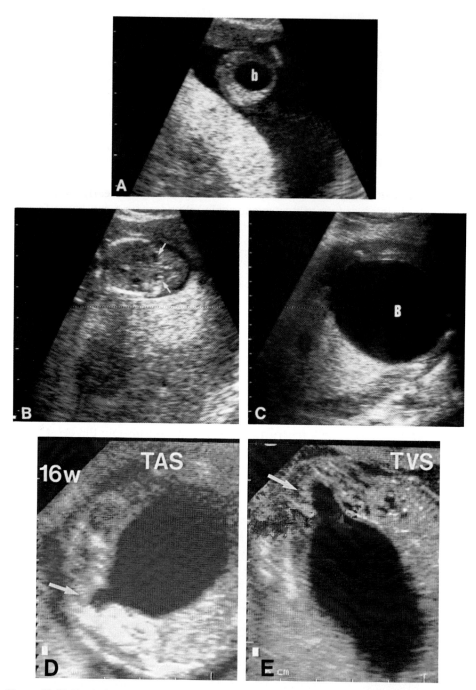

Figure 13.17 Fetal obstructive uropathy diagnosed transvaginally at 12 weeks of pregnancy. (**A**) The distended bladder (b) is evident. (**B**) Longitudinal scan through the fetal abdomen at 12 weeks demonstrating bilateral dilatation of the renal pelvis (arrows). (**C**) Longitudinal scan of the same fetus at 16 weeks gestation. The lack of amniotic fluid was evident. The distended fetal bladder (B) occupies most of the abdomen. The abortus had the classical appearance of Prune-Belly Syndrome. (**D**) Bladder outlet obstruction at 16 weeks; an image with the transabdominal probe. (**E**) Transvaginal probe demonstrating the thick bladder wall and the typical keyhole appearance of the bladder. (Figures A–C, courtesy of Dr. Israel Meizner. Soroka Medical Center, Beer Sheba, Israel.)

The renal parenchyma has a large number of sonolucent cystic structures leading to enlargement of the kidney. Usually the fetal bladder is not imaged and oligohydramnios is present or will develop. This disease may be unilateral (in this case there is amniotic fluid produced by the contralateral kidney) or bilateral. The contralateral kidney may be slightly hydronephrotic due to a compensating overproduction of urine.[40] In the second trimester a gradual enlargement of the abdominal girth is noticed. This represents an association of anomalies with MKD, such as cardiovascular anomalies, CNS abnormalities (mostly NTDs) diaphragmatic hernia, cleft palate, duodenal stenosis, imperforate anus, and tracheoesophageal fistula. Similarly, an increased number of anomalies was found in association with unilateral MKD.[41,42] The time of insult is early: between 8 and 11 weeks; therefore the diagnosis of the pathology may be aided by TVS. This early diagnosis is important since early first-trimester chorionic villus sampling can be performed for genetic workup. The termination of the pregnancy can be offered to the patient in the early second trimester.

An infantile type polycystic kidney at 14 weeks is shown in Figure 13.18.

ABDOMINAL WALL DEFECTS

Abdominal wall defects constitute a group of anomalies such as diaphragmatic hernia, omphalocele, gastroschisis, body stalk anomaly, and a more complex anomaly of the anterior midline, the pentalogy of Cantrell, and extrophy of the bladder.

The Diaphragmatic Hernia

This condition consists of a protrusion of abdominal organs into the chest cavity through a defect in the diaphragm. The diaphragm closes by the ninth week of gestation. Incomplete closure of the diaphragm at 10 weeks allows the herniation of abdominal organs into the thoracic cavity. The diagnosis is made by imaging the

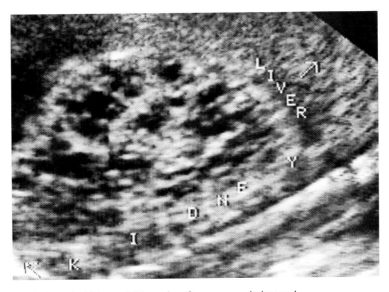

Figure 13.18 Polycystic kidney at 14 weeks of pregnancy is imaged.

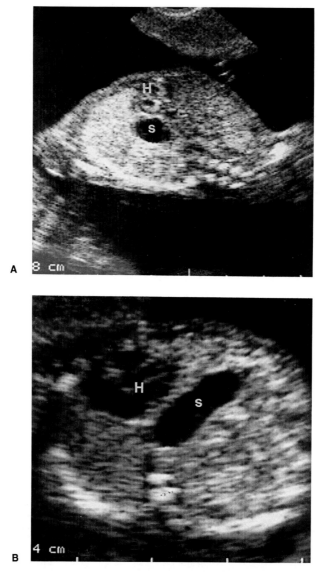

Figure 13.19 Diaphragmatic hernia. (**A**) Longitudinal scan of the trunk. (**B**) Cross section of the thorax in a fetus with diaphragmatic hernia at 16 weeks. Note that the stomach (s) is in the chest at the same level as the heart.

transverse section of the chest with both the heart and the herniated bowel on the same scanning plane. The stomach and loops of bowel displace the heart to the right. The earliest diagnosis of a diaphragmatic hernia by TVS has been made as soon as 16 weeks (Fig 13.19).[43] Our feeling is that the diagnosis could potentially be made earlier, probably at or after 13–14 weeks.

Hypoplastic lungs and malrotation of the gut are present in almost all cases. In addition to this, the number of cases with associated anomalies is high (50–57%) and includes those of several large groups of malformations, such as the nervous system, gastrointestinal, skeletal, cardiovascular, genitourinary, and others.[44,45] The association of diaphragmatic hernia with chromosomal abnormalities (mainly trisomy 21 but also 18) was also reported.[44–47]

Omphalocele

Omphalocele represents a ventral wall defect in which content of the abdominal cavity is herniated into a sac in close proximity to the umbilical cord and covered with a limiting membrane: the amnio-peritoneal membrane. If the anomaly of the ventral wall is more extensive and, in addition to the herniation of the umbilical area, the sternum, the diaphragm and the pericardium are involved, the anomaly is called *pentalogy of Cantrell*. In this "cephalic fold defect," the heart is in an ectopic position. The "caudal fold defect," which is the area below the umbilicus, is defective and contains the bladder extrophy. Figure 13.20**A** depicts the Cantrell anomaly at 11 weeks gestation. Before the early diagnosis of an omphalocele is considered one must be familiar with the physiologic midgut herniation which subsides at 12 weeks. It is easy to image and recognize the herniated midgut between 9 and 14 weeks by high-frequency TVS.[48] The hyperechoic nature of the still-nonfunctional bowel in early pregnancy can immediately be seen; however, its width at the level of the abdominal wall insertion rarely exceeds 1.5–2.0 times the width of the cord itself (Fig 11.33). If the omphalocele does not contain the liver it is difficult to make the diagnosis before 12 weeks because the bowel physiologically migrates into and returns from the cord by 12 weeks gestation. It is conceivable, therefore, that the normal ventral hernia is confused with and misdiagnosed as an omphalocele. If, however, with its typical echogenic properties the liver is seen within the sac, and knowing that the liver never "migrates" outside the permanent place below the diaphragm, we can make the diagnosis of a "liver-containing" omphalocele before 12 weeks (Fig 13.20**B**). Later, the detection of omphalocele by TVS does not present a problem (Fig 13.20**C,D**). This view is supported by the observations of Curtis and Watson.[49] From the literature it is evident that a basic difference exists between the "nonliver-containing" and the

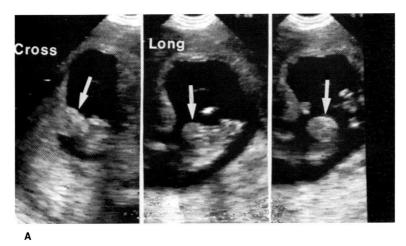

A

Figure 13.20 Ventral wall defects. (**A**) Pentology of Cantrell. Note that the heart (white arrow) is seen floating in the amniotic fluid on the cross and longitudinal sections. (Courtesy of L. B. Zielin, Rochester, New York.) (**B**) Omphalocele at 9½ weeks. The liver (marked by arrows) is seen to bulge into the physiologic midgut herniation. (**C**) The abdominal cross-sectional image of the same patient at 16 weeks demonstrating the membrane-covered liver (small arrows) as well as the stomach (S). (**D**) Omphalocele at 14 weeks. Note the membrane covering the liver (arrow). (Courtesy of Dr. I. Meizner, Soroka Medical Center, Beer Sheba, Israel.)

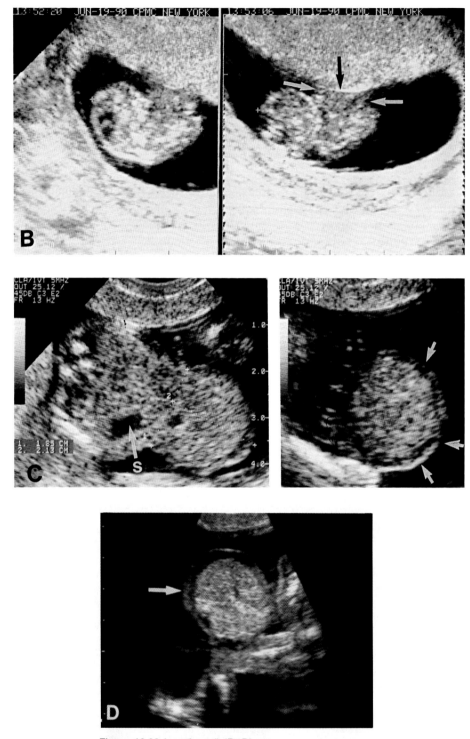

Figure 13.20 (*continued*) (B–D).

"liver-containing" omphalocele; the former having a larger association, the latter almost no association with chromosomal abnormalities.[50] Trisomy 18 and 13 are the more common chromosomal abnormalities associated with omphalocele. Others are trisomy 21, 45X0 and triploidies.[50,51]

The earliest reported diagnosis of omphalocele by TVS was at 13 weeks.[39]

The omphalocele (mostly the "nonliver-containing" type) must be differentiated from another entity which bears a very close "sonographical relationship" to the omphalocele.

Gastroschisis

Gastroschisis is the usually right-sided paraumbilical defect of the abdominal wall, probably resulting from a very early occlusion of the right umbilical or the omphalomesenteric vessel.[52] Through this opening the abdominal organs—usually only small bowel (the liver is very rarely found herniating in this anomaly)—protrude into the amniotic fluid without being covered with a limiting membrane. The gut may appear edematous and thickened because of the chemical exposure to the urine-containing amniotic fluid.[54]

The diagnosis of gastroschisis by TVS at 12 weeks and 3 days was reported.[53] The author concluded that this diagnosis can be made even before 12 weeks due to the technological advances (TVS) and the clear anatomic appearance of the free-floating bowel, which is not covered by membrane (Fig 13.23).

Abdominal Cysts

These cysts, sometimes of unknown origin, appear as large sonolucent cystic structures, and can at times be imaged in the abdominal cavity in the early second trimester. Figures 13.22**A** and **B** show a large intra-abdominal cyst at 14 weeks which vanished at around 20 weeks. The origin of the cysts, which disappeared

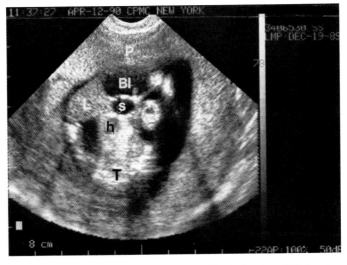

Figure 13.21 Body stalk anomaly at 16 weeks. The liver (L), the bladder (Bl), the stomach (s), and the heart (h) are found outside the trunk (T) and are in close proximity to the area of the placenta (P).

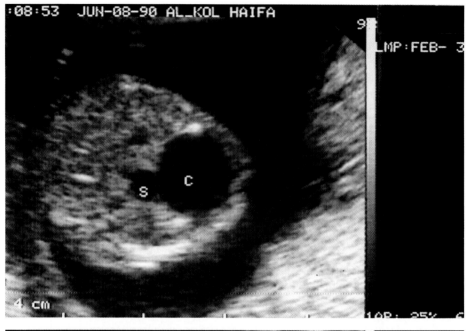

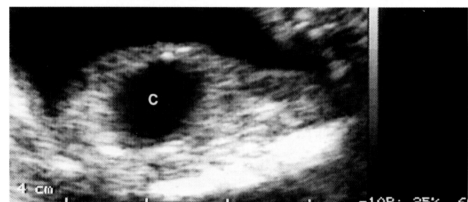

Figure 13.22 Abdominal cyst of unknown origin. (**A**) Longitudinal section. (**B**) Cross section of the fetal abdomen at 14 weeks. Note the abdominal cyst (C) and the stomach (S). Amniocentesis at 16 weeks revealed normal karyotype. The structure resolved at 20 weeks. A normal-term neonate was born.

after several weeks, could not be tracked down as belonging to any organ system such as kidney, ovary, or vitelline duct. The neonate was considered normal by the neonatologists.

Body Stalk Anomaly

This is an extensive abnormality of the anterior wall due to failure of the umbilical cord development. It is a rare disorder.[55] The amnion and part of the placenta in this anomaly cover the ectopically located abdominal organs in such a manner that the fetus appears to be connected directly to the placenta. The diagnosis of a body stalk anomaly was done at 16 weeks by TVS (Fig 13.21). Potentially, this malformation could be detected as early as 8–10 weeks.

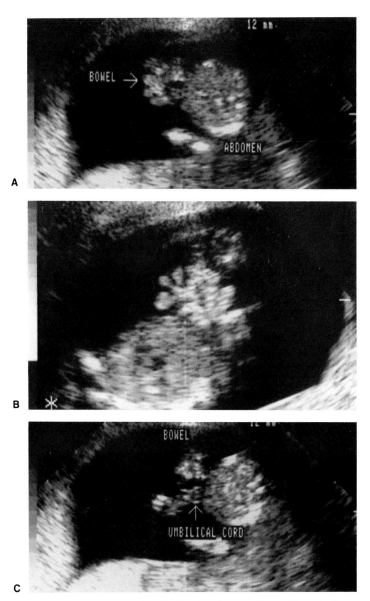

Figure 13.23 Gastroschisis at 12 weeks. (**A**) The free loops of bowel float in the amniotic fluid. (**B**) A magnified picture of the digit-like prothroganthis representing the free-floating bowel loops. (**C**) Note the insertion of the umbilical cord at a small distance from the right-sided ventral wall defect, enabling the bowel protrusion into the amniotic fluid. (Reprinted by permission from Guzman; Am J Obstet Gyn 1990;162:1253, The Mosby Co.).[53]

PATHOLOGY OF THE UMBILICAL CORD

Three kinds of structural anomalies are attributed to the umbilical cord.

Single Umbilical Artery

This, the most common pathological finding of the cord (0.2–1.0%) in all pregnancies,[55–58] probably results from degeneration of one of the two umbilical arteries. Its most important association is with congenital anomalies such as skeletal, cardiovascular, gastrointestinal, genitourinary, and CNS.[5,6,57–59] Of the commonly associated chromosomal anomalies, trisomy 18 and 13 were reported.[59–61] Based on the observations made, antenatal chromosomal studies seem indicated in cases where the detection of at least one additional anomaly to that of the single umbilical artery is found.[62] Transvaginal sonography enabled us to detect a cord with a single umbilical artery at 13 weeks (Fig 13.24).

Omphalomesenteric Cysts

Also called simply *umbilical cord cysts*, these are remnants of the omphalomesenteric duct which are lined with epithelium originating in the gastrointestinal tract. Their size is variable, and sonographically they appear sonolucent and thin-walled. Only a few cases were reported in the literature.[63] They are usually found close to the fetal insertion of the cord, are generally asymptomatic, and the prognosis is good. They may disappear in the second half of the pregnancy. Figures 13.18 and 13.25 depict umbilical cord cysts revealed by TVS at 10 weeks and 14 weeks, respectively. The one detected at 10 weeks was rescanned at 14 weeks during the malformation workup. The cysts at that time were smaller, and at 20 weeks could no longer be detected. The infant was normal at birth. The umbilical cord cyst may be associated with omphalocele, cardiac defects, trisomy 21, spina bifida, and cleft lip.[64]

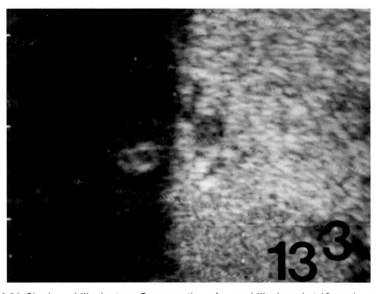

Figure 13.24 Single umbilical artery. Cross section of an umbilical cord at 13 weeks and 3 days.

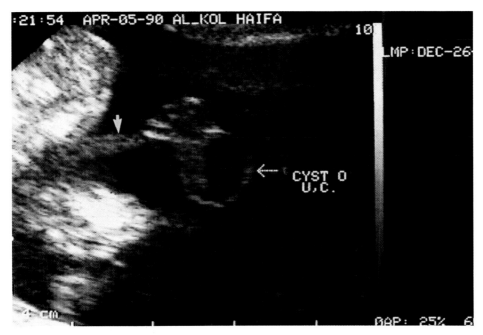

Figure 13.25 Umbilical cord cyst at 14 weeks and 2 days. The arrow points to the umbilical cord.

The Allantoid Cyst

This is an allantoid remnant lined with flattened epithelium and usually located close to the fetus, sometimes within its abdominal cavity. One case has been published in the literature.[65] A series of allantoid cysts of 1–1.5 cm were detected by TVS lying in close proximity to the abdominal wall and within the abdominal cavity at 12 weeks (Fig 13.26). A careful scan should be done to rule out genito-urinary anomalies and mechanical pressure on the cord or on other intra-abdominal organs.

FACE AND NECK ANOMALIES

The developing fetal face approaches final shape at 13–14 weeks. Starting at the tenth week, the fetal head gradually ''straightens up'' and extends slowly from its previous flexed position that prevented the study of the face with the use of high-frequency ultrasound equipment. Some of the important structures, the orbits, the palate, the mandible, can be targeted by TVS as early as 13–14 weeks.[7,8,66] The palate completes its midline closure only at 13 weeks.[67–69] The use of a high-frequency transvaginal probe, and the fact that the key anatomic structures to be scanned for possible malformations are in their final developmental stage at this point, resulted in the inclusion of the face and palate into the scheduled malformation workup at 13–15 weeks.[39,70] The earliest image of a cleft lip and palate was obtained at 15 weeks by one of the authors (MB) (Fig 13.27). Recently, the diagnosis of low-set ears was reported.[70]

Excellent and exhaustive reviews of sonographic evaluation of the face and

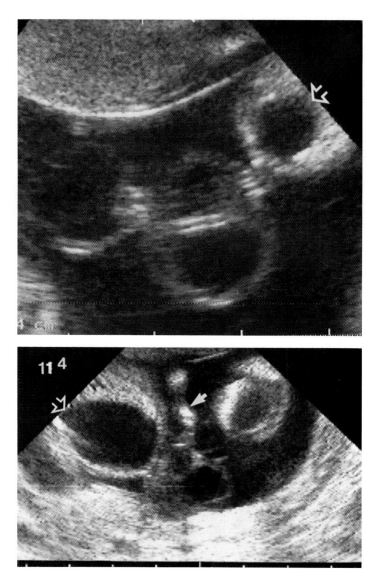

Figure 13.26 Allantoid cyst at 11 weeks and 4 days. One of the cysts (open arrow) is found within the abdominal cavity. The arrow marks the umbilical cord.

neck are available;[5,6] therefore, an attempt to discuss all anomalies detected by TAS here seems impractical. However, it it our belief that early detection of face and neck anomalies will soon follow in increasing numbers.

The Neck

The most common anomaly involving the neck is the *cystic hygroma colli* (CHC), reported to have an incidence of 1 in 120–6000 pregnancies.[71–93] The lesion probably arises from failure of the lymphatic drainage of the neck to connect with the internal jugular veins.

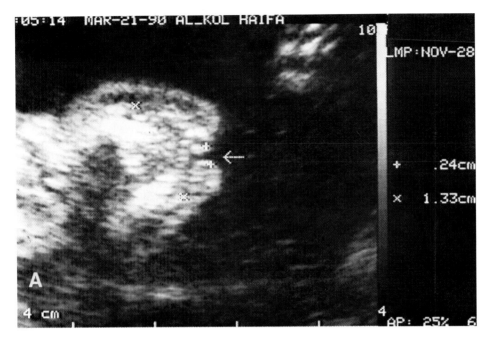

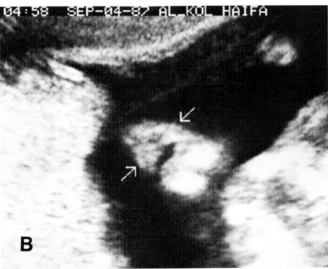

Figure 13.27 (**A**) Cleft lip and palate (arrow). Axial view at 15 weeks. (**B**) Normal lips for comparison.

Because of the relatively early appearance of the thickened nuchal fold, TVS has the distinct advantage of *detecting this structural anomaly very early*.[39,70,74–76] The natural course of these thick nuchal folds/cysts is now under extensive scrutiny. From the data available at the time of this writing, it appears that not all fetuses demonstrating this thick, sonolucent "fold," or "nuchal cysts" continue and result in a full-blown "cervical or nuchal cystic hygroma," heralding or being associated with a chromosomal disease (trisomy 21, 18, 13 or monosomy X).[76,77,121] Some of these elongated sonolucent nuchal structures found on the upper posterior sagittal contours of the fetus at 9–11 weeks disappear during the next several weeks. In the material studied by Pirrone et al[77] 20 out of 133 fetuses scanned before chorionic villus sampling (CVS) at 9 to 12 weeks had a thick nuchal fold. Seven of the 17 karyotypes obtained were normal, 2 fetuses no longer had heart activity at the time of the scan, and 1 patient did not return for CVS. All ten patients with normal karyotype continued the pregnancy, and in all fetuses the nuchal fold resolved. There seems to be a structural difference between repeated and nonseptated cystic hygromas (Fig 13.28). Bronshtein et al supported the concept of different prognosis for the CHC with or without septae.[76] In their eight cases, four with septae had a bad outcome as opposed to four without septae which resolved by midpregnancy and resulted in healthy neonates. In contrast, in a series of 30 cases the imaged thick nuchal fold/cysts were analyzed as to their outcome by the anatomic location (nuchal, cervical, lateral) and the chromosomal workup. The incidence of aneuploidy in the 30 cases was 53% and was found to be unrelated to their location or the presence of septae in the hygroma.[78]

Because of the at least 50% chance to detect a fetus with aneuploidy in the presence of a CHC which was found before 12–14 weeks, it now seems reasonable to offer immediate fetal karyotyping to the patient.

The findings associated with CHC are aneuploidy (mostly monosomy X and trisomy 21, 18, and 13), hydrops (about 75%), oligohydramnios (about 50–60%), and polyhydramnios.[73,79–82] If scanning is done in the first or early second trimester, remember that observations of CHC associations were made by late second- and third-trimester sonography.

The differential diagnosis of CHC in the first and early second trimester included the following:

1. A variant of the normal development.[65,121]
2. A temporary, resolving pathology of the lymphatic drainage. This theory is not yet supported in the literature but it may be a valid speculation based on observations of the natural course of this entity.
3. Local, more exaggerated expression of a generalized edema. A case of extensive edema of the fetal head and neck are shown in Figure 13.29.
4. Posterior meningocele or cephalocele.[73,83,84] However, TVS should be able to resolve the differential diagnosis clearly at 10–14 weeks due to high-resolution imaging of the nuchal area. Figure 13.6 depicts an occipital encephalocele and demonstrates the structural pathology to be differentiated from CHC.

Figure 13.28 Pathology of the nuchal-occipital area. (**A**) An axial section of the head showing nuchal cystic structure (H) at 11 weeks and 4 days. The karyotype was normal (c = choroid plexus). (**B**) Nuchal cystic structure shown on the longitudinal end cross-sectional planes at 10 weeks and 4 days. Karyotype was normal and the fetus was born normal. (Courtesy of Vickie Mahoney, Sonography Specialists, Virginia Beach, Virginia.) (**C**) Nuchal hygroma at 12 weeks with septum (arrow). The karyotype shows trisomy 21.

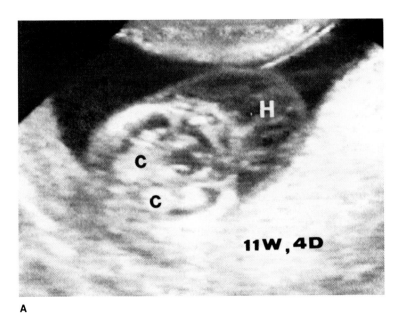

A

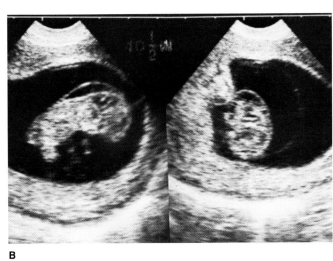

B

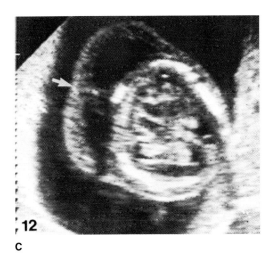

C

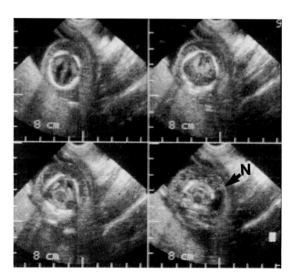

Figure 13.29 Three axial sections of the head and a section of the neck (N) showing extensive edema at 13 weeks. The CVS resulted in trisomy 21.

SKELETAL ANOMALIES

Transvaginal sonographic scanning of the skeletal system introduced a new dimension in imaging the first- and early second-trimester fetus. Chapter 11 of this book contains a description of the normal skeletal anatomy seen by TVS that is necessary to understand and scrutinize structural anomalies at an early fetal age.

The ossification of the maxilla, mandible, and clavicle begins at 8–9 weeks.[85,86] Transabdominal imaging and detailed description of the fetal extremities were reported by Mahony et al.[87] Some of the anomalies in which the skeletal system was involved will be discussed here.

Caudal Regression Syndrome

Also known as phocomelic diabetic embryopathy, this condition occurs in about 1 in 350 infants from diabetic mothers, representing a 200-fold increase over the rate seen in the general population.[88] The lesion probably originates in the midposterior-axis mesoderm of the embryo, causing an absence or dysplasia of the sacrum and associated anomalies.[89] It is also termed sacral agenesis. Baxi et al[90] and Meizner[91] reported on the detection of the caudal regression syndrome and its sonographic features from 9 to 17 weeks (Fig 13.30). Another spinal deformity is the *kyphoscoliosis* which was seen at 9 weeks and 4 days (Fig 13.15) in conjunction with a grossly abnormal appearance of the brain.

Conjoined Twins

This is not strictly a skeletal abnormality. Conjoined twins originate in failure of normal cleavage of the embryonic cell mass in a monozygotic twin. Transvaginal sonographic detection by the tenth week presents no problem (Fig 13.31). For an extensive review, the interested reader is referred to the pertinent literature.[92–100]

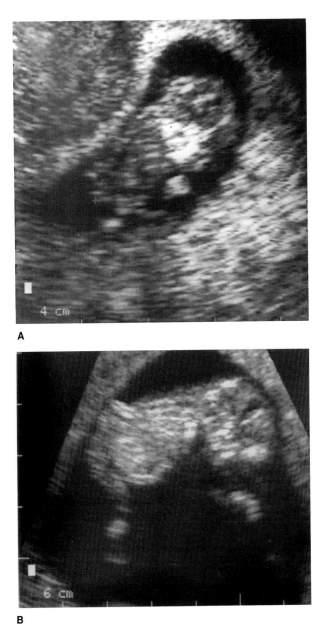

Figure 13.30 Caudal regression syndrome. (**A**) The crown-rump length showed stunted growth at 9 weeks and 4 days lagging 3–4 days behind a certain menstrual age. (**B**) The sagittal section of the spinal column at 11 weeks. (**C**) The spinal column and the deformity of the lower sacral area at 14 weeks. (**D**) The aborted specimen and its x-ray study at the seventeenth week. (Reprinted by permission; Baxi et al: Obstet Gynecol 1990;75:486, Elsevier Science Publishing Co.).[90]

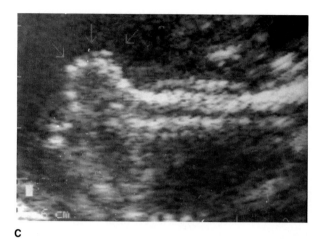

C

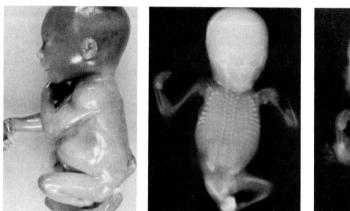
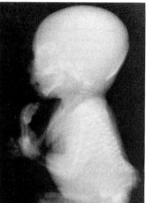

D

Figure 13.30 *(continued)* (C–D).

Anomalies of Extremities

These are common and can be examined by TVS as early as 11 weeks. Their sonographic diagnosis should not present technical problems.[8]

Clubfoot

Clubfoot and pes equinovarus were reportedly diagnosed at 13 weeks[39,39a]; images of these anomalies at 16 weeks are shown in Figures 13.32**A** and **B**.

Rockerbottom Foot

This was diagnosed by TVS at 16 weeks (Fig 13.33) in a fetus with trisomy 18.

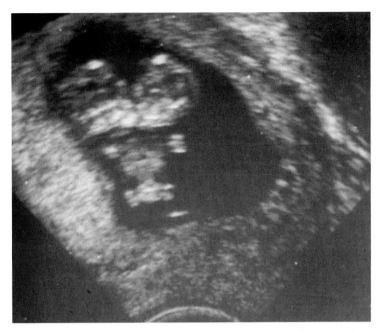

Figure 13.31 Conjoined twins with two heads, two upper, and two lower limbs are shown. One single heart was common to the two fetuses at 10 weeks gestational age. (Courtesy of D. Kepple, RDMS, University of Tennessee, Nashville, Tennessee.)

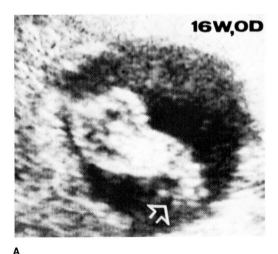

A

Figure 13.32 (**A**) Pes equinovarus at 16 weeks. (Reprinted by permission; Rottem et al: J Clin Ultrasound, 1990;18:307.)

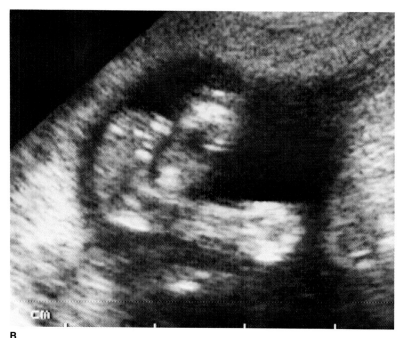

B
Figure 13.32 (*continued*) (B) Clubfoot at 16 weeks.

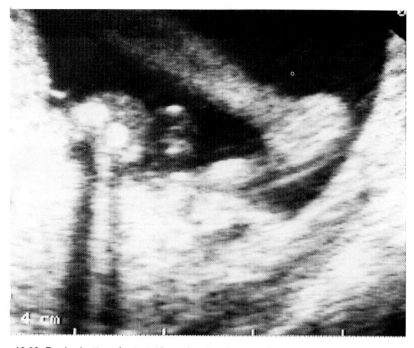

Figure 13.33 Rockerbottom foot at 16 weeks. Amniocentesis revealed trisomy 18.

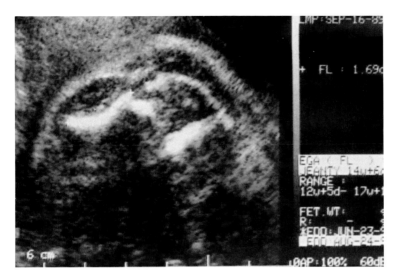

Figure 13.34 Short femur of a thanatophoric dwarf, measuring 1.69 cm at 23 weeks. Note the telephone receiver–shaped femur, which is typical for this dysplasia.

Skeletal Dysplasias

Transvaginal sonography can help define the subtle pathological features of long bones in cases of skeletal dysplasias. This is in addition to an early and very accurate measurement of the long bones. Figure 13.34 represents a picture of the femur in a fetus with *thanatophoric dysplasia* showing a femur of 1.69 cm with extensive bowing ("telephone receiver" shape).

Since the ratio of the femur length to the foot length is constant (1.0) from 14 weeks,[101] and the foot as well as the femur can easily be measured from 13 weeks on by TVS, the ratio should be used for a very early detection of short limb sequences.

CONGENITAL HEART DISEASE

Early detection of fetuses with congenital cardiac defects is important as the incidence of these abnormalities is 3 to 9 per 1000 live births, and nearly half of these fetuses have an associated extracardiac or chromosomal anomaly.[102–104]

The risk factors include:

1. *Family history:* The risk of congenital heart disease (CHD) recurring is about 1 in 50 if one previous sibling was affected, and one in 10 if two siblings had CHD.[105–107]
2. *Maternal diabetes:* This raises the risk of CHD five times over that of the general population.[108] Miller reported on a direct relationship between the maternal glycosilated hemoglobin (A_{1C}) levels and the risk of CHD.[109]
3. *Chromosomal abnormalities:* Detected in fetuses, these should raise the suspicion of CHD since the risk for it is significantly increased.[106] Trisomies have a particularly high incidence of CHD.[106,110]
4. *Teratogens:* Teratogens, such as oral contraceptives, alcohol, lithium, and anticonvulsants, were implicated in the association with CHD.

5. *Fetal hydrops and/or fetal arrhythmia:* When diagnosed, this is one of the possible causes for the development of CHD.[111,112]
6. *Other malformations:* If an anomaly rather than CHD is detected, a meticulous search for heart anomaly should be undertaken since there is a higher risk for genitourinary, CNS, and gastrointestinal anomalies with CHD.[113]

From the time Kleinman[114] reported on the possibility of accurately defining anomalies of the heart in utero, the use of ultrasonographic workup for the fetal heart has continuously increased.

Transabdominal imaging of cardiac anatomy and structural abnormalities is usually not possible before 16 weeks of gestation. There is only one case report on the detection of ventricular septal defect, hypertrophied ventricular walls, and pericardial effusion in a fetus of 14 weeks gestation.[115] With the constant improvement of equipment, as well as the advent of higher frequency TVS, the gestational age at which fetal CHD can be detected is steadily pushed back toward the beginning of the second trimester.

With the transvaginal technique, the four-chamber view of the fetal heart can be obtained in some cases as early as 11 weeks gestation, and in all fetuses at 13 weeks gestation.[8,70,116,117]

Previous studies have shown that the four-chamber view is a useful screen for the presence of congenital heart disease. Approximately 80% of heart abnormalities were detected in fetuses with an abnormal four-chamber view.[102,118] Recently, cardiac growth charts have been established for fetuses at 12–16 weeks gestation. The ventricles were found to be of equal size, and in a linear correlation to gestational age.[117] Gembruch et al[116] detected a complete arterioventricular canal defect and complete heart block in a fetus of 11 weeks gestation. Bronshtein et al[117] reported on five cardiac anomalies detected at 12–16 weeks gestation:

1. Ventricular septal defect and overriding aorta
2. Ventricular septal defect and pericardial effusion
3. Hypoplastic left heart
4. Cardiomegaly and pericardial effusion
5. Transposition of great arteries and ventricular septal defect (Fig 13.35)

Figure 13.36 represents a normal four-chamber view as well as a double outlet right ventricle diagnosed by one of the authors (Moshe Bronshtein).

The increasingly superb findings with the use of TVS will undoubtedly enable the detection of cardiac anomalies at the end of the first and beginning of the second trimester.

COMMENTS

There is no doubt that the introduction of transvaginal probes operating at higher frequencies can yield crisp images for diagnostic use in the first- and early second-trimester fetus. The natural questions that arise are: Do we have sufficient experience to offer malformation workup to pregnant women? To whom should this be offered and when should the scan be done?

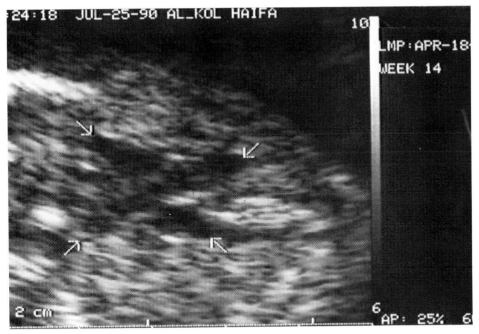

A

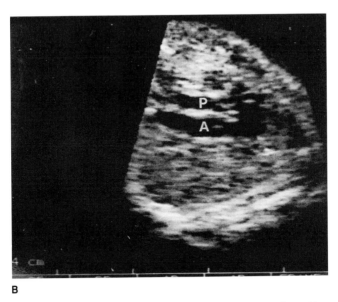

B

Figure 13.35 Transposition of the great vessels. (**A**) The normal cross-shaped image of the great vessels (arrows) at 14 weeks. (**B**) Parallel position of the pulmonary artery (P) and the dilated aorta (A).

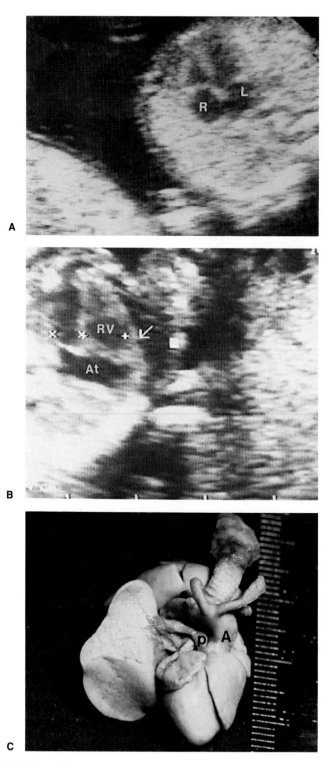

Figure 13.36 Double outlet right ventricle. (**A**) For comparison, a normal four-chamber view is shown at 14 weeks. Note the symmetrical sizes of the left and right heart which are marked. (**B**) The enlarged right ventricle (RV) and the unilocular atrium (At) are shown. (**C**) A pathologic specimen (A = aorta that is widened. p = pulmonary artery). Both emerge from the right ventricle.

Experience

The amount of information concerning TVS is continuously mounting. The foundation for a meaningful malformation workup is laid by the systemic studies on normal structural anatomy imaged by TVS.

The material presented in Chapter 11 and this chapter attests to the fact that normal anatomy and anomalies can be recognized, described, and defined. This can be done partially by TAS and more effectively by high-frequency TVS. The earlier the gestational age, the better TVS "performs." The increasing number of case reports on new and early detections of fetal anomalies contributes to the growing data base and builds the necessary experience to understand fetal dysmorphism.[119,120]

Who Should Be Scanned?

There is no doubt that patients who are at high risk for malformation, who have a child with an anomaly, or who have a malformation themselves should be offered the benefits of an early malformation workup. It is our firm belief that as time advances and the necessary knowledge increases (as well as the numbers of sophisticated equipment and those who receive TVS training during their residency programs), the scanning of all early pregnancies will be undertaken. This may be several years away; however, it seems to be unavoidable and most probably will become the standard of care.

When to Scan?

If a comprehensive scan has to be performed, it should be offered at a time when most of the organs can be scrutinized. Most centers performing extensive malformation workup feel that 13–15 weeks is the optimal time to take advantage of the vaginal probe and examine the largest possible number of organs or systems.

However, if a single organ or body part is targeted, this can undoubtedly be performed earlier at a time when the specific structure can consistently be imaged by TVS.

There are too few studies large enough to prove the statistical significance and the cost/benefit ratio of an early second-trimester malformation workup by TVS. The results achieved and presented at meetings and conferences, or published at the time of this writing, are encouraging as to the practical value of TVS in the early and comprehensive perinatal management of the pregnant patient.

REFERENCES

1. Shepard TH: Human teratogenicity. Adv Pediatr 1986;33:225.
2. Beckman DA, Brent RL: Mechanism of known environmental teratogens: drugs and chemicals. Clin Perinatol 1986;13:649.
3. Oakley GP: Frequency of human congenital malformation. Clin Perinatol 1986;13:545.
4. Campbell S, Johnstone FD, Holm EM, et al: Anencephaly: early ultrasonic diagnosis and active management. Lancet 1972;2:1226.
5. Romero R, Pilu G, Jeanty P, Ghidini A, Hobbins JC (eds): Prenatal Diagnosis of Congenital Anomalies. E. Norwalk, CT, Appleton & Lange, 1988, pp 255–301.
6. Nyberg DA, Mahony BS, Pretorius DA (eds): Diagnostic ultrasound of fetal anomalies: Text and Atlas. Chicago, Ill., Yearbook Medical Publishers, Inc., 1990, pp 433–491.

7. Rottem S: Targeted organ study of developmental anatomy from 4 to 14 weeks using a 6.5 MHz transvaginal probe. DSc Thesis. Technion-Israel Institute of Technology, Haifa, Israel, 1989.

8. Rottem S, Bronshtein M, Thaler I, Brandes JM: First trimester transvaginal sonographic diagnosis of fetal anomalies. Lancet 1989;1:444–445.

9. Kennedy KA, Flick KJ, Thurmond AS: First-trimester diagnosis of exencephaly. Am J Obstet Gynecol 1990;162:461–463.

10. Shoham ZS, Caspi B, Chemke J, Dagani R, Lancet M: Inicencephaly: prenatal ultrasonographic diagnosis—a case report. J Perinat Med 1988;16:139.

11. Cullen MT, Athanassidiasis AP, Romero R: Prenatal diagnosis of anterior parietal encephalocele with transvaginal sonography. Obstet Gynecol 1990;75:489.

12. Chi JG, Dooling EC, Gilles FH: Gyral development of the human brain. Ann Neurol 1977;1:86–93.

12a. Kushnir O, Shalev J, Bronshtein M, et al: Fetal intracranial anatomy in the first trimester of pregnancy: transvaginal ultrasonographic evaluation. Neuroradiology 1989;31:222–225.

13. Kirkinen P, Jouppila P, Valkeakari E, et al: Ultrasonic evaluation of the Dandy-Walker syndrome. Obstet Gynecol 1982;59:185.

14. Fileni A, Colosimo C, Mirk P: Dandy-Walker syndrome: diagnosis in utero by means of ultrasound and CT correlations. Neuroradiology 1983;24:233.

15. Taylor GA, Sanders RC: Dandy-Walker syndrome: recognition by sonography. AJNR 1983;4:1203.

16. Nyberg DA, Cyr DR, Mack LA, et al: The Dandy-Walker malformation prenatal sonographic diagnosis and its clinical significance. J Ultrasound Med 1988;7:65.

17. Reuss PD, Pretorius DH, Johnson MJ: Dandy-Walker syndrome: a review of fifteen cases evaluated by prenatal sonography. Am J Obstet Gynecol 1989;161:401.

18. Achiron R, Tadmor O, Abulafia Y, et al: Advantages of transvaginal ultrasonography in detecting fetal anomalies during the first trimester pregnancy. Proceedings of the Seventh Congress of the EUROSON, Jerusalem, Israel, 1990, A8.

19. Shuangshoti S, Netsky MG: Neuroepithelial (colloid) cysts of the nervous system: further observations on pathogenesis, location, incidence and histochemistry. Neurology 1966;16:887.

20. Chudleigh P, Pearce JM, Campbell S: The prenatal diagnosis of transient cysts of the fetal choroid plexus. Prenat Diagn 1984;4:135.

21. Friday RO, Schwartz DB, Tuffli GA: Spontaneous intrauterine resolution of intraventricular cystic masses. J Ultrasound Med 1985;4:385.

22. Bundy AL, Saltzman DH, Pober B, et al: Antenatal sonographic findings in trisomy 18. J Ultrasound Med 1986;5:361.

23. Chitkara U, Cogswell C, Norton K, et al: Choroid plexus cysts in the fetus: a benign anatomic variant or pathologic entity? Report of 41 cases and review of the literature. Obstet Gynecol 1988;72:185.

24. Benacerraf BR: Asymptomatic cysts of the fetal choroid plexus in the second trimester. J Ultrasound Med 1987;6:475.

25. Farhood AI, Morris JH, Bieber FR: Transient cysts of the fetal choroid plexus: morphology and histogenesis. Am J Med Genet 1987;27:977.

26. DeRoo TR, Harris RD, Sargent SK, et al: Fetal choroid plexus cysts: prevalence, clinical significance and sonographic appearance. AJR 1988;151:1179.

27. Clark SL, DeVore GR, Sabey PL: Prenatal diagnosis of cysts of the fetal choroid plexus. Obstet Gynecol 1988;72:585.

28. Benacerraf BR, Laboda L: Cyst of the fetal choroid plexus: a normal variant. Am J Obstet Gynecol 1989;160:319.

29. Chan L, Hixson JL, Laifer SA, et al: A sonographic and karyotypic study of second-trimester fetal choroid plexus cysts. Obstet Gynecol 1989;73:703.

30. Hertzberg BS, Kay HH, Bowie JD: Fetal choroid plexus lesions: relationships of antenatal sonographic appearance to clinical outcome. J Ultrasound Med 1989;8:77.

31. Fitzsimmons J, Silson D, Pascoe-Mason J, et al: Choroid plexus cysts in fetuses with trisomy 18. Obstet Gynecol 1989;73:257.

32. Nicolaides KH, Rodek CH, Gosden CM: Rapid karyotyping in non-lethal fetal malformation. Lancet 1986;1:283.

33. Jones KL: Smith's Recognizable Patterns of Human Malformation, 4th ed. Philadelphia, WB Saunders, 1988, pp 16.

34. Benacerraf BR: The antenatal sonographic diagnosis of congenital clubfoot: a possible indication for amniocentesis. J Clin Ultrasound 1986;14:703.

35. Benacerraf BR, Adzick S: Fetal diaphragmatic hernia: ultrasound diagnosis and clinical outcome in 19 cases. Am J Obstet Gynecol 1987;156:573.

36. Benacerraf BR, Miller WA, Frigoletto FD: Sonographic detection of fetuses with trisomy 13 and 18: accuracy and limitations. Am J Obstet Gynecol 1988;168:404.

37. Mahoney BS, Filly RA: The genitourinary system in utero. Clin Diagn Ultrasound 1986;18:1.

38. Hadlock FP, Deter RL, Carpenter R, et al: Sonography of fetal urinary tract anomalies. AJR 1981;137:261.

39. Rottem S, Bronshtein M: Transvaginal sonographic diagnosis of congenital anomalies between 9 weeks and 16 weeks, menstrual age. J Clin Ultrasound 1990;18:307–314.

39a. Bronshtein M, Zimmer E: Transvaginal ultrasound diagnosis of fetal clubfeet at 13 weeks menstrual age. J Clin Ultrasound 1989;17:518–520.

40. Sanders RC, Hartman DS: The sonographic distinction between neonatal mulicystic kidney and hydronephrosis. Radiology 1984;154:621.

41. Bearman SP, Hine PL, Sanders RC: Multicystic kidney: a sonographic pattern. Radiology 1976;118:685.

42. Greene LF, Feinzaig W, Dahlin DC: Multicystic dysplasia of the kidney: with special reference to the contralateral kidney. J Urol 1971;103:482.

43. Bronshtein M. Personal communication.

44. David TJ, Illingworth CA: Diaphragmatic hernia in the southwest of England. J Med Genet 1976;13:253.

45. Butler NR, Claireaux AE: Congenital diaphragmatic hernia as a cause of perinatal mortality. Lancet 1962;1:586.

46. Hansen J, James S, Burrington J, et al: The decreasing incidence of pneumothorax and improving survival of infants with congenital diaphragmatic hernia. J Pediatr Surg 1984;19:305.

47. Harrison MR, Golbus MS, Filly RA: The Unborn Patient: Prenatal Diagnosis and Treatment. Orlando, Fl., Gruen & Stratton, 1984, pp 257–275.

48. Timor-Tritsch IE, Warren WB, Peisner DB, Pirrone E: First trimester midgut herniation: a high frequency transvaginal sonographic study. Am J Obstet Gynecol 1989;161:831–833.

49. Curtis JA, Watson L: Sonographic diagnosis of omphalocele in the first trimester of fetal gestation. J Ultrasound Med 1988;7:97–100.

50. Nyberg DA, Fitzsimmons J, Mack LA, et al: Chromosomal abnormalities in fetuses with omphalocele: significance of omphalocele contents. J Ultrasound Med 1989;8:299–308.

51. Gilbert WM, Nicolaides KH: Fetal omphalocele: associated malformations and chromosomal defects. Obstet Gynecol 1987;70:633–635.

52. Hoyme HE, Higginbottom MC, Jones KL: The vascular pathogenesis of gastroschisis: intrauterine interruption of the omphalomesenteric artery. J Pediatr 1981;98:228.

53. Guzman ER: Early prenatal diagnosis of gastroschisis with transvaginal ultrasonography. Am J Obstet Gynecol 1990;162:1253–1254.

54. Kluck P, Tibboel D, Van Der Kamp AWM, et al: The effect of fetal urine on the development of bowel in gastroschisis. J Pediatr Surg 1983;18:47–50.

55. Mann L, Ferguson-Smith MA, Desai M, et al: Prenatal assessment of anterior abdominal wall defects and their prognosis. Prenata Diagn 4;427:1984.

56. Faierman E: The significance of one umbilical artery. Arch Dis Child 1960;35:285–288.

57. Froehlich LA, Fukikura T: Significance of a single umbilical artery: report from the collaborative study of cerebral palsy. Am J Obstet Gynecol 1966;94:274–279.

58. Benirschke K, Bourne GL: The incidence and prognostic implication of congenital absence of one umbilical artery. Am J Obstet Gynecol 1960;79:251–254.

59. Byrne J, Blane WA: Malformations and chromosome anomalies in spontaneously aborted fetuses with single umbilical artery. Am J Obstet Gynecol 1985;1:340–342.

60. Lenoski EF, Medovy H: Single umbilical artery: incidence, clinical significance and relation to autosomal trisomy. Can Med Assoc J 1962;87:1229–1231.

61. Vlietinck RF, Thiery M, Orye E, et al: Significance of the single umbilical artery. Arch Dis Child 1972;47:639–642.

62. Nyberg DA, Shephard T, Mack LA, et al: Significance of a single umbilical artery in fetuses with CNS malformations. J Ultrasound Med 1988;7:265–273.

63. Heifetz SA, Rueda-Pedraza ME: Omphalomesenteric cyst of the umbilical cord. Pediatr Pathol 1983;1:325.

64. Doscher C: The patient omphalomesenteric duct. Illinois Medical Journal 1971;493–496.

65. Hertzberg BS, Bowie JD, Carroll BS, Killam AP, Ruiz P: Normal sonographic appearance of the fetal neck late in first trimester: the pseudomembrane. Radiology 1989;171:427–429.

66. Timor-Tritsch IE, Farine D, Rosen MG: A close look at early embryonic development with the high frequency transvaginal transducer. Am J Obstet Gynecol 1988;159:676–681.

67. England AM: Color Atlas of Life Before Birth: Normal Fetal Development. Chicago Year Book Medical, 1983.

68. Moore KL: The developing human. Philadelphia, W. B. Saunders, 1988.

69. Crelin ES: Development of the musculo skeletal system. Clin Symp 1981;33:1.

70. Cullen MT, Green J, Whetham J, Solofia C, Gabrielli S, Hobbins JC: Transvaginal ultrasonographic detection of congenital anomalies in the first trimester. Am J Obstet Gynecol 1990;163:466–476.

71. Rahmani MR, Fong KW, Connor TP: The varied sonographic appearance of cystic hygroma in utero. J Ultrasound Med 1986;5:165–168.

72. Byrne J, Blanc WA, Warburton D, et al: The significance of cystic hygroma in fetuses. Hum Pathol 1984;15:61–67.

73. Pearce JM, Griffin D, Campbell S: Cystic hygroma in trisomy 18 and 21. Prenat Diagn 1984;4:371–375.

74. Exalto N, Van Zalen R, Van Brandenburg WJA: Early prenatal diagnosis of cystic hygroma by real-time ultrasound. J Clin Ultrasound 1985;13:655–668.

75. Reuss A, Pijpers L, van Swaaij E, Jahoda MGJ, Wladimiroff JW: First-trimester diagnosis of recurrence of cystic hygroma using a vaginal ultrasound transducer. Eur J Obstet Gynecol Reprod Biol 1987;26:71–73.

76. Bronshtein M, Rottem S, Yoffe N, Blumenfeld Z: First-trimester and early second-trimester diagnosis of nuchal cystic hygroma by transvaginal sonography: diverse prognosis of the septated from the nonseptated lesion. Am J Obstet Gynecol 1989;161:78–84.

77. Pirrone EC, Timor-Tritsch IE: Clinical significance of the thickened nuchal fold in the first trimester fetus (submitted for publication).

78. Cullen MT, Gabrielli S, Green JJ, et al: Diagnosis and significance of cystic hygroma in the first trimester. Prenat Diagn 1990 (in press).

79. Chervenak FA, Isaacson G, Blakemore KJ, et al: Fetal cystic hygroma: cause and natural history. N Engl Med 1983;308:822–825.

80. Garden AS, Benzie RJ, Miskin M, et al: Fetal cystic hygroma colli: antenatal diagnosis, significance and management. Am J Obstet Gynecol 1986;154:221–225.

81. Pijpers L, Reuss A, Stewart PA, et al: Fetal cystic hygroma: prenatal diagnosis and management. Obstet Gynecol 1988;72:223–224.

82. Brown BSJ, Thompson DL: Ultrasonographic features of the fetal Turner syndrome. J Can Assoc Radiol 1984;35:40–46.

83. Bieber FR, Petres RE, Biebar JM, et al: Prenatal definition of a familial nuchal bleb simulating encephalocele. Birth Defects 1979;15:51–61.

84. Nevin NC, Nevin J, Thompson W, et al: Cystic hygroma simulating an encephalocele. Prenat Diagn 1983;3:249–252.

85. O'Rahilly R, Gardner E: The initial appearance of ossification in staged human embryos. Am J Anat 1972;134:291–308.

86. Chinn DH, Bolding DB, Callen PW, et al: Ultrasonographic identification of fetal lower extremity epiphyseal ossification centers. Radiology 1983;147:815–818.

87. Mahony BS, Filly RA: High-resolution sonographic assessment of the fetal extremities. J Ultrasound Med 1984;3:489–498.

88. Mills JL: Malformations in infants of diabetic mothers. Teratology 1984;25:385–394.

89. Gabbe SG, Cohen AW: Diabetes mellitus in pregnancy, in Bologneses RJ, Schwarz RH, Schneider J (eds): Perinatal Medicine: Management of the High Risk Fetus and Neonate. Baltimore, Williams and Wilkins, 1982, pp 336–347.

90. Baxi L, Waren W, Collins MH, Timor-Tritsch IE: Early detection of caudal regression syndrome with transvaginal scanning. Obstet Gynecol 1990;75:486–489.

91. Meizner I. Personal communication.

92. Schmidt W, Heberling D, Kubli F: Antepartum ultrasonographic diagnosis of conjoined twins in early pregnancy. Am J Obstet Gynecol 1981;139:961.

93. Siegfried MS, Koptik GF: Prenatal sonographic diagnosis of conjoined twins. Postgrad Med 1983;73:317.

94. Edmonds LD, Layde PM: Conjoined twins in the United States, 1970–1977. Teratology 1982;25:301.

95. Herbert NP, Cephalo RC, Koontz WL: Perinatal management of conjoined twins. Am J Perinatol 1983;1:58.

96. Maggio M, Callan NA, Hamod KA, et al: The first trimester ultrasonographic diagnosis of conjoined twins. Am J Obstet Gynecol 1985;152:883.
97. Sanders SP, Chin AJ, Parness IA, et al: Prenatal diagnosis of congenital heart defects in thoracoabdominally conjoined twins. N Engl J Med 1985;313:370.
98. Filler RM: Conjoined twins and their separation. Semin Perinatol 1986;10:82.
99. Somasundaram K, Wong KS: Ischiopagus tetrapus conjoined twins. Br J Surg 1986;73:738.
100. Votteler TP: Conjoined twins, in Welch KJ, Randolph JG, Ravitch MM, et al (eds): Pediatric Surgery. Chicago, Year Book, 1986, pp 771–779.
101. Campbell J, Henderson A, Campbell S: The fetal femur/foot ratio: a new parameter to assess dysplastic limb reduction. Obstet Gynecol 1988;72:181–184.
102. Allan LD, Crawford DC, Chita SK, Tynan MJ: Prenatal screening for congenital heart disease. Brit Med J 1986;292:1717–1719.
103. Berg KA, Clark EB, Astemborski JA, Bonghman JA: Detection of cardiovascular malformations by echocardiography: an indication for cytogenetic evaluation. Am J Obstet Gynecol 1988;159:477–481.
104. Ferencz C, Neill CA, Gonghman JA, Rubni JD, Brenner JI, Perry LW: Congenital cardiovascular malformations associated with chromosome abnormalities: an epidemiologic study. J Pediat 1989;114:79–86.
105. Copel JA, Pilu G, Kleinman CS: Congenital heart disease and extracardiac anomalies: associations and indications for fetal echocardiography. Am J Obstet Gynecol 1986;154:1121–1132.
106. Ferencz C, Rubin JD, McCarte RJ, et al: Cardiac and non-cardiac malformations: observations in a population-based study. Teratology 1987;35:367–378.
107. Boughman JA, Berg KA, Astemborski JA, et al: Familial risks of congenital heart defect assessed in a population-based epidemiologic study. Am J Med Genet 1987;26:839–849.
108. Rowland TW, Hubbell JP Jr, Nadas AS: Congenital heart disease in infants of diabetic mothers. J Pediatr 1973;83:815–820.
109. Miller E, Hare JW, Cloherty JP, et al: Elevated maternal hemoglobin A_{1C} in early pregnancy and major congenital anomalies in infants of diabetic mothers. N Engl J Med 1981;304:1331–1334.
110. Row RD, Uchida IA: Cardiac malformations in mongolism. Am J Med 1961;31:726–735.
111. Allan LD, Tynan M, Campbell S, et al: Identification of congenital cardiac malformations by echocardiography in the midtrimester fetus. Br Heart J 1981;46:358–362.
112. Crawford D, Chapman M, Allan LD: The assessment of persistent bradycardia in prenatal life. Br J Obstet Gynecol 1985;92:941–944.
113. Crawford DC, Chita SK, Allan LD: Prenatal detection of congenital heart disease: factors affecting obstetric management and survival. Am J Obstet Gynecol 1988;159:352–356.
114. Kleinman CS, Hobbins JC, Jaffe CC, et al: Echocardiographic studies of the fetal human fetus: prenatal diagnosis of congenital heart disease and cardiac dysrhythmias. Pediatrics 1980;65:1059–1065.
115. DeVore GR, Steiger RM, Larson EJ: Fetal echocardiography: the prenatal diagnosis of a ventricular septal defect in a 14-week fetus with pulmonary artery hypoplasia. Obstet Gynecol 1987;69:494–497.
116. Gembruch V, Knopfe G, Chatterjee M, Beld R, Hensmann M: First trimester diagnosis of fetal congenital heart disease of transvaginal two-dimensional and Doppler echocardiography. Obstet Gynecol 1990;75:496–498.
117. Bronshtein M, Sigler E, Zimmer EZ, Brandes JM, Blumenfeld Z: Cardiac anomalies: detection and establishment of nomograms at 12–16 weeks gestation by a high frequency transvaginal probe. Proceedings of the Third World Congress of Vaginosonography in Gynecology. San Antonio, Texas, 1990, pp 6–7.
118. Copel JA, Pilu G, Green J, Hobbins JC, Kleinman CS: Fetal echocardiographic screening for congenital heart disease: the importance of the four-chamber view. Am J Obstet Gynecol 1987;157:648–655.
119. Benacerraf BR: Examination of the second trimester fetus with severe oligohydramnios using transvaginal scanning. Obstet Gynecol 1990;75:491–493.
120. Weber TM, Hertzberg BS, Bowie JD: Use of endovaginal ultrasound to optimize visualization of the distal fetal spine in breech presentations. J Ultrasound Med 1990;9:519–524.
121. Tarantal FA, Hendrickx AG, O'Rahilly R: First trimester conceptus. Letter to the editor, J Ultrasound Med 1990;9:614–615.

CHAPTER 14

Think Ectopic

Shraga Rottem, MD, DSc
Ilan E. Timor-Tritsch, MD

EPIDEMIOLOGY

Reports indicate that during the last 15 years, there has been a marked increase in ectopic pregnancies throughout the world. In Sivin and Cooper's study[1] of 35,496 American women, the rate of ectopic pregnancy (EP) almost doubled between 1965 and 1976. Rubin et al[2] described an increase in rate from 4.5 to 9.4 per 1000 reported pregnancies. In Sweden, the rate of EP increased from 5.8 to 11.1 per 1000 conceptions in 15 years,[3] and in Great Britain, the rate per 1000 live births and therapeutic abortions increased from 3.2 to 4.3.

Ectopic pregnancy accounts for a significant rate of maternal death (26% of all maternal deaths in the United States), a fetal wastage of nearly 100%, and a high incidence of maternal morbidity.[4]

In 1980, a 3-week delay in making the correct diagnosis was reported in 14.4% of cases.[5] We believe it is possible to shorten this diagnostic delay time with the use of higher resolution ultrasound equipment together with the βhCG assay which is available most hours of the day. Nevertheless, the diagnostic and therapeutic problems of ectopic pregnancy are far from being solved.

The basic reason for the increase in the rate of EP is the fact that more adolescent girls are sexually active; with this comes sexually transmitted disease as well as pregnancy. The microorganisms causing ectopic pregnancy are usually the chlamydiae and *Neisseria gonorrhoeae*, but other microbes may be implicated in the resulting salpingitis as well. Therefore, it becomes increasingly important to consider ectopic pregnancy in the differential diagnosis of a teenager presenting with abdominal pain and irregular vaginal bleeding.

The chance of recurrence after one EP varies from 5% to 20%. Some women with a previous EP develop problems of infertility and never deliver a living child. According to Curran's projection, by the year 2000 at least 10% of all females of reproductive age will become involuntarily sterile as a result of the sequelae of pelvic inflammatory disease; more than 3% will experience an ectopic pregnancy.[6]

NONINVASIVE DIAGNOSIS OF ECTOPIC PREGNANCY

The noninvasive diagnostic "triad" of the "think ectopic" concept consists of clinical presentation, laboratory tests, and ultrasonographic scanning, detailed as follows.

Clinical Presentation

It is well known that the patient suspected of having an ectopic gestation presents with the triad of pain, abnormal vaginal bleeding, and pelvic mass; however, these signs are nonspecific and frequently misleading. Only 45% of a group of 245 patients suspected of ectopic pregnancy had the above-mentioned "classic triad."[7] Even in accordance with modern trends, it is not superfluous to mention the statement of Howard Kelly: "If one is confronted with a pelvic condition which follows no rules and conforms to no standards one should think of ectopic pregnancy, particularly if she has any menstrual irregularity and has incurred the risk of pregnancy." Other clinical signs may be amenorrhea, which is usually followed by irregular vaginal bleeding; shoulder pain; an enlarged soft uterus; vertigo; fainting; and shock. Symptoms need not always be present and are insufficiently precise to enable the diagnosis of an early ectopic pregnancy before rupture and intraperitoneal bleeding and their devastating consequences.

Pregnancy Tests

These tests are based on the determination of human chorionic gonadotropin (hCG). The amount of hCG doubles every 2 days, reaching a peak of 100 IU/mL at a gestational age of 6 weeks.[8] The first commercially available tests for hCG were immunological tests performed on blood or urine samples. The frequent false positive and false negative results, as well as the fact that they become positive about a week after a missed period, limited their effectiveness.[8] The hCG molecule cross-reacts with other hormones and medications and shows a false positive result in hematuria, in proteinuria, and, to add to the confusion, in tubo-ovarian abscess.[9] The cross-reactivity of hCG in ectopic pregnancy and in cases of tubo-ovarian abscesses was particularly worrisome because of the clinical closeness of the two entities.

The false negative results of the hCG assay in EP probably result from the low titer of hormone produced by the relatively small amount of trophoblastic tissue.[10]

Because of the limited value of the immunological hCG assay in differentiating between a normal intrauterine pregnancy and a very early EP (low sensitivity and specificity), clinicians sought more accurate ways of determining low titers of hCG. Introduction of the radioimmunoassay made possible measurement of levels of 0.1 IU.[11] The test is specific for the β chain of the hormone and, therefore, does not cross-react with other hormones or chemical compounds.

The levels of βhCG are closely correlated to the normally developing gestation, and because a negative result excluded pregnancy with 100% confidence,[10] this pregnancy test came into widespread use. Modifications of the laboratory procedure significantly reduced the time in which a result could be obtained by the clinician.[12] As a result of these advances, determination of the β-subunit of hCG became one of the cornerstones of correct diagnosis of ectopic pregnancy.[7,13,14]

Several laboratory methods are available to measure the level of βhCG in the serum. They basically reflect the purity of the reagents used. The most used reference values are the First International Reference Preparation (IRP) and the Second International Reference Preparation (SIR). About 1.8 mIU/mL IRP are equal to 1 mIU/mL of the IRP. For more information on the use of the various "discriminatory zones," the reader is referred to Chapter 6.

Sonography

The third noninvasive clinical tool in the workup of the patient with suspected faulty implantation of the embryo is sonography. A vast amount of literature deals with various aspects of the sonographic diagnosis of ectopic gestation. The diagnosis was usually made by viewing an empty but slightly enlarged uterus along with an adnexal mass and, sometimes, fluid in the cul-de-sac.[15] Over the years it became obvious that the "classic" sonographic findings of EP were not always present[15,16]; despite notable technical advances made in the last decade, transabdominal-transvesical sonography did not provide the expected solutions to the diagnostic problem presented by ectopic gestation. A significant contribution to the earliest possible diagnosis of ectopic gestation, using transabdominal ultrasound in conjunction with determination of βhCG levels, was made by Kadar et al in 1981.[17] They introduced the "discriminatory zone" of 6500 mIU/mL at which a normal intrauterine gestational sac should be detected. Nyberg et al, using more advanced sonographic equipment, reduced this "discriminatory zone" to 1800 mIU/mL or greater, levels at which they were first able to detect a normal intrauterine pregnancy.[18]

Unfortunately, transabdominal (transvesical) sonography (TAS) reaches diagnostic accuracy only by the seventh postmenstrual week of gestation. The false positive rate of diagnosis ranges between 3% and 30% (mean 16%); the false negative rate is lower: 2–35% (mean 5%).[19] Since diagnosis of ectopic pregnancy is reached before the seventh week in more than half the cases, only a few remaining patients with EP will benefit from the conventional, transabdominal sonographic examination.

Transvaginal sonography (TVS) is certain to overcome some of these limitations because of the high-resolution transducer and the conjecture that proximity to structures is involved in the process of diagnosing ectopic gestation.

INVASIVE DIAGNOSIS OF ECTOPIC PREGNANCY

The "invasive" diagnostic procedures for diagnosing an ectopic pregnancy are the *D&C, culdocentesis,* and *laparoscopy.*

In a "stable" patient with vaginal bleeding, an undefined intrauterine finding on transabdominal sonography, and a serum hCG level lower than 6500 mIU/mL and where the pregnancy is unwanted, a D&C may help confirm the diagnosis.[17] For its historical merit, culdocentesis must be mentioned here. This invasive technique is losing popularity because of its high false positive rate in cases of bleeding ovarian cysts as well as its high false negative rate in cases of unruptured "early" ectopic pregnancy; it is being replaced by noninvasive sonography coupled with βhCG determination.

In order to prove the redundant nature of culdocentesis in the management of ectopic pregnancy, we have to expand on the study performed by Vermesh et al.[20] In that study, the operative findings of 297 women undergoing surgical procedures for ectopic pregnancy were reviewed. In 252 cases culdocentesis was done prior to surgery. Of the 252 patients, 210 (83%) had a positive test and 42 (17%) had negative results. Aspiration of blood correctly predicted a ruptured ectopic in half of the cases; in 58% negative tests predicted an unruptured ectopic pregnancy. *Six patients without an ectopic pregnancy underwent unnecessary surgery for a positive culdocentesis, and 27 patients were discharged from the emergency room after negative test results but were subsequently found to have ectopic pregnancies.*

This study clearly demonstrates the "limited value of culdocentesis in a clinical setting where sensitive, rapid testing and pelvic ultrasonography are used."[20] ("Pelvic sonography" in this instance, refers to TVS.)

Laparoscopy, the third and last of the invasive techniques used to diagnose ectopic gestation, is well established; its use in diagnosing tubal pregnancies will continue until sonographic diagnosis becomes more reliable. The advantage of laparoscopy is its versatility. In cases of unruptured tubal gestation, the diagnostic procedure can continue as a therapeutic–surgical one. The need for hospitalization and anesthesia should not deter the managing team. Despite its high accuracy, laparoscopy may miss the diagnosis of a pregnancy if the fallopian tube is only slightly distended by a 0.5 cm gestational sac, or if technical difficulties are encountered in viewing the tubes, even though the false positive and false negative rates are low, both being about 3%.

The use of laparoscopy becomes extremely important in surgical management if an unruptured tubal gestation is diagnosed and the patient desires future pregnancies.[21] In the last few years, conservative laparoscopic procedures have been performed to extract the products of conception while preserving the tube.

USE OF THE TRANSVAGINAL PROBE IN THE WORKUP OF ECTOPIC PREGNANCY

A large body of information became available in the last few years dealing with the transvaginal sonographic imaging and diagnosis of ectopic pregnancy.[27-43] If possible, the sonographic workup should always start with a transvaginal scan. If the urinary bladder of the patient is full, one may proceed first to abdominal scanning. As mentioned before, a slightly reversed Trendelenburg position should be maintained throughout the examination.

A systematic approach is advised. Scan the uterus first, then the fallopian tube and the cul-de-sac, and, finally, look for rare but possible alternate sites of an ectopic gestation.

The procedures to be performed are discussed below in detail:

Uterus

Intrauterine Pregnancies. Intrauterine pregnancies can be documented with absolute reliability as early as 5 weeks from the LMP, regardless of patient obesity or position of the uterus. Very early imaging of embryonic and extraembryonic structures enhances the reliability of diagnosing a normal or abnormal intrauterine gestation. (For a detailed description the reader is referred to Chapters 11 and 12.) Once intrauterine pregnancy has been diagnosed, one may, with high confidence, discard the suspicion of ectopic pregnancy.

Endometrial Response to Extrauterine Pregnancy. The endometrium responds to adequate hormonal stimulation of the growing extrauterine gestation. Transvaginal sonography may demonstrate a highly echogenic, thickened endometrium. Eventually the ectopic and immature trophoblast ceases to secrete, leading to decidual degeneration and bleeding (Fig 14.1). This bleeding may have been what various authors[22-24] described as the "pseudogestational sac" (PGS) of ectopic

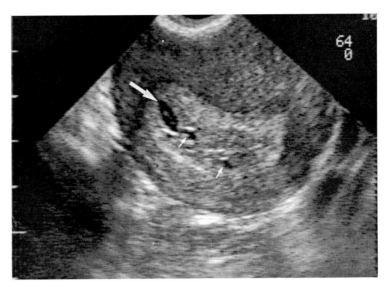

Figure 14.1 Transverse section of the uterus in a case of ectopic gestation. Note the thick endometrium with a clearly defined sonolucent area (large arrow) that is devoid of the decidual double ring of a normal gestation. The cavity line (small arrows) is marked by small sonolucent structures all of which may represent bleeding. The patient had vaginal spotting.

pregnancy. This PGS is primarily located symmetrically in the center of the uterus, outlining its cavity. If TVS detects an ectopic gestation early enough (at a time when no decidual degeneration has yet occurred), no intracavital bleeding occurs. Hence, no pseudogestational sac should be seen. Later, as mentioned earlier, hormonal support of the endometrium decreases and occult intracavital bleeding is imminent. Therefore, it is our feeling that this concealed bleeding was defined in classic transabdominal examinations as the pseudogestational sac. Appearance of this PGS may precede overt vaginal bleeding by several hours or days.

A *normal* or *true gestational sac* must show two distinct features easily demonstrated by TVS: first, a *double-contoured gestational sac* previously described by transabdominal sonography[24,25]; second, peculiar lacunar structures with a distinct flow appearing at one pole of the gestational sac (Fig 14.2**A**). These structures have not yet been described by others in the sonographic literature.[26] The lacunar formations can be demonstrated only by TVS and may be forerunners of the placental site. We believe that maternal blood flow to the site of implantation produces this picture. This flow was seen to persist around the gestational sac for several days after cessation of a previously detected fetal heartbeat in the case of abnormal gestations. If a pseudogestational sac was observed, no such flow could be visualized by transvaginal sonography. We had the impression that in a small number of tubal gestations these lacunar "lakes" showing blood flow could be seen (Fig. 14.2**B**).

Fallopian Tube

The Progressing Tubal Pregnancy. In the case of a live tubal pregnancy, the embryo will continue to grow until the tubal epithelium is able to "sustain" the

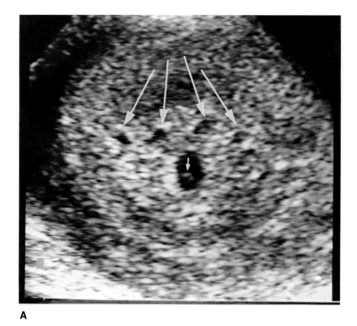

A

B

Figure 14.2 (**A**) A 5-week 2-day *intrauterine* gestation; the small arrow points to the yolk sac. The four long arrows point to lacunar structures. During real-time scan, flow is seen in these places. (**B**) Cross section of the fallopian tube at the level of the ampulla outlined by small arrows. Tubal wall is "invaded" by a trophoblast. Lacunar structures (large arrows) showing flow under real time can be observed. The gestational sac contains a live embryo (7 weeks gestation from the LMP).

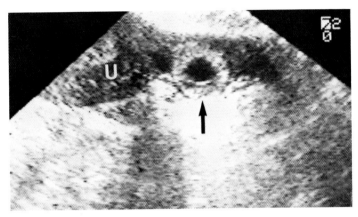

Figure 14.3 An ectopic, tubal chorionic sac at 5 weeks. No fetal pole or yolk sac was seen at this time.

already implanted sac. The similarity between the lacunar (maternal?) blood flow of a very early tubal gestation and the previously described lacunar blood flow of an intrauterine gestation (Fig 14.2**B**) is worth mentioning. In this early stage, development of the embryo and extraembryonic structures is similar to that in intrauterine gestation. At first, at 4½–5 weeks only a chorionic sac is seen in the tube (Fig 14.3). The ectopic gestational sac with a visible heartbeat, adjacent to the fetal pole, is revealed by transvaginal scanning (Fig 14.4). The advantage of the high-frequency transvaginal probe lies in its ability to visualize a live tubal pregnancy before its rupture or before tubal abortion occurs. Embryonic structures, such as the fetal pole with heartbeats, or extraembryonic structures, such as the yolk sac and the tiny placenta, may be recognized by the attentive sonographer (Figs 14.2–14.5). Once the diagnosis of tubal gestation has been made, exact location of the cyesis along the tube may be attempted.

During an analysis of cases of tubal pregnancy in which the diagnosis had been made by transvaginal sonography, it was noted that in most cases of *unruptured* tubal pregnancy (*with or without* the detection of fetal heartbeats) the tubal wall containing the sac was thickened, measuring 4–6 mm (Figs 14.2**B**, 14.3–14.7). As against the term ''adnexal ring'' used in TAS, we propose the more precise description *tubal ring*. Sometimes the blood clot fills the tube stretching its wall. In these cases the tubal ring may become thin (Fig 14.8).

Tubal Abortion. The ectopic and immature trophoblast in the tube may not secrete adequate quantities of hCG to sustain a normal corpus luteum. Corpus luteum insufficiency occurs and the embryo dies.

Development of the ''tubal embryo'' is dependent not only on the levels of secreted hormones but also on the trophoblast's ability to ''invade'' the underlying tissue to ensure blood support. Since this trophoblast will not be able to find an adequate decidual–placental bed, it will have to invade the muscular wall of the tube. This muscular wall is then weakened and eroded by the ingrowing chorionic tissue in search of supporting blood vessels. The stretching and erosion of the tubal wall result in bleeding into the sac as well as between the tubal wall and the gestational sac.

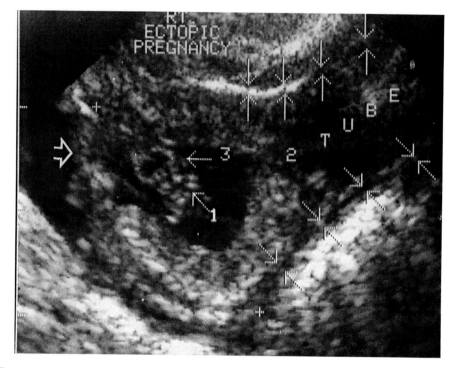

Figure 14.4 Unruptured right ampullar (2) pregnancy, 6 weeks and 3 days from the LMP. Fetal pole (1) and yolk sac (3) are evident. Arrows point to tubal contours. The open arrow points to the distal end of the tube (fimbrioplasty was performed 20 months prior to this ectopic pregnancy).

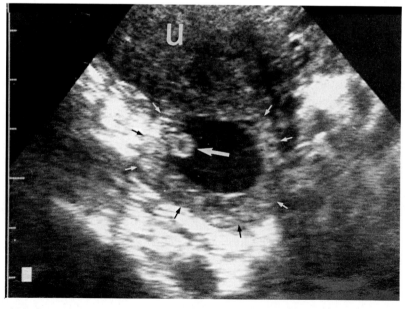

Figure 14.5 Cross section of an intact left tube (note its thick wall marked by small arrows) containing the gestational sac was visualized in the cul-de-sac below the uterus (u). This section shows the yolk sac (large arrow). The fetal pole with heartbeats was seen on a subsequent section.

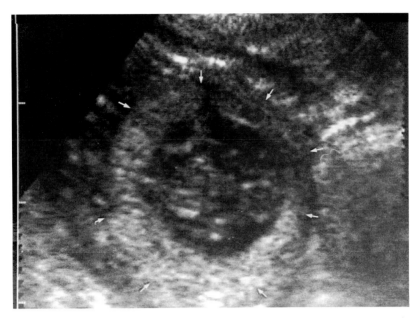

Figure 14.6 Cross section of the right salpinx is outlined by arrows. An irregularly echogenic substance was noted to fill its lumen. At surgery, a blood clot was extracted, along with the products of conception, from the unruptured ampullar section of the tube.

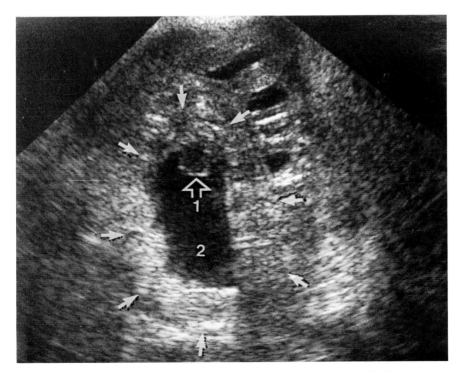

Figure 14.7 Arrows outline the cross section for a tube with gestational sac (2). The open arrow (1) points to the shrunken, amorphous fetal pole. No heartbeats were observed in this 6½-week ectopic gestation.

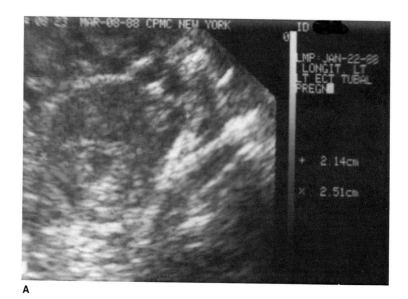

A

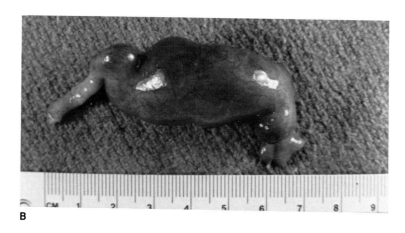

B

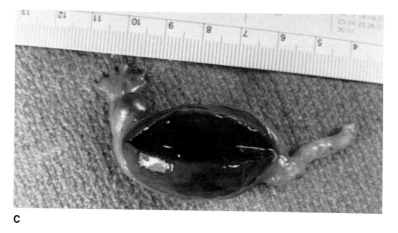

C

Figure 14.8 (**A**) The cross section of a thin tubal ring (arrows) contains mixed echoes. (**B**) The resected tube is distended by a blood clot (**C**) This is a type II tubal echogenic pregnancy.

Once the gestational sac has separated from the tubal wall, four events may occur[44]:

1. Rupture of the sac into the lumen of the tube (Fig 14.6)
2. Absorption of the gestation (Fig 14.7)
3. Abortion into the pelvis (extrusion of the ectopic gestation through the fimbrial end into the peritoneal cavity)
4. A slow blood leak or rupture of the tube leading to pelvic intraperitoneal fluid collection (Fig 14.9)

Cul-de-sac

Careful examination of the space posterior to the uterus may provide us with two important pieces of information:

(a) The *presence* of *free fluid* in an amount larger than normally detected, with or without blood clots (Fig 14.9). The blood clots are depicted as a bizarre-shaped mass of irregularly echogenic substance. They may float freely; thin chords of fibrin are attached to their surface. If the probe is gently moved in and out or the patient is asked to tilt her pelvis to the right and the left several times, the blood clots may be observed to move. When free fluid is detected one may search the tubes for more detailed information concerning the presence or absence of the tubal contents. As described in Chapter 3, this fluid creates optimal contrast for visualization of the tube, improving diagnostic accuracy. The importance of placing the patient in a reversed Trendelenburg position cannot be overstressed. If the

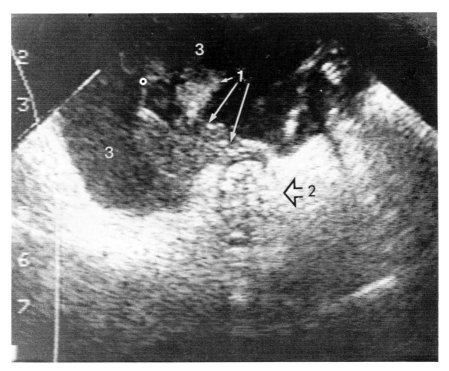

Figure 14.9 Irregularly shaped blood clots (1) surrounded by fluid (3), most probably blood, in the Douglas space anterior to the cross section of the rectum (2).

patient can stand up, she should do so and wait about 1 minute before assuming the proper position for the transvaginal scan. The examiner should patiently wait longer in anticipation of a possible slow appearance of fluid before making the diagnosis that ''no free fluid was detected in the pelvis.'' It is difficult to estimate large amounts of blood loss based on sonographic imaging of free blood and blood clots in the cul-de-sac. Other areas in the abdominal cavity should be scanned with TAS.

(b) *The absence of free fluid* excludes the possibility of active bleeding into the pelvis. In this case, the sonographer's attention must be directed to the uterus and the tubes as well as to other clinical and laboratory data to provide evidence for or rule out EP.

HOW CAN TRANSVAGINAL SONOGRAPHY HELP IN THE DIAGNOSIS AND MANAGEMENT OF ECTOPIC PREGNANCY?

Obviously, the diagnostic power of the transvaginal probe in general, and the 6.5 MHz probe in particular, lies in the superior imaging resulting from the high resolution. The diagnosis or exclusion of an ectopic gestation depends heavily on a combination of two or more of the following features:

Documentation of the Intrauterine Pregnancy and Extraembryonic Structures at a Very Early Stage

1. Appearance of the gestational sac at less than 5 weeks from the LMP
2. Early diagnosis of the typical echogenic chorionic ring of a normal gestation with lacunar flow adjacent to the gestation (described in Chapter 11)
3. Appearance and outlining of the yolk sac 5 weeks from the LMP
4. Detection of fetal heartbeats as early as 6 weeks from the LMP

Exclusion of Intrauterine Pregnancy by Documentation of the Lack of a Gestational Sac in the Uterus

In other words, TVS makes it possible to distinguish between a true gestational sac and an endometrial response to an ectopic gestation (eg, pseudogestational sac). Although it occurs rarely, a concomitant intrauterine and extrauterine pregnancy should always be kept in mind and ruled out.

Sonographic Documentation of Tubal Pregnancy

The diagnosis of *adnexal ring* (made prior to the use of TVS by abdominal scanning) can now be replaced by the more specific *tubal ring*. Imaging the typical ''tubal ring'' in cases of unruptured tubal EP is of the utmost importance. Embryonic structures (fetal pole, fetal heartbeats) and extraembryonic structures (yolk sac, cord, membranes, trophoblastic layers) are recognized with a great deal of accuracy in cases of progressing unruptured tubal gestation.

Fluid in Cul-de-sac

Precise and reliable evaluation of the cul-de-sac for presence or absence of fluid, with or without blood clots, is an important component of the diagnostic algorithm in cases of "leaking," unruptured, and/or ruptured tubal gestations.

THE DIFFERENTIAL DIAGNOSIS OF TUBAL PREGNANCY

The most prevalent and important images that mimic the tubal ring are the following.

1. *The Graafian follicle of the ovary.* Its wall is usually thin, thinner than that of a tubal ring. It is typically found within the ovary, surrounded by ovarian tissue of various thickness. The differential diagnostic problem usually arises when a static film is read.

2. *The corpus luteum of pregnancy.* If there is any particular structure that can be misdiagnosed as a tubal ring then the corpus luteum is the one. It usually presents as a ring-like structure but it has various shapes (Fig 7.5**A–F,** Chapter 7). Its size is from 2 to 4 cm in diameter and it usually has a 3–4 mm thick wall. It may or may not contain internal echoes just like a blood clot–containing tube. To try to differentiate it from a real tubal ring, multiple sections in various planes should be performed. Here are three useful features that differentiate the corpus luteum from a tubal ring:

   a. The first is that the *ovarian tissue is less echoic* than the tubal ring (Fig 14.10).

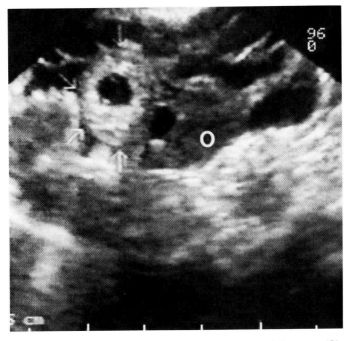

Figure 14.10 There is a clear difference between the echogenicity of the ovary (O) and the tubal ring containing a yolk sac (arrows).

   b. The second observation is that the tubal ring usually contains a *peculiar blood flow within the adjacent lacunar structures* of the ectopic placenta (Fig 14.2). This flow is better seen if the scanning frame rate is increased. If color flow Doppler is available, the trophoblastic tissue will show a much more increased flow than in the case of a corpus luteum.

   c. The third means to differentiate the corpus luteum from the tubal ring is based on the fact that they originate in different structures such as the tube and ovary which usually move freely in the pelvis. Therefore, if by the tip of the probe or the abdominal hand, these two structures are gently pushed, *they should show a sliding motion related to each other* (see Chapter 3). If in doubt, one should rely on the criteria of the different echogenicity between the tubal ring and the ovarian tissue.

4. *The small bowel.* This problem usually arises if a static film is read. On real time, the relatively fast peristalsis of the small bowel is readily observed.

5. *Other tubal pathology.* An example would be the cross section of a full fluid-filled tube (hydrosalpinx). Longitudinal sections should be attempted in order to observe the pear-shaped, evenly sonolucent hydrosalpinges.

6. *Uterine malformations.* An example would be bicornuate uterus. An intra-uterine pregnancy situated in one of the horns with decidual reaction and a small pseudogestational sac in the other horn may raise the false impression of a tubal ring with an ectopic gestation and an empty uterus holding a decidual cast.

7. *Nabothian cyst.* The novice sonographer may be confused by a dilated cervical gland. However, this structure is usually centrally located along or very close to the cervical canal and it is far from the adnexae. One should be extremely careful not to overlook the very rare case of cervical pregnancy and misdiagnose that structure as a Nabothian cyst.

The Transvaginal Sonographic Criteria for the Diagnosis of Ectopic Pregnancy

After the previously discussed "building blocks" of transvaginal sonographic findings, which help in the diagnosis of the ectopic gestation, we will propose the criteria for vaginal sonographic diagnosis of ectopic pregnancy.

These criteria were developed after scanning 1150 patients suspected of having an ectopic gestation.[45]

The transvaginal sonographic assessment of tubal pregnancy and its differential diagnosis were based on *six criteria:*

1. The presence or the absence of gestational structures within the Fallopian tubes. This includes the presence of the yolk sac, the fetal heartbeat, and the embryonic or fetal pole.

2. The presence or the absence of amorphous material (most probably blood clot) in a moderately or severely dilated Fallopian tube (Figure 14.8).

3. The presence or the absence of an indirect sign of ectopic pregnancy such as blood or blood clots in the pelvis.

4. The higher echogenicity of the suspected finding such as the tubal ring or its remnants relative to the ovary which has a relatively lower echogenicity (Figure 14.10).

5. The presence or absence of flow within the suspected sonographic finding of the tubal ring. Once again, color blood flow imaging can be of help in these instances.

6. The movement of the ovary containing the corpus luteum in relation to the suspected tubal ring. This can only be tested if they are on the same side. If gently pushed by the vaginal probe or the abdominal examining hand, they can be moved apart or may slide separately indicating that they are different structures.

MANAGEMENT OF THE TUBAL ECTOPIC GESTATION

Classification

By applying the previous imaging criteria to diagnose the tubal ectopic pregnancy, one can arrive at the practical classification of the ectopic pregnancies.

Type I—all those tubal ectopic pregnancies in which a fetal heartbeat and/or distinct embryonic and extraembryonic structures are seen in a discrete tubal ring with intensive blood flow in the trophoblastic tissue. If the gestational age is known and it was calculated that it is 5–5½ weeks or less, and within the tubal ring only a gestational or yolk sac can be seen, this should still be classified as type I in spite of the fact that no heart beats were seen.

The clinical meaning of the type I tubal ectopic pregnancy is *alive* and *unruptured tubal ectopic gestation.* Figures 14.2, 14.3, 14.5, 14.10, and 14.11 represent type I tubal ectopic gestations.

Type II—In the patients belonging to this group *a tubal ring of various thickness may be seen which may or may not show extraembryonic structures;* however, the distinguishing feature is that *no fetal heartbeats can be observed.* As said before, an ectopic pregnancy of 5 weeks, containing a chorionic sac or a yolk sac, is still classified as type I. The *clinical equivalent of the type II tubal ectopic pregnancy is a missed tubal ectopic pregnancy which contains a nonviable embryo or fetus and/or a blood clot.* Sometimes a small amount of free blood is found in the cul-de-sac. Figures 14.6, 14.7, and 14.8 depict type II tubal ectopic pregnancies.

Type III—this category of patients doesn't demonstrate a clear tubal ring and/or embryonic or extraembryonic structures. They have an empty uterus and a various amount of blood and blood clots in the cul-de-sac. Figure 14.9 represents a typical picture of type III tubal ectopic gestation. Clinically this patient has a ruptured or a severely bleeding tubal ectopic pregnancy. The importance of classifying the pictures, or tubal ectopic pregnancies, has an important practical aspect. By determining the type of ectopic pregnancy one can apply different kinds of treatment or management to these patients.

Management

Type I, the live tubal ectopic gestation, may be treated by the classical means of laparotomy and salpingostomy or by salpingectomy depending upon the clinical circumstances. Pelvicscopic and laser surgery were also applied to these patients avoiding more extensive abdominal intervention.[47,50] In the last years, an additional conservative treatment was suggested. Feichtinger and Kemeter[51] have pioneered this semi-invasive puncture procedure, treating an unruptured tubal gestation by injecting 10 mg of methotrexate in 1 ml of solution after aspirating the fluid contents of a gestational sac. A number of centers treated tubal ectopic gestations by salpingocentesis.[51–60] Salpingocentesis is extensively discussed in

Chapter 16. A rare case of twin tubal ectopic gestation is shown in Fig 14.11. The two yolk sacs in the two chorionic sacs were clearly seen in a patient having ascites due to Dranan hyperstimulation.

Type II, the nonlive, missed tubal ectopic gestation, can be treated in various ways. Laparotomy can be performed; however, this intervention is performed

Figure 14.11 A twin tubal ectopic gestation (arrows). (**A**) The two tubal rings contain a chorionic sac with yolk sacs and are surrounded by ascites. (**B**) The tube in situ at the laparotomy. (**C**) The resected tube is opened to show the two gestations it contains.

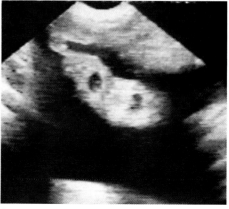

A

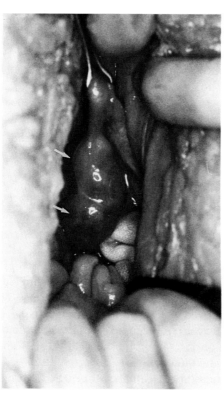

B

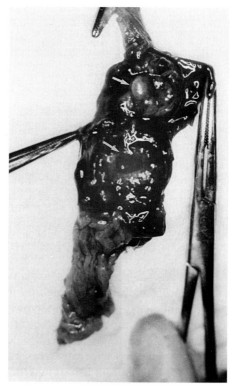

C

less and less due to alternate treatment modalities. Pelviscopic surgery can easily treat these tubal ectopic pregnancies. However, lately, patients having nonlive tubal ectopic gestations were successfully monitored and followed up by means of serial quantitative βhCG and transvaginal sonographic imaging.[61,62]

Type III, as mentioned before, is a *bleeding or ruptured ectopic pregnancy*. The classical treatment is still emergency laparotomy and control of the bleeding by salpingectomy for the partially or totally destroyed tube. Some skilled pelviscopic surgeons are able to manage these patients through the pelviscope.

OTHER POSSIBLE SITES OF ECTOPIC PREGNANCY

About 95% of ectopic pregnancies occur in the tube. However, one should always keep in mind the possibility of other ectopic sites such as *interstitial, ovarian, cornual, cervical,* and *abdominal pregnancies*. These relatively rare sites of implantation should not present a special diagnostic problem for TVS. In the last few years, cervical pregnancies were imaged by slowly withdrawing the probe after its contact with the cervix and at a distance of 2–3 cm. From the external os, the anterior and posterior lips as well as the cervical canal should be scrutinized.

A gestational sac partially surrounded by typical ovarian tissue should arouse suspicion of an ovarian pregnancy. Nevertheless, this diagnosis requires a very careful and prolonged examination and the prerequisite of this diagnosis should be that the gestational sac is surrounded by ovarian tissue.

The diagnosis of abdominal pregnancy is theoretically feasible provided that the implantation occurs within the pelvis inside the reach of the hectifocal range of the probe. Transabdominal sonography in these cases may help. Abdominal pregnancies however, occur at a very low rate (1.6% of ectopic pregnancies).

CONCLUDING REMARKS

The widespread use of TVS with the introduction of the high-frequency probes changed the gynecological practice. It is quite interesting to review the literature spanning the last three years. At first, the articles were reporting on the comparison of the new transvaginal method of diagnosing ectopic pregnancies with that of the golden standard used before, ie, the transabdominal sonographic method. In the last two years, however, the clinicians finally recognized the value of the transvaginal probe. This is reflected in the literature. An abundance of articles were reaching the obstetrical, gynecological, radiological, and ultrasonography journals, reporting on basically the same success rate in diagnosing the ectopic pregnancy. The specificity and sensitivity of the TVS in diagnosing and ruling out ectopic pregnancy were as high as 99.1% and 99%, respectively; whereas the positive and negative values of the past achieved 98.8% and 99.1%, respectively.[34]

As the articles are reviewed, fewer and fewer references are made to the use of the βhCG. However, the βhCG would still be an important laboratory tool to be used in conjunction with ultrasonographic methods to successfully manage these patients. It is clear today that the early diagnosis and treatment of ectopic pregnancy is based on the first line diagnostic test for any patient who is suspected of having an ectopic gestation and that is *transvaginal sonography*.

REFERENCES

1. Sivin I, Cooper T: IUD use and ectopic pregnancy rates in the United States. Contraception 1979;19:151–173.
2. Rubin GL, Peterson HB, Dorfman SF, et al: Ectopic pregnancy in the United States, 1970 through 1978. JAMA 1983;249:1725–1729.
3. Westrom L, Bengtsson L, Mardh PA: Incidence, trends and risks of ectopic pregnancy in a population of women. Br Med J 1981;282:15–18.
4. Tancer ML, Delke I, Veridiano NP: A fifteen year experience with ectopic pregnancy. Surg Gynecol Obstet 1981;152:179–183.
5. Hazelkamp JT: Ectopic pregnancy: diagnostic dilemma and delay. Int J Gynaecol Obstet 1980;17:598–601.
6. Curran JW: Economic consequences of pelvic inflammatory disease in the United States. Am J Obstet Gynecol 1980;138:848–851.
7. Schwartz RD, DiPietro DL: βhCG as a diagnostic aid for suspected ectopic pregnancy. Obstet Gynecol 1980;56:197–201.
8. Derman R, Edelman DA, Berger GS: Current status of immunologic pregnancy tests. Int J Gynaecol Obstet 1979;17:190–198.
9. Jacobson E, Rothe D: False positive hemagglutination tests for pregnancy with tubo-ovarian abscess. Int J Gynaecol Obstet 1980;17:307–312.
10. Rasor FL, Braunstein GD: A rapid modification of the βhCG radioimmunoassay. Use as an aid in the diagnosis of ectopic pregnancy. Obstet Gynecol 1977;50:553–557.
11. Vaitukaitis FL, Braunstein GD, Ross GT: Radioimmunoassay which specifically measures human chorionic gonadotrophin in the presence of luteinizing hormone. Am J Obstet Gynecol 1972;113:751–758.
12. Seppala M, Tontiti K, Ranta T, et al: Use of a rapid hCG beta-subunit radioimmunoassay in acute gynaecological emergencies. Lancet 1980;1:165–167.
13. Ackerman R, Deutsch S, Krumholtz B: Levels of human chorionic gonadotropin in unruptured and ruptured ectopic pregnancy. Obstet Gynecol 1982;60:13–16.
14. Kadar N, Taylor KJW, Rosenfield AT: Combined use of serum hCG and sonography in the diagnosis of ectopic pregnancy. Am J Roentgenol 1983;141:609–615.
15. Lawson, TL: Ectopic pregnancy, criteria and accuracy of ultrasonic diagnosis. Am J Roentgenol 1978;131:153–158.
16. Brown TW, Filly RA, Laing FC, et al: Analysis of ultrasonographic criteria in the evaluation for ectopic pregnancy. Am J Roentgenol 1978;131:967–971.
17. Kadar N, DeVore G, Romero R: Discriminatory hCG zone. Its use in sonographic evaluation for ectopic pregnancy. Obstet Gynecol 1981;58:156–161.
18. Nyberg DA, Filly RA, Mahoney BS, et al: Correlation of hCG levels and sonographic identification. Am J Roentgenol 1985;144:951–954.
19. Levi S, Leblicq P: The diagnostic value of ultrasonography in 342 suspected cases of ectopic pregnancy. Acta Obstet Gynecol Scand 1980;59:29–36.
20. Vermesh M, Graczykowsky JW, Sauer M: Reevaluation of the role of culdocentesis in the management of ectopic pregnancy. Am J Obstet Gynecol, 1990;162:411–413.
21. Stangel J: Newer methods of treatment of ectopic pregnancy, in De Cherney AH (ed): Ectopic Pregnancy. Rockville, Md, Aspen Publishers Inc, 1986, pp 89–102.
22. Weiner C: The pseudogestational sac in ectopic pregnancy. Am J Obstet Gynecol 1981;139:959–961.
23. Abramovici H, Auslender R, Lewin A, et al: Gestational–pseudogestational sac: A new ultrasonic criterion for differential diagnosis. Am J Obstet Gynecol 1983;145:377–379.
24. Nyberg DA, Laing FC, Filly RA, et al: Ultrasonic differentiation of the gestational sac of early pregnancy from the pseudogestational sac of ectopic pregnancy. Radiology 1978;146:755–759.
25. Bradley WC, Fiske CE, Filly RA: The double sac sign of early intrauterine pregnancy: Use in exclusion of ectopic pregnancy. Radiology 1982;143:223–226.
26. Timor-Tritsch IE, Rottem S: Transvaginal sonographic study of the Fallopian tube. Gynecol Obstet, 1987;70:424.
27. Nyberg DA, Mack LA, Jeffrey RB, Laing FC: Endovaginal sonographic evaluation of ectopic pregnancy prospective study. AJR, 1987;149:1181–1186.
28. Loong EP, Lee HC: Transvaginal ultrasonographic imaging of ectopic pregnancy. Aust NZJ Obstet Gynecol 1987;27:346–348.

29. deCrepigny LC: Demonstration of ectopic pregnancy by transvaginal ultrasound. Br J Obstet Gynecol 1988;95(12):1253–1256.

30. Shapiro BS, Cullen M, Taylor KJ, DeCherney AH: Transvaginal ultrasonography for the diagnosis of ectopic pregnancy. Fertil Steril 1988;50(3):425–429.

31. Dashefsky SM, Lyons EA, Levi CS, Lindsay DJ: Suspected ectopic pregnancy: endovaginal and transvesicle US. Radiology 1988;169(1):181–184.

32. Degenhardt F: Endosconography in extrauterine pregnancy. Geburtshilfe Grauenheilkd 1988;48(5):352–354 (German).

33. Funk A, Fendel H: Improved diagnosis of extrauterine pregnancy by endosonography. Z Geburtshilfe Preinatol 1988;192(2):49–53 (German).

34. Timor-Tritsch IE, Yeh MN, Peisner DB, Lesser KB, Slavik TAL: The use of transvaginal ultrasonography in the diagnosis of ectopic pregnancy. Am J Obstet Gynecol 1989;161(1):157–161.

35. Timor-Tritsch IE, Rottem S: Diagnosis and management of ectopic pregnancy using transvaginal sonography, in Fredericks CM (ed): Ectopic Pregnancy, Pathophysiology and Clinical Management. New York, Hemisphere Publishing Corp., 1989.

36. Russel JB, Cutler LR: Transvaginal detection of primary ovarian pregnancy with laparoscopic removal: a case report. Fertil Steril 1989;51(6):1055–1056.

37. Neiger R, Bailey S, Wall AM, Palmisano G: Diagnosis of ectopic using transvaginal ultrasound. J Reprod Med 1989;34(1):52–54.

38. Mattox JH, Kolb DJ, Goggin MW, Thomas WE: Heterotopic pregnancy diagnosed by endovaginal scanning. J Clin Ultrasound 1989;17(a):523–526.

39. Hill LM, Kilak S, Martin JG: Transvaginal sonographic detection of the pseudogestational sac associated with ectopic pregnancy. Obstet Gynecol 1990;75:986–988.

40. Kirikosky AL, Martin CM, Smeltzer JS: Transabdominal and transvaginal ultrasonography in the diagnosis of ectopic pregnancy: a comparative study. Am J Obstet Gynecol 1990;163:123–128.

41. Bateman BG, Nunley EC Jr, Kolp LA, Kitchin JD III, Felder R: Vaginal sonography findings and hCG dynamics of early intrauterine and tubal pregnancies. Obstet Gynecol 1990;75(3):421–427.

42. Goswamy RK, Williams G, Macnamee M: Two years experience using vaginal ultrasound as a diagnostic and therapeutic tool in the management of ectopic pregnancies. Human Reproduction 1988 3(supp 1). Abstract #241 from the fourth meeting of ESHRE.

43. Jansen RPS, Elliott PM: Angular intrauterine pregnancy. Obstet Gynecol 1981;58(2):167–175.

44. Parsons L, Sommers SC: Ectopic Pregnancy in Gynecology. Philadelphia, WB Saunders Co, 1978, pp 500–526.

45. Rottem S, Thaler I, Levron J, et al: Criteria for transvaginal sonographic diagnosis of ectopic pregnancy. J Clin Ultrasound 1990;18:274–279.

46. De Cherney AH, Romero R, Naftolin F: Surgical management of unruptured ectopic pregnancy. Fertil Steril 1981;35:21–24.

47. Shapiro HI, Adler DH: Excision of ectopic pregnancy through the laparoscope. Am J Obstet Gynecol 1973;1217:290.

48. Semm K: Advances in pelviscopic surgery. Prog Clin Biol Res 1982;112:127.

49. De Cherney AH, Diamond MP: Laparoscopic salpingostomy for ectopic pregnancy. Obstet Gynecol 1987;70:948.

50. Paulson JD, Asmar P: Use of CO_2 laser surgery in the treatment of tubal pregnancy, in Fredericks CM, Paulson JD, Holtz G (eds): Ectopic Pregnancy, Pathophysiology and Clinical Management. New York, Hemisphere Publishing Corp., 1989, pp 141–152.

51. Feichtinger W, Kemeter P: Conservative treatment of ectopic pregnancy by transvaginal aspiration under sonographic control and methotrexate injection. Lancet 1987;1:381.

52. Leeton J, Davison G: Nonsurgical management of unruptured tubal pregnancy with intraamniotic methotrexate: preliminary report of two cases. Fertil Steril 1988;50(1):167–169.

53. Timor-Tritsch IE, Baxi L, Peisner DB: Transvaginal salpingocentesis: a new technique for treating ectopic pregnancy. Am J Obstet Gynecol 1989;160(2):459–461.

54. Feichtinger W, Kemeter P: Treatment of unruptured ectopic pregnancy by needling of sac and injection of methotrexate or PG E_2 under transvaginal sonographic control. Arch Gynecol Obstet 1989;246:85–89.

55. Jeng CJ, Yang YG, Lan CC: Transvaginal ultrasound guided salpingocentesis with methotrexate injection: a minimally invasive treatment for early ectopic pregnancy. Proceedings of the Third World Congress on Vaginosonography in Gynecology, June 15, 1990, San Antonio, Tex.

56. Jansen CAM, Brandsma G, Cleveringa LM, Schats R, Vroegop I, Lankhorst PFC: Vaginal ultrasound puncture in the management of early ectopic pregnancy. Human Reproduction 1988 3(supp 1) Abstract #238 from the fourth meeting of ESHRE.

57. Popp L: Personal communication.
58. Gosswamy RK: Personal communication.
59. Kurjak A: Personal communication.
60. Menard A, Crequat J, Mandelbrot L, et al: Treatment of unruptured tubal pregnancy by local injection of methotrexate under transvaginal sonographic control. Fertil Steril 1990;54:47–50.
61. Mashiach S, Carp HJA, Serr DM: Nonoperative management of ectopic pregnancy: a preliminary report. J Reprod Med 1982;27:127.
62. Adoni A, Milwidsky A, Hurwitz A: Declining hCG levels: an indicator for expectant approach in ectopic pregnancy. Int J Fertil 1986;31:40.
63. Hinton A, Bea CH, Winfield AC, Entman SS: Carcinoma of the Fallopian tube. Urol Radiol 1988;10:113–115.

CHAPTER 15

Transvaginal Sonography of the Second- and Third-Trimester Fetal Brain

Ana Monteagudo, MD
Ilan E. Timor-Tritsch, MD
M. Lynne Reuss, MD
Mortimer G. Rosen, MD

INTRODUCTION

Anomalies of the central nervous system are among the most common and devastating malformations affecting the developing fetus. Since the first ultrasonographic diagnosis and active management of anencephaly by Campbell et al in 1972[1] our ability to diagnose congenital abnormalities has greatly improved. This improvement is mostly attributed to advances in ultrasonographic technology over the past three decades. Despite these technological advances, anomalies during the second and early third trimester of pregnancy can be missed, especially in cases where the malformation is subtle or the exam is suboptimal due to maternal (obesity, abdominal wall scars, etc) or fetal (position, etc) factors.

Prenatal diagnosis of fetal malformations during the first trimester has greatly benefited from the advent of high-frequency transvaginal sonography.[2] Transvaginal scanning of the late second and third trimester fetus has not been widely performed because of limitations in the focal range of the high frequency vaginal probes. However, transvaginal sonography (TVS) beyond the first trimester is possible and yields valuable information if specific organs or fetal parts are targeted for imaging. During the latter half of pregnancy the fetus is commonly in the cephalic presentation; therefore, TVS provides us with an ideal new tool for examining the fetal head. Early prenatal diagnosis and treatment of a potentially devastating fetal brain anomaly is possible and should no longer be missed due to a suboptimal transabdominal examination.

In the literature there are few published reports in which the use of TVS during the second and third trimester of pregnancy is described. In 1987, Chayen et al[3] reported a case of third-trimester cephalocentesis of a hydrocephalic fetus performed successfully under transvaginal sonographic guidance. Farine et al[4] in 1988 described the use of transvaginal sonography to evaluate and diagnose placenta previa. The following year, Benacerraf et al[5] further expanded the applications of TVS to include imaging and measuring of the low fetal head, deep in the pelvis. Recently, Hilpert et al[6] reported a case of agenesis of the corpus callosum (ACC), in which TVS permitted coronal and sagittal sections of the fetal brain to be obtained, thus diagnosing correctly the intracranial anomaly.

In this chapter we will describe a new approach for the evaluation of the normal and abnormal fetal brain anatomy. The technique is a modification of the neonatal exam which is performed transvaginally through the anterior fontanelle.

DEVELOPING A MODEL

A greater understanding of the developing fetal brain has emerged from the experience gained with neurosonographic imaging of the preterm neonate. The evolution of the neurosonographic exam of the fetus duplicates that of the neonatal exam. The preterm neonate was initially scanned in axial sections,[7-14] with low-frequency transducers through the fetal cranium, which is the now present routine used for the fetus. As high-frequency sector scanners became available, neonatal ultrasonographers improved the resolution of their images by using the anterior fontanelle as an acoustic window.[15-25]

In obstetrics, high-frequency transvaginal probes are now available. Therefore, we can increase the resolution of fetal brain images by using the acoustic window provided by the anterior fontanelle. Similar to the scanning of neonates, this new approach requires that the fetal brain be studied in sagittal and coronal sections. In a preliminary study 70 normal fetuses were scanned by the technique described in this chapter.[26]

SCANNING TECHNIQUE

Using the same safety guidelines employed for the use of a speculum or the bimanual examination during pregnancy, TVS can be safely performed in the second and third trimesters. The fetus must be in a cephalic presentation. In a few cases of a breech presentation with suspected intracranial malformation the transabdominal exam may be suboptimal, and sagittal and coronal views may be technically difficult to obtain. Such cases may benefit from an external cephalic version in order to obtain sagittal and coronal sections transvaginally.

A 5.0–6.5 MHz transvaginal probe (preferably an end-firing probe) is prepared for transvaginal scanning (see Chapter 3). The probe is advanced slowly into the vagina until the entire fetal head is imaged. Once the head is imaged, the aim is to obtain a clear image of the brain structures. This is accomplished by aligning the anterior fontanelle of the fetal head with the tip of the probe. In order to achieve this alignment, the probe can be angled anteriorly/posteriorly, moved up/down or side-to-side over the fetal head until a clear image appears. Occasionally, a combination of these probe maneuvers is necessary in order to locate the fontanelle. In addition to maneuvering the probe, the examiner's free hand can be used to gently manipulate the fetal head into position through the maternal abdomen (Fig 15.1). The free hand is placed over the abdomen just above the symphysis pubis. The fetal head can gently be flexed or moved side-to-side until a sharp image appears. Also, a very active fetus can be held in place for the duration of the exam.

OBTAINING THE SCANNING PLANES

The scanning planes obtained with transvaginal sonography are dependent on the position of the fetal head. A flexed head (common in the late second and third trimesters) will allow the coronal and sagittal planes to be imaged. Rotating the probe 90° around its axis over the anterior fontanelle will produce sagittal and coronal sections (Figs 15.1 and 15.2). If a coronal section is apparent, subsequent

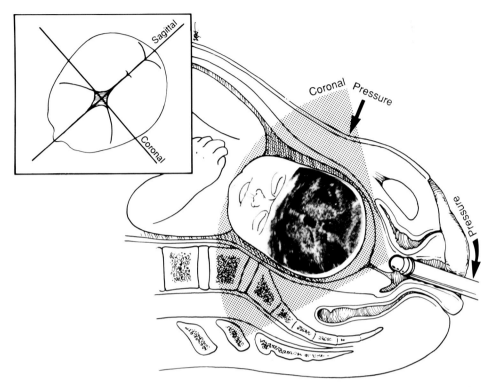

Figure 15.1 Schematic drawing depicting the technique of transvaginal sonography during the second and third trimesters. Inset: The relationship of the anterior fontanelle to the transvaginal transducer is demonstrated. (Reprinted by permission, A. Monteagudo et al., Obstet Gynecol 1991;77:27.)[26]

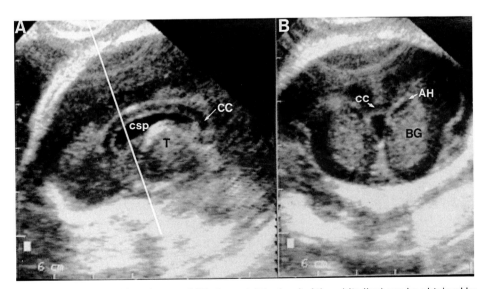

Figure 15.2 Sagittal (**A**) and coronal (**B**) planes (at the level of the white line) can be obtained by rotating the probe 90° around its axis in the anterior fontanelle. csp = cavum septi pellucidi; CC = corpus callosum; T = thalamus; AH = anterior horn of the lateral ventricle; BG = basal ganglia.

serial coronal planes are obtained by slowly aiming the probe away from the face
and toward the occiput or vice versa. Sagittal sections are obtained by turning the
probe 90° from the coronal sections. By angling the probe laterally toward the fetal
ears, right or left parasagittal sections are possible.

NORMAL FETAL INTRACRANIAL ANATOMY

At times it is virtually impossible to obtain ''clean'' and ''perfect'' sections of the
described planes. This is due to limited mobility of the probe within the vagina, the
less than perfect positioning of the fetal head, and the constant fetal movements.

Coronal Sections

The coronal anatomy will be described through a series of consecutive sections
from anterior to posterior (Figs 15.3 and 15.4).

The *first section* is anterior to the *corpus callosum*. The *interhemispheric fis-*

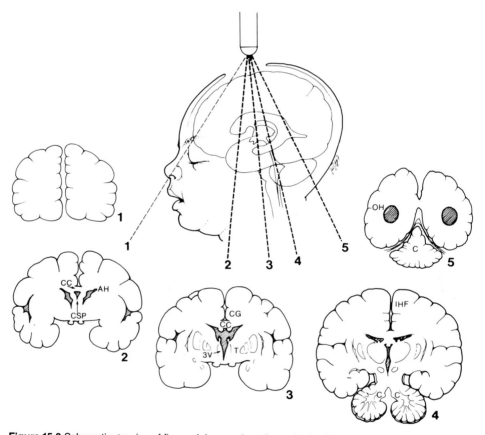

Figure 15.3 Schematic drawing of five serial coronal sections obtained through the anterior fontanelle.
Plane 1 anterior to the corpus callosum. *Plane 2* at the level of the anterior horns of the lateral ventricle.
Plane 3 at the level of the third ventricle. *Plane 4* posterior plane through the peduncules. *Plane 5* the most
posterior coronal plane through the occipital horns. IHF = interhemispheric fissure; CC = corpus
callosum; AH = anterior horns of the lateral ventricle; CSP = cavum septi pellucidi; 3V = third ventricle;
C = cerebellum; OH = occipital horn of the lateral ventricle; CG = cingulate gyrus.

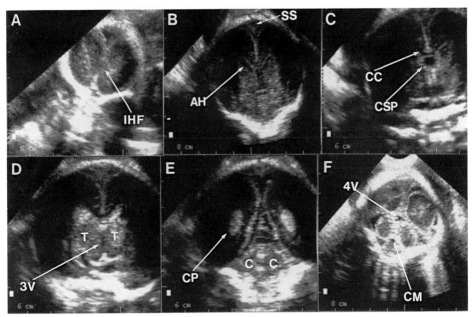

Figure 15.4 Serial sonographic sections corresponding to Figure 15.3 (except **B**, which is not represented on the schematic sections). (**A**) Plane 1, between the two frontal lobes the interhemispheric fissure (IHF) is seen. (**B**) Slightly posterior section to **A**. (**C**) Plane 2. The anterior horns (AH) of the lateral ventricles are seen below the hypoechoic corpus callosum (CC). The cavum septi pellucidi (CSP) appears as a prominent anechoic structure in the midline. (**D**) Plane 3, between the thalami (T) the third ventricle (3V) with its small transverse diameter is seen. (**E**) Plane 4, the choroid plexus (CP) fills the cross-sectional diameter of the lateral ventricle. In the posterior fossa the cerebellum is imaged. (**F**) Plane 5, a most posterior section in which the cerebellum (C) is imaged between the fourth ventricle (4V) and the cisterna magna (CM). SS = superior sagittal sinus.

sure is seen as a bright midline echo between the cerebral tissue of the frontal lobes. Early in the second trimester this fissure appears relatively straight. With advancing gestational age, as new gyri and sulci develop, the interhemispheric fissure becomes progressively irregular (Figs 15.3(1), 15.4**A**, 15.5).

Below the bright echogenic rim of the skull, the *superior sagittal sinus* appears as a slightly triangular structure through which, using a high frame rate or color Doppler, blood flow can be imaged. The *subarachnoid space* appears as a hypoechoic area between the skull and the cerebral cortex. During the second trimester, the subarachnoid space appears prominent but with advancing gestational age the cerebral hemispheres grow, filling the cranial vault. The *falx cerebri* is seen in the midline arising from the inferior surface of the superior sagittal sinus, traverses the subarachnoid space, and continues through the interhemispheric fissure (Fig 15.6).

The *second section* is an anterior section through the anterior horns of the *lateral ventricles*. At the base of the interhemispheric fissure and at right angles to it, the hypoechoic corpus callosum can be seen crossing the midline. Below and to the right and left side of the corpus callosum the anterior horns of the lateral ventricles appear as bilateral fluid-filled structures which are concave laterally. As the fetus matures the anterior horns become progressively narrower, becoming slit-like and sometimes difficult to image. The *cingulate gyrus* can be seen in the

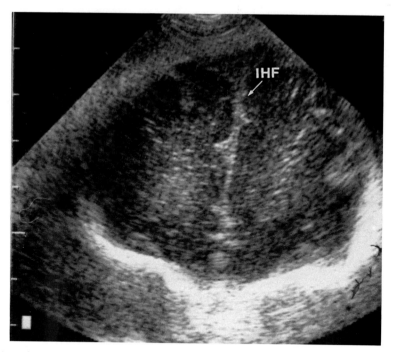

Figure 15.5 Coronal section anterior to the corpus callosum (Plane 1 in Fig 15.3). The interhemispheric fissure (IHF) is seen between the frontal lobes.

midline above the corpus callosum. Between the anterior horns, in the midline, the sonolucent *cavum septi pellucidi* is present. Posterior and adjacent to the anterior horns, the *caudate nucleus* of the *basal ganglia* can be imaged. The pulsations of the *middle cerebral artery* may be seen arising below the caudate nucleus and heading laterally toward the Sylvian fissure (Figs 15.3(2), 15-4**C**, 15.7).

The *third section* is a midcoronal section and passes through the level of the *third ventricle*. The bodies of the lateral ventricle approximate each other in the midline. The echogenic *choroid plexus* may be seen as a bright echo lining the most inferior wall of the lateral ventricle. The *corpus callosum* is imaged crossing the midline. Between the *thalami* in the midline the *third ventricle* is occasionally imaged. This lack of visualization of the third ventricle is due to its normal but small transverse diameter (Figs 15.3(3), 15.4**D**, 15.8).

The *fourth section* images the *posterior horns* of the lateral ventricles. The *cerebellum* or the *midbrain* structures may also be imaged depending on the angle of the coronal section, the frequency of the probe, and the gestational age of the fetus (Figs 15.3(4), 15.4**E**, 15.9).

The *fifth section* is the most posterior coronal section, which can sometimes be imaged. In this section the occipital horns of the lateral ventricle appear as rounded sonolucent structures. The cerebellum is imaged between two sonolucent structures: above the *fourth ventricle* and below the *cisterna magna* (Figs 15.3–5, 15.4**F**, 15.10).

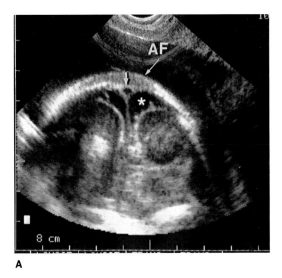

A

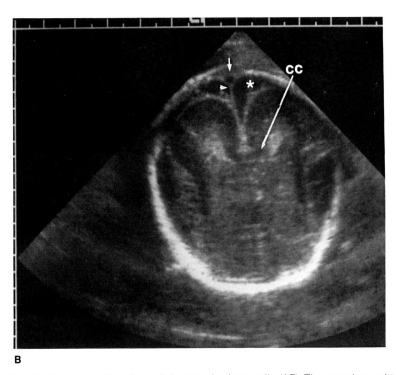

B

Figure 15.6 (**A**) Coronal section through the anterior fontanelle (AF). The superior sagittal sinus (small arrow) is seen just below the fontanelle. (**B**) Coronal-semi-axial section corpus callosum (CC) is seen at the base of the interhemispheric fissure. The falx cerebri (arrowhead) and the subarachnoid space (*) are imaged in this 21-week fetus.

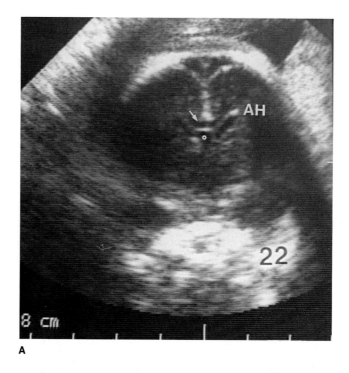

A

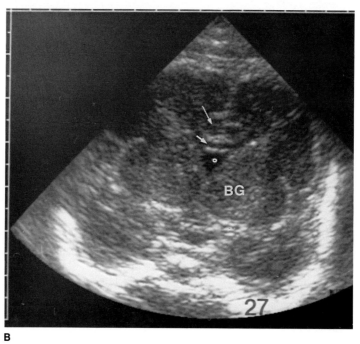

B

Figure 15.7 (A, B) Coronal sections through the anterior horns (AH) of the lateral ventricles corresponding to Plane 2 (in Fig. 15.3). Twenty-two- and 27-week gestations, respectively. Small arrow = corpus callosum; open circle = cavum septi pellucidi; long arrow = cingulate gyrus; BG = basal ganglia.

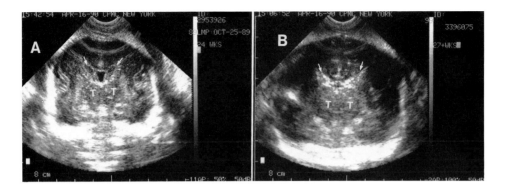

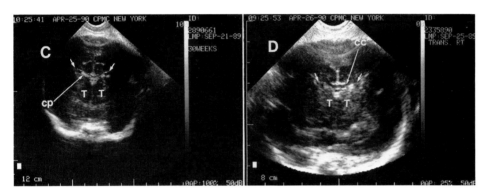

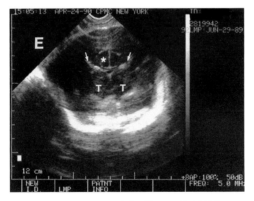

Figure 15.8 Midline coronal sections. Plane 3 (in Fig. 15.3). (**A**) The anterior horns (small arrows) are seen to each side of the triangularly shaped cavum septi pellucidi in this 24-week fetus. (**B, C, D, E**) 27 weeks, 30 weeks, 31 weeks, and 35 weeks, respectively. In the midline between the thalami occasionally the third ventricle is imaged due to its narrow, but normal, transverse diameter. The anterior horns, as pregnancy progresses, become slit-like. The cavum septi pellucidi begins to close in utero and by term is barely visible. Cingulate gyrus (∗) is clearly imaged in **C** and **E**.

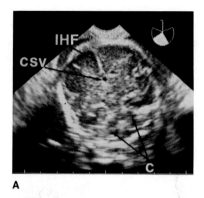

A

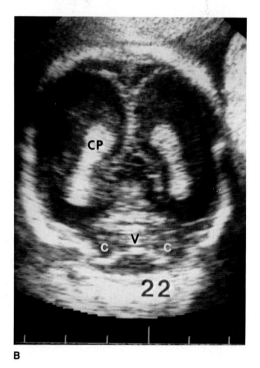

B

Figure 15.9 (A, B) Posterior coronal sections. (**A**) The vermis (V) appears as an echogenic structure between the two lobes of the cerebellum (C). (**B**) A semi-axial coronal section showing the echogenic choroid plexus (CP) filling the lateral ventricle. IHF = interhemispheric fissure; CSV = cavum septi vergae.

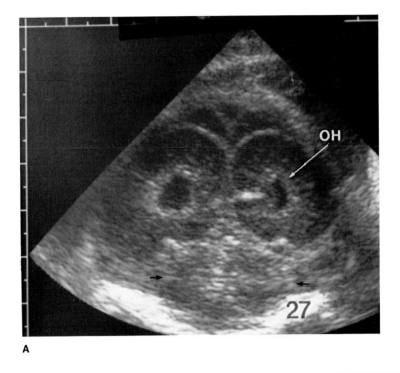

A

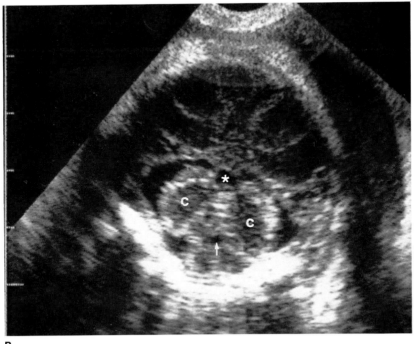

B

Figure 15.10 (**A, B**) Very posterior coronal sections (Plane 5, in Fig. 15.3). (**A**) The occipital horns (OH) appear as symmetrical anechoic round structures. The transverse diameter of the cerebellum (black arrows) can be easily measured in this section. (**B**) Slightly more posterior section than **A**. The cerebellum is seen between the fourth ventricle (∗) and the cisterna magna (arrow).

Sagittal and Parasagittal Sections

A *midsagittal section* reveals several important but simple to locate structures such as the *corpus callosum* and the sonolucent *cavum septi pellucidi*. The corpus callosum is a prominent hypoechoic, semilunar midline structure located above the cavum septi pellucidi. The corpus callosum is fully developed by 18–20 weeks gestation and is composed of three parts: *the genu* (anterior), *body* (middle), and *splenium* (posterior) (Figs 15.11, 15.12**B**–**E**). The *cingulate gyrus* is evident above the corpus callosum especially as gestation nears term. Above the thalamus the bright echogenic *tela choroidea* of the third ventricle can be imaged. The cerebellum appears in the posterior fossa as a hyperechoic structure indented by the

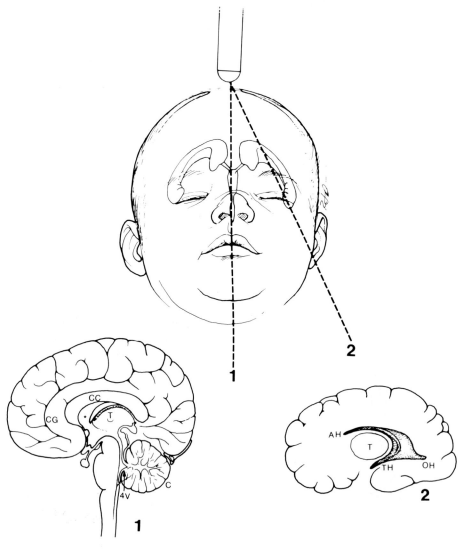

Figure 15.11 Schematic drawing of the two sagittal planes. Plane 1: midline sagittal section. Plane 2: parasagittal section. CC = corpus callosum; CG = cingulate gyrus; T = thalamus; C = cerebellum; 4V = fourth ventricle; AH = anterior horns; OH = occipital horns; TH = temporal horns. (Reprinted by permission, Monteagudo et al., Obstet Gynecol 1991;77:27–32).[26]

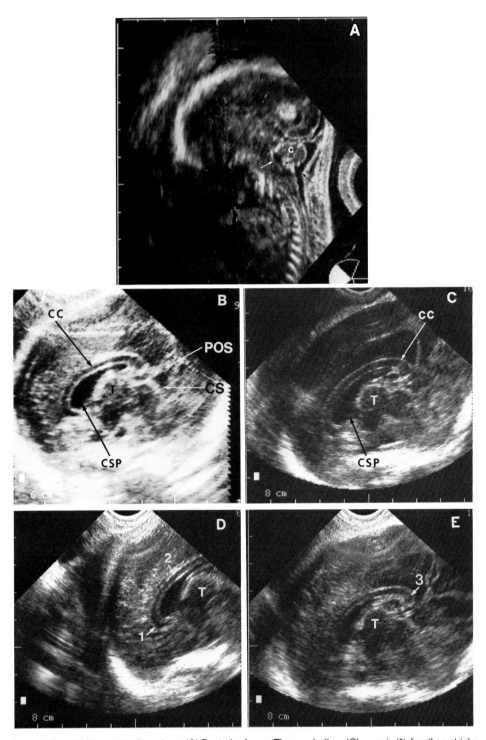

Figure 15.12 Midline sagittal sections. (**A**) Posterior fossa. The cerebellum (C), vermis (*), fourth ventricle (white arrow), and the cisterna magna (black arrow) are imaged. (**B**, **C**) The corpus callosum (CC), cavum septi pellucidi (CSP), thalamus (T), parieto-occipital sulcus (POS), and calcarine sulcus (CS) are imaged in a 23-week and 27-week fetus, respectively. (**D**, **E**) The genu (1), body (2), and splenium (3) of the corpus callosum are imaged in a 30-week fetus.

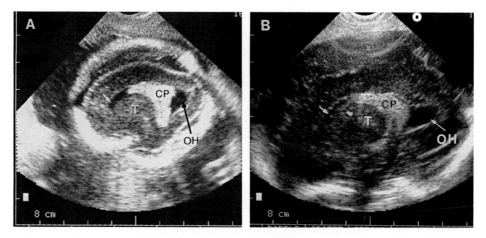

Figure 15.13 Parasagittal sections. (**A**) 20-week fetus. Note the smooth surface of the brain and the large subarachnoid space typical of this gestational age. (**B**) 30-week fetus. The caudothalamic groove is not clearly imaged in this section, but the arrowhead points to the area where it is usually seen. Arrow = anterior horn; OH = occipital horn; CP = choroid plexus; T = thalmus.

sonolucent fourth ventricle. The *cisterna magna* is another sonolucent structure located below the cerebellum (Figs 15.11(1), 15.12**A**).

A *parasagittal section* reveals portions of the *anterior horn* and body of the lateral ventricles which appears as the mirror image of the letter C, the open end of which points toward the fetal face. *All the segments of the lateral ventricle (anterior, body, posterior, and temporal horns) may be imaged in the same section only if dilatation of the ventricle is present.* The homogeneous and echogenic choroid plexus extends anteriorly from the atria into the body of the lateral ventricles, but does not extend into the frontal horns. Medially, the choroid plexus passes through the *foramen of Monroe* into the third ventricle. The *caudothalamic groove* appears as a bright echogenic arc that separates the head of the caudate nucleus anteriorly from the more posterior thalamus. The germinal matrix is a highly vascular tissue located inferior and lateral to the ependyma lining the floor of the lateral ventricle and just anterior to the caudothalamic groove. This germinal matrix is the site of origin for the vast majority of intracranial hemorrhages in the preterm neonate. However, as gestation nears term, involution of the germinal matrix tissue takes place (Figs 15.11(2), 15.13).

In our material (70 fetuses) we documented a learning curve to master the technique; however, we were able to image all planes in approximately 75% of the fetuses. The posterior coronal sections were the most difficult to obtain, imaged in approximately 59% of the fetuses.[26]

Imaging the Gyri

This imaging is possible through a midline sagittal section when the flat interhemispheric surface is tangentially scanned. The surface of the cerebral hemispheres during the second trimester is smooth due to the lack of gyri and sulci present. Due to the fetal brain growth spurts that occur between 28 and 30 weeks of gestation, many new *gyri* and *sulci* develop.[27,28] As a result, the sonographic appearance of the developing brain changes from smooth to one with an increasingly complex pattern of echodense lines covering the cerebral surfaces (Fig 15.14).

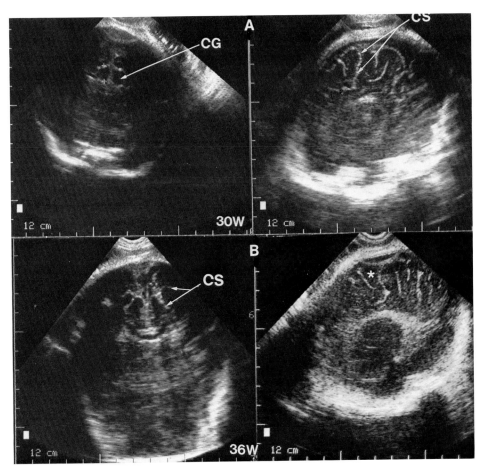

Figure 15.14 Sulci and gyri are imaged in coronal and parasagittal sections. (**A**) 30-week gestation. (**B**) 36-week gestation. Note the convoluted appearance of the fetal brain at this gestation. CG = cingulate gyrus; CS = cingulate sulcus; * = precentral lobe.

CONGENITAL BRAIN ABNORMALITIES

Congenital brain abnormalities can result from alterations in the morphogenesis or the histogenesis of the neural tissue, or from developmental failures occurring in associated structures.[29] These anomalies may be due to exogenous factors such as congenital infections (rubella, toxoplasmosis, cytomegalovirus etc), radiation or chemical agents (fetal alcohol syndrome), genetic or chromosomal factors (trisomies), or a combination of several factors (Table 15.1).

The images presented in this section were all obtained by transvaginal imaging. We had the opportunity to detect and scan a variety of brain abnormalities. However, it should be clear that these are but a few of those mentioned in this chapter.

DISORDERS OF NEURAL TUBE CLOSURE

Anencephaly, Exencephaly, Iniencephaly, Encephalocele

Failure of the rostral neuropore to close during the fourth week of development results in an abnormal development of the skull and malformation of the brain and meninges. When the cranial defect is large the resulting forebrain develops par-

TABLE 15.1 Congenital Brain Malformations

I. Disorders of Neural Tube Closure (fourth week of gestation)
   1. Anencephaly
   2. Exencephaly
   3. Iniencephaly
   4. Encephalocele
II. Disorder of Ventral Induction (fifth–sixth week of gestation)
   1. Holoprosencephaly —Alobar
                        —Semilobar
                        —Lobar
III. Disorders of Agenesis and Dysgenesis (eighth–twenty-fourth week of gestation)
   1. Cerebral Abnormalities
      a. Microcephaly —Primary
                      —Secondary
      b. Schizencephaly
      c. Hydranencephaly
   2. Commissural Abnormalities
      a. Agenesis of the Corpus Callosum
      b. Septal Agenesis
IV. Disorders of Cortex (twelfth–twenty-fourth week of gestation)
   1. Lissencephaly or Agyria
   2. Pachygyria
   3. Microgyria and Polymicrogyria
   4. Heterotopias
V. Disorders of Size
   1. Congenital Hydrocephalus
      a. Aqueductal Stenosis
      b. Communicating
      c. Dandy-Walker Syndrome
      d. Other
   2. Megalocephaly
VI. Others
   1. Choroid Plexus Cysts
   2. Arachnoid Cysts
   3. Aneurysms of Vein of Galen
   4. Intracranial Tumors

tially and then degenerates.[29] If the cranial defect is small, it results in varying degrees of herniation of the brain or the meninges.

Acrania or *exencephaly* is defined as absence of the entire or a substantial portion of the cranium in the presence of the cerebral hemispheres. This condition is theorized to be the embryologic predecessor of anencephaly in man.[29–31] *Anencephaly* is the most common of these disorders, occurring in about 1 per 1000 births.[29,32,33] The female fetus is affected four times as often as the male.[29,34] This condition is lethal with about 75% of the fetuses being stillborn and the rest dying shortly after birth. Polyhydramnios is present in approximately 50% of the cases during the second and third trimesters due to decreased fetal swallowing.[29,34,35] Anencephaly was the first anomaly diagnosed by transvaginal sonography by Rottem et al.[36] The sonographic findings of an anencephalus are absence of the cranium above the prominent orbits with preservation of the base of the skull and facial features.[37] Transvaginal sonography during the second and third trimesters does not add significantly to the diagnosis of anencephaly except in obese women

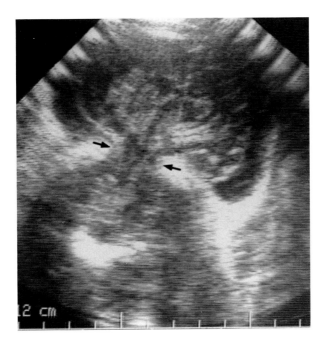

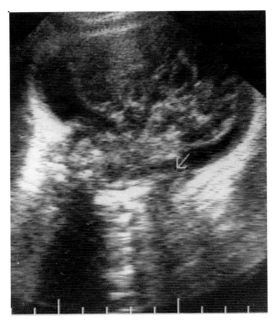

Figure 15.15 Two views of a posterior encephalocele with transvaginal sonography. Note the defect in the skull (black arrows) and the gyri and sulci in the herniated sac.

with a suboptimal abdominal exam, or who have a deeply engaged fetal head.

    Encephalocele are midline herniations of the brain and/or meninges that involve the occipital portion of the head in about 75% of the cases, but may be found in the frontal, parietal, orbital, nasal, or nasopharyngeal region.[33,35,38,39] The incidence has been estimated to be 1 in 2500 births.[35] Sonographic findings include defects in the bony skull with a protruding sac-like structure, the contents of which may be cystic or solid with obvious brain tissue or a combination of

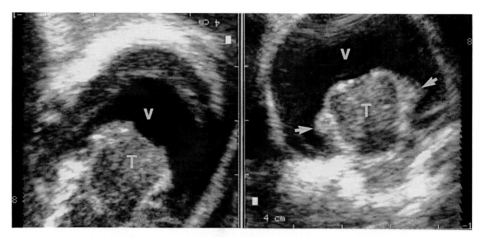

Figure 15.16 Alobar holoprosencephaly at 19 weeks gestátion. Coronal sections in which single ventricle (V) and fused thalami (T) are imaged. Arrowhead = choroid plexus. Note the absence of the corpus callosum and cavum septi pellucidi.

both[37,38,40] (Fig 15.15). Other associated brain sonographic findings that may be present include *hydrocephalus* (85–95%), *agenesis of the corpus callosum,* and *Dandy-Walker syndrome.*[35,38] Transvaginal sonography can help differentiate between encephalocele from cystic hygromas, hemangiomas, teratomas and branchial clefts which may have similar transabdominal appearances.

Iniencephaly is a rare, lethal developmental neural tube defect, characterized by a defect in the occiput involving the foramen magnum with retroflexion of the fetal head in association with cervical and thoracic spine defect.[41,46,47] The malformation results from a developmental arrest of the embryo during the third week of gestation, resulting in persistence of the embryonic cervical retroflexion which leads to failure of the neural groove to close in the area of the cervical spine or upper thorax.[41–44] In 84% of the fetuses with iniencephaly multiple anomalies are present.[45] The anomalies include hydrocephalus, microcephalus, ventricular atresia, holoprosencephaly, polymicrogyria, agenesis of the cerebellar vermis, occipital encephalocele, diaphragmatic hernia, thoracic cage deformities, urinary tract anomalies, cleft lip and palate, and omphalocele.[41,42,46,47] Typical sonographic findings include retroflexion of the fetal head with short neck and trunk and open cervical and thoracic spinal defects. The short neck and trunk may lead to a very early size-date discrepancy. In one of our cases of iniencephaly, the crown-rump length (CRL) was only 80% of expected value at 9 weeks, and by 11 weeks, only 70% of the expected value. This suggests that discrepancies in the expected CRL may be the first clue to the presence of a fetal malformation that affects the length of the fetus (see Chapter 13).

DISORDERS OF VENTRAL INDUCTION

Holoprosencephaly

Holoprosencephaly results from failure of the prosencephalon to differentiate into the cerebral hemispheres and lateral ventricles between the fourth and eighth weeks of gestation.[48,49] A spectrum of the anomaly exists which ranges from complete to partial failure of cleavage of the prosencephalon. *Three types* are described: *alobar, semilobar,* and *lobar holoprosencephaly,* depending on the degree of failed differentiation. The incidence in abortuses has been reported to be

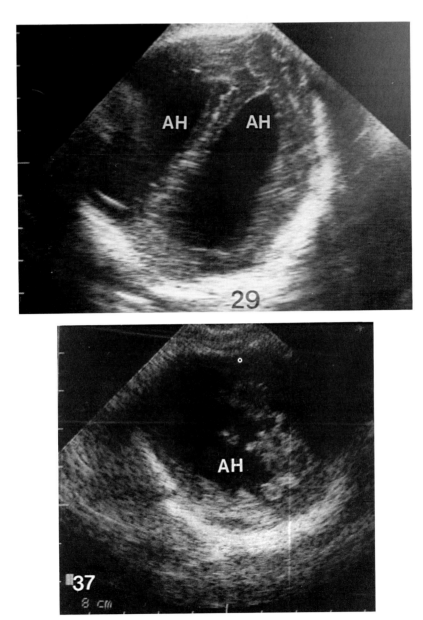

Figure 15.17 (A, B) Anterior coronal section (see Fig 15.3, Plane 1). Severe ventriculomegaly of a 29- and 37-week fetus. The latter also had microcephaly and in utero infection with cytomegalovirus (CMV). AH = anterior horn.

0.4 per 1,000 with a lower incidence in live births of 0.6 per 1000.[33] Alobar holoprosencephaly, in which no cleavage has taken place, is the most extreme type consisting of a single ventricle, small cerebrum, fused thalami, and agenesis of the corpus callosum and falx cerebri.[40,41] Facial anomalies include cyclopia, ethmocephaly, cebocephaly, hypertelorism, and other midline facial defects.[33] Sonographic findings include absence of midline structures (falx cerebri, interhemispheric fissure, absence of the corpus callosum), single ventricle with communicating dorsal cyst, fused thalami, and facial defects (Fig 15.16). In semilobar holoprosencephaly, some cleavage has occurred, the ventricles and the cerebral hemispheres are partially separated posteriorly, there is incomplete separation of the thalami, but anteriorly there is still a single ventricular cavity.[40] In the lobar type, the interhemispheric fissure is present, and the basal ganglia, thalamus, cingulate gyrus, and frontal horns may be properly divided or show a variable spectrum of fusion.[48,49]

DISORDERS OF AGENESIS AND DYSGENESIS

Cerebral Abnormalities

Microcephaly

This condition is usually diagnosed when the fetal head size falls at least below three standard deviations from the mean.[53,54,58] Microcephaly can occur as a result of an autosomal recessive trait, as part of a chromosomal syndrome (eg, trisomies 13, 18), due to environmental factors such as infections (CMV), intrauterine alcohol exposure, intrauterine anoxia, maternal metabolic diseases, or abnormality of the skull (eg, craniosynostosis).[44,53-57] Microcephaly is usually present in cases of lissencephaly, porencephaly, and holoprosencephaly. Agenesis of the corpus callosum and ventriculomegaly secondary to brain atrophy are often found with microcephaly.[53,57] In cases of microcephaly TVS can assess the brain structures and rule out associated brain anomalies. The prognosis of a microcephalic fetus relates to severity of associated anomalies and to the size of the head. Unfortunately, isolated microcephaly may not be diagnosed until the late second or third trimester when the growth of the fetal head slows down significantly.[55]

Schizencephaly

These disorders represent a spectrum of destructive lesions affecting the brain. Schizencephaly or porencephalic cysts are a rare congenital malformation in which bilateral and nearly symmetric clefts are usually present in the brain.[49-51] Two types have been described.[50] Type I has small symmetrical clefts in which the lips of the clefts are fused within a pia-ependymal seam that is continuous with the ependyma of the lateral ventricle. Type 2 has more extensive clefts which extend from the ventricle to the surface of the brain.[49-51] The clefts are wedge-shaped and extend outward to reach the bones of the skull. Their pathogenesis is not clear but they are believed to arise from an in utero ischemic event. Sonographic findings include the presence of bilateral brain clefts as well as ventriculomegaly. No such pathology was seen by us using TVS.

Hydranencephaly

This is believed to be the result of either an in utero cerebral brain infarction due to a bilateral carotid artery occlusion, or primary agenesis of the neural wall.[35,52] The cerebellum, midbrain, thalami, and basal ganglia are usually preserved. Sonographic findings include macrocephaly, a large fluid-filled intracranial cavity with variable amounts of echogenicity. No cerebral cortex is present, but there is partial preservation of portions of the occipital lobe. The falx cerebri is usually intact. The midbrain and basal ganglia are variably preserved. Polyhydramnios is usually present.

Commissural Abnormalities

Agenesis of the Corpus Callosum

The corpus callosum begins to develop anterior to the foramen of Monroe at about 12 weeks of gestation.[59] Growth of the corpus callosum continues upward and backward, in a C shape, as the primitive cerebral hemispheres grow laterally and then posteriorly.[49,60,61] First, the genu of the corpus callosum develops followed by the corpus, and lastly, the splenium is formed.[62] Agenesis of the corpus callosum can be complete or partial depending on the stage of development at which growth was arrested. Complete or primary agenesis can result from a primary vascular or inflammatory insult occurring before the twelfth week of gestation. Agenesis of the corpus callosum can occur as an isolated anomaly, but 80% of the cases have other associated malformations such as polymicrogyria, heterotopias, interhemispheric arachnoid cysts, lipomas, microcephaly, Dandy-Walker malformation, Arnold-Chiari malformation, holoprosencephaly, and hydrocephalus.[59,60,62,63] Secondary dysgenesis can result from partial or complete destruction occurring in a normally formed corpus callosum. This secondary destruction usually occurs toward the latter half of gestation when the callosum is partly or completely formed due to a vascular or inflammatory process. Partial agenesis usually involves the posterior portion of the callosum, since embryologically it develops in a cranial-caudal fashion.[64] It may be associated with microcephaly, hydrocephalus, and porencephaly. By 18 to 20 weeks gestation the corpus callosum has achieved its adult morphology. Most cases of agenesis of the corpus callosum are sporadic, but several genetic disorders as well as chromosomal disorders have been associated with its absence.[64] Transvaginal sonography can easily and reliably diagnose in utero agenesis of the corpus callosum.[6] Sonographic findings on a midsagittal section demonstrate the complete absence of the characteristic normal corpus callosum, pericallosal cistern, and cingulate gyri.[63,65-68] The gyri and sulci on the flat medial surface of the hemispheres have a typical radial ("sunburst") orientation.[6,60,63] On a parasagittal section the frontal horns appear narrow and laterally displaced, and the atria and occipital horn appear slightly dilated.[63] The coronal section demonstrates a wide interhemispheric fissure, absence of the corpus callosum, and a high position of the third ventricle between the lateral ventricle.

DISORDERS OF THE CORTEX

Lissencephaly, Pachygyria, Microgyria, and Heterotopias

These disorders result from disturbances in migration of the neuroblasts to the forming cerebral cortex. Depending on when the disturbance or insult occurred, the resulting cortex will completely lack gyri and sulci (lissencephaly), may have few gyri (pachygyria), may have multiple small gyri (microgyria), or have names of gray matter present in an abnormal location of the brain (heterotopias).[49,56] All children with this type of migrational disorder are severely neurologically impaired.[56,69,70]

Lissencephaly or agyria is a rare developmental anomaly of the brain characterized by incomplete or failure of neuronal migration to occur during 12 to 24 weeks of gestation, resulting in a lack of gyri and sulci development. Microcephaly, ventriculomegaly, wide Sylvian fissures, and little operculation of the insula are found with lissencephaly. Complete or partial agenesis of the corpus callosum is often associated with lissencephaly as well.[49,69,70] Transvaginal sonography allows imaging of the surface of the cerebral hemispheres and can facilitate the in utero diagnosis of lissencephaly. However, no such reports are yet available. In cases of lissencephaly the brain surface appears smooth on coronal and parasagittal sections. The interhemispheric fissure will appear as a relatively straight midline echo. The subarachnoid space and the Sylvian grooves will appear wide, similar to the appearance of the fetal brain before 20 weeks gestation (Figs 15.4**A**, 15.7**A**, 15.13**A**). Ventricular dilatation is apparent in both coronal and parasagittal sections with lissencephaly.[49] Prenatal diagnosis of lissencephaly cannot be reliably made until 26 to 28 weeks gestation, when the normal gyri and sulci become well defined, since up to this time the normal fetal brain has a smooth appearance.[26]

DISORDERS OF SIZE
Congenital Hydrocephalus

Aqueductal Stenosis, Communicating Hydrocephalus

This is defined as dilatation of the ventricular system with or without enlargement of the skull not due to primary atrophy of the brain. The overall incidence of congenital hydrocephalus has been estimated to be between 0.5 to 3 per 1000 live births and the incidence of isolated hydrocephalus, between 0.39 and 0.87 per live births.[71] The three most common types of isolated congenital hydrocephalus are aqueductal stenosis, which accounts for 43% of the cases, communicating hydrocephalus (38%), Dandy-Walker malformation (13%), and other causes (6%), which include agenesis of the corpus callosum, arachnoid cysts, and aneurysm of the vein of Galen (Figs 15.17, see p. 429; and Figs 15.18–15.22).[72] Polyhydramnios is resent in 30% of the cases.[73]

The flow of cerebrospinal fluid is unidirectional. The cerebrospinal fluid is produced by the choroid plexus of the lateral ventricle. The cerebrospinal fluid flows through the third ventricle, aqueduct of Sylvius, fourth ventricle, through the foramina of Magendie or Luschka to the basal cisterns, and eventually to the subarachnoid space to be absorbed across the arachnoid granulations. Obstruc-

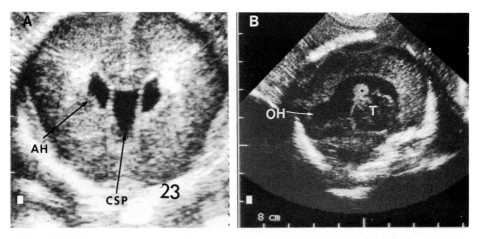

Figure 15.18 (**A**) Anterior coronal section (see Fig 15.3, Plane 2) of 23 weeks with fetus showing ventriculomegaly. This fetus in addition had a cystic hygroma. (**B**) Parasagittal section (Fig 15.8, Plane 2). The choroid plexus (∗) is distorted and widely separated from the superior wall of the ventricle. Note: The conventional orientation in this image is reversed. T = thalamus.

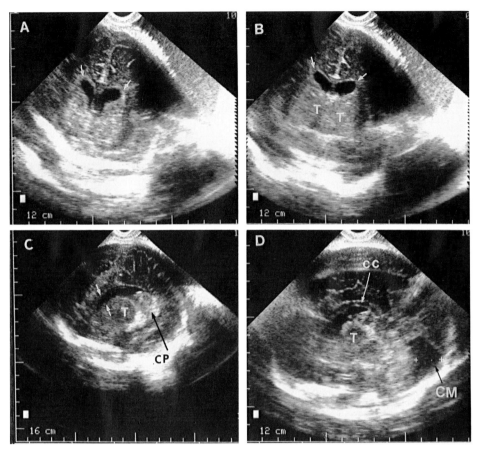

Figure 15.19 Coronal and sagittal sections of a full-term fetus with ventriculomegaly. (**A**) Anterior coronal section (see Fig 15.3, Plane 2). The anterior horn has a tear shape (arrow). The taper end points toward the thalamus (T). (**B**) Midline coronal section (see Fig 15.3, Plane 3). (**C**) Angled parasagittal (Fig 15.8, Plane 2) demonstrating the dilatation of the anterior horns. (**D**) Midsagittal section (see Fig 15.8, Plane 2) with enlarged cisterna magna (CM). CC = corpus callosum; CP = choroid plexus.

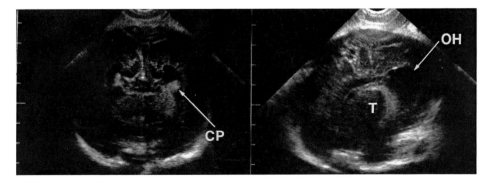

Figure 15.20 Posterior coronal and parasagittal section (see Fig 15.8, Plane 2) of a full-term fetus with trisomy 21 showing dilatation of the posterior horn of the lateral ventricle. CP = choroid plexus; OH = occipital horn; T = thalamus.

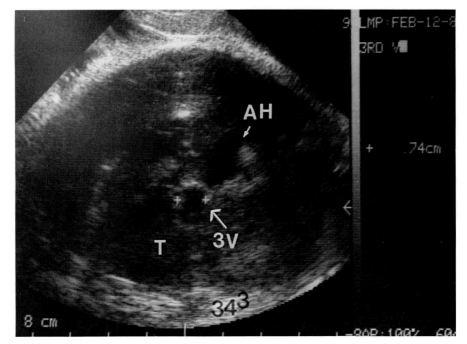

Figure 15.21 Midline coronal section (see Fig 15.3, Plane 3) showing dilatation of the anterior horn (AH) of the lateral ventricle and the third ventricle (3V) at 34 weeks and 3 days. T = thalamus.

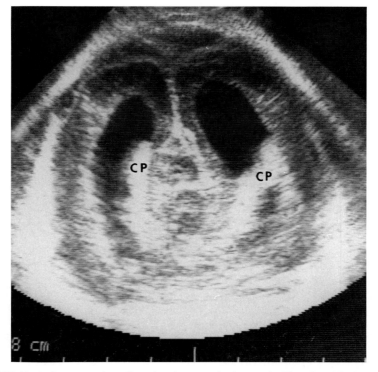

Figure 15.22 Posterior coronal section showing ventriculomegaly. The choroid plexus (CP) is detached from the medial wall on the right and falls over the outer wall.

tion to flow along this pathway will result in hydrocephalus. *Aqueductal stenosis* is the most common form of *noncommunicating hydrocephalus* and can be the result of genetic diseases, infections, or exposures to teratogens.

Dandi-Walker Malformations (DWM)

These result from a cystic dilatation of the fourth ventricle associated with dysgenesis or complete agenesis of the vermis of the cerebellum and, frequently, hydrocephalus.[74–79] The pathogenesis of DWM is not certain. The original theory was postulated to be secondary to atresia of the foramen of Magendie, and Luschka resulting in a noncommunicating hydrocephalus. However, often these apertures are found to be open. Recently, evidence suggests that DWM represent a complex developmental anomaly of the fourth ventricle occurring at around the sixth and seventh weeks of gestation, which accounts for the concurrent anomalies present in this syndrome.[53,74,75] Sonographic findings of the coronal and sagittal planes include a large posterior fossa cyst contiguous with the fourth ventricle, an elevated tentorium, and dilatation of the third and lateral ventricles. Differentiation between a Dandy-Walker and posterior fossa arachnoid cyst relies on the demonstration of a hypoplastic vermis and a connection of the cyst with the fourth ventricle[63,109] (Figs 15.23, 15.24).

Early recognition of hydrocephalus still remains a diagnostic dilemma. Transvaginal sonography, because of its superior resolution and ability to image the fetal brain in the coronal and sagittal planes, has allowed us to gain a better understanding of the ventricular developmental changes occurring during the late

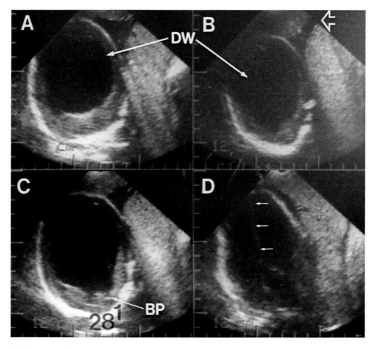

Figure 15.23 Serial axial sections of a Dandy-Walker malformation (DWM) at 28 weeks. BP = brain parenchyma; small arrows = midline; open arrow = cervix.

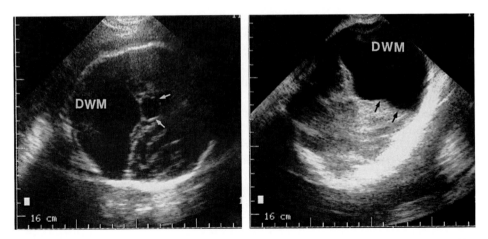

Figure 15.24 Two axial sections of a Dandy-Walker malformation (DWM) at 34 weeks. The tentorium (black arrows) is clearly demarcated and the third ventricle (white arrows) is prominent due to agenesis of the corpus callosum.

first and early second trimester of pregnancy. Also, TVS allows us to employ the criteria used in neonates for early detection of mild ventriculomegaly.

Sonographic findings of ventriculomegaly can be defined by quantitative or qualitative methods.[80–84] Quantitative *measurements of ventricular size* using the transfontanelle approach have been reported for preterm infants.[80–82] In the coronal plane, at the level of the bodies of the lateral ventricles in a plane that includes the third ventricle, *two measurements can be done.* The *midline-lateral dimension* was defined by measuring the distance from the midline to the most lateral aspect of the ventricle. The normal limit of this distance was found to be ≤ 12 mm. *Ventricular depth* was defined as the widest measurement perpendicular to the longest axis of the lateral ventricle and was found to be ≤ 4 mm. An increase in the ventricular depth was found earlier in mild ventriculomegaly than the increase in the midline-lateral dimension.[81,83] The *third ventricle* on coronal sections normally is not evident or appears slit-like due to its normal but small transverse diameter. The *fourth ventricle* is best imaged in the midsagittal plane and appears as a triangular anechoic structure whose apex, the fastigium, indents the vermis of the cerebellum.[84]

Qualitative methods for assessing ventriculomegaly include: (1) *on the coronal plane,* progressive rounding and bulging of the superior and lateral angles of the frontal horns with inferior pointing; and (2) *on the parasagittal plane,* dilatation of the occipital horns of the lateral ventricles.[85–87]

OTHER BRAIN MALFORMATIONS

Choroid Plexus Cysts

The choroid plexus cysts first appear at about 6 to 7 weeks of gestation. The growth of the choroid plexus is fast and by 9 weeks gestation fills 75% of the lateral ventricle. The adult appearance is reached by 20 weeks gestation.[88,89] Choroid plexus cysts are commonly found during sonography and may be unilateral, bilateral, single, or multiple, and may completely disappear nearing the twenty-fourth week of gestation. Reportedly, up to 1% of all second-trimester fetuses have choroid plexus cysts during the second trimester.[88,90,91] Small cysts of the choroid plexus have been found in infants and adults with an incidence of 57% reported in some adult autopsy series.[92] The pathogenesis of the cyst is not clear but is thought to be due to filling of the neuroepithelial folds with cerebrospinal fluid.[92] The choroid plexus cysts are usually small, less than 1 cm in size, asymptomatic, and benign.[93–96] Isolated cysts are transient and have been associated with normal fetal karyotype.[90,91,94,96–99] In the presence of choroid plexus cysts and other anomalies, Benacerraf found that 77% of those fetuses had trisomy 18. The associated anomalies are those that are frequently seen in trisomy 18 (eg, omphaloceles, diaphragmatic hernia, neural tube defects). Therefore, genetic amniocentesis was recommended in cases of choroid plexus cysts if associated with other congenital anomalies.[90] The sonographic appearance is that of a distinct anechoic cystic area within the choroid plexus (Fig 15.25).

Arachnoid Cysts

Arachnoid cysts are collections of cerebrospinal fluid within the layers of the arachnoid membrane which may or may not communicate with the subarachnoid space.[49] The cysts are located on the surface of the brain, most commonly at the level of the cerebral fissures and within the anterior, middle, and posterior fossa. Primary cysts arise from an abnormal developmental process of the leptomeningeal formation. Secondary or acquired arachnoid cysts are the result of cerebral spinal fluid entrapment within arachnoid adhesions.[35,100–102] The arachnoid cyst has been reported to account for 1% of all intracranial cystic structures during childhood.[100,102] A large cyst can cause hydrocephalus occurring from the mass effect, causing obstruction of flow of the cerebrospinal fluid.[100,101] Sonographic findings include an anechoic structure with thin, smooth walls lying adjacent to the cerebral hemispheres, cerebellum, or brain stem.[35] Ventriculomegaly may occasionally be present.

Aneurysms of the Vein of Galen

Aneurysms of the vein of Galen are rare arteriovenous malformations of the brain. The aneurysm has been reported to be detected by prenatal sonography.[104–107] On sonographic pictures the aneurysm appears as a large, well-defined, supratentorial, midline, nonpulsatile structure. Doppler sonography demonstrated turbulent flow within the dilated cavity.[104,105,108] The aneurysm of the vein of Galen may cause obstruction of the aqueduct of Sylvius, resulting in hydrocephalus.[109] Other associated findings include polyhydramnios, nonimmune hydrops, hepatomegaly, and cardiomegaly. The prognosis depends on the severity and time of presentation of the cardiovascular symptomatology. Development of high output failure in utero or before 3 months of life is usually lethal despite medical and surgical treatments.[49,106,110]

Intracranial Tumors

Intracranial tumors occurring during fetal life are rare. When they occur they are usually associated with hydrocephalus and polyhydramnios. The prognosis is very poor, with most neonates dying shortly after birth.[112–122]

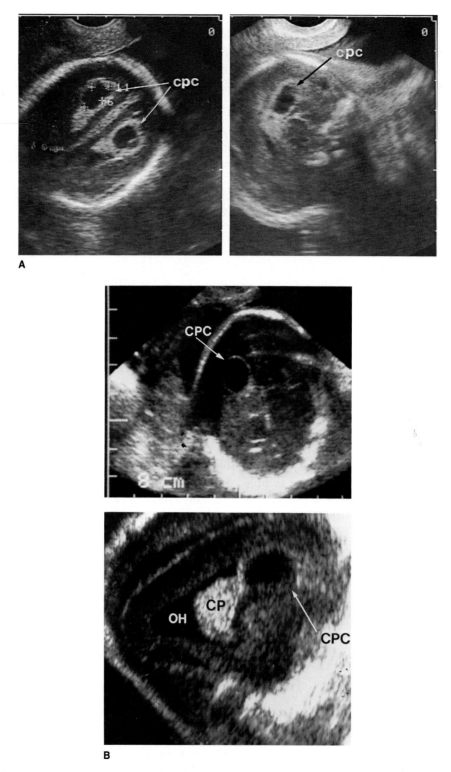

Figure 15.25 Axial and parasagittal sections at 20 and 23 weeks gestation, respectively, with choroid plexus cysts (CPC) and no other congenital abnormalities. (**A**) Bilateral choroid plexus cysts. (**B**) Unilateral cyst. CP = choroid plexus; OH = occipital horn.

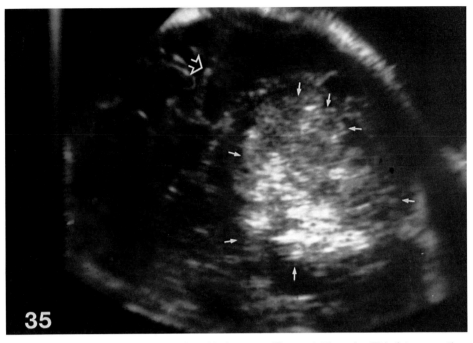

Figure 15.26 Coronal section of a choroid plexus papilloma at 35 weeks. This fetus over time developed ventriculomegaly. Note the echogenic nature of the mass. The small arrows point to the papillary edge of the mass. Open arrow = shifted midline.

Choroid Plexus Papilloma

This is a rare benign tumor of the choroid plexus.[111,112] The tumor may occur anywhere the choroid plexus is present, but most commonly is unilateral and located in the atria of the lateral ventricle. Polyhydramnios and communicating hydrocephalus is usually present. Hydrocephalus may result from an overproduction of cerebrospinal fluid by the choroid plexus or an obstruction to the flow caused by the mass.[113–116] The sonographic appearance is that of a large, lobulated, highly echogenic mass within the lateral ventricle. Transvaginal sonography can further characterize the mass as well as demonstrating the papillary nature of the tumor (Fig 15.26).

CONCLUSION

Transvaginal sonography during the second and third trimesters of pregnancy allows high-resolution imaging of the fetal intracranial structures in the sagittal and coronal planes. Although the coronal and sagittal planes can be obtained with transabdominal sonography, often the planes are technically difficult to image due to maternal or fetal factors precluding adequate imaging. We believe this new approach will become part of the routine fetal neuro-exam, especially when a previous history of a fetal nervous system anomaly or predisposing factors for such conditions are present. Early prenatal detection of such abnormalities may have an impact in the management of the pregnancy.

REFERENCES

1. Campbell S, Johnstone FD, Holt EM, May P: Anencephalus: early ultrasonic diagnosis and active management. Lancet 1972;2:1226.
2. Rottem S, Bronshtein M: Transvaginal sonographic diagnosis of congenital anomalies between 9 weeks and 16 weeks, menstrual age. J Clin Ultrasound 1990;18:307.
3. Chayen B, Rifkin MD: Cephalocentesis: guidance with an endovaginal probe and endovaginal needle placement. J Ultrasound Med 1987;6:221.
4. Farine D, Fox HE, Jakobson S, Timor-Tritsch IE: Vaginal ultrasound for diagnosis of placenta previa. Am J Obstet Gynecol 1988;159:566.
5. Benacerraf BR, Estroff JA: Transvaginal sonographic imaging of the low fetal head in the second trimester. J Ultrasound Med 1989;8:325.
6. Hilpert PL, Kurtz AB: Prenatal diagnosis of agenesis of the corpus callosum using endovaginal ultrasound. J Ultrasound Med 1990;9:363.
7. Kossoff G, Garret WJ, Radavanovich G: Ultrasonic atlas normal brain of infant. Ultrasound Med Biol 1974;1:259–266.
8. Garret WJ, Kossoff G, Jones RF: Ultrasonic cross-sectional visualization of hydrocephalus in infants. Neuroradiology 1975;8:279–288.
9. Lees RF, Harrison RB, Sims TL: Gray scale ultrasonography in the evaluation of hydrocephalus and associated abnormalities in infants. Am J Dis Child 1978;132:376–378.
10. Babcock DS, Han BK, LeQuesne GW: B-mode gray scale ultrasound of the head in the newborn and young infant. AJR 1980;134:457–468.
11. Skolnick ML, Rosenbaum AE, Matzuk T, et al: Detection of dilated cerebral ventricle in infants: a correlative study between ultrasound and computed tomography. Radiology 1979;131:447–451.
12. Haber K, Wachter RD, Christenson PC, et al: Ultrasonic evaluation of intracranial pathology in infants: a new technique. Radiology 1980;134:173–178.
13. Vlieger M: Evaluation of echoencephalography. J Clin Ultrasound 1980;8:38.
14. Johnson ML, Rumack CM: Ultrasonic evaluation of the neonatal brain. Radiol Clin North America 1980;18:117–131.
15. Slovis TL, Kuhns LR: Real-time sonography of the brain through the anterior fontanelle. AJR 1981;136:277–286.
16. Ben-Ora A, Eddy L, Hatch G, Solida B: The anterior fontanelle as an acoustic window to the neonatal ventricular system. J Clin Ultrasound 1980;8:65–67.
17. Dewbury KC, Aluwihare APR: The anterior fontanelle as an ultrasound window for study of the brain: a preliminary report. Br J Radiol 1980;53:81–84.
18. Cremin BJ, Chilton SJ, Peacock WJ: Anatomical landmarks in anterior fontanelle ultrasonography. Br J Radiol 1983:56:517.
19. Naidich TP, Yousefzadeh DK, Gusnard DA. II: The neonatal head. Sonography of the normal neonatal head. Supratentorial structures: State-of-the-art imaging. Neuroradiology 1986;28:408–427.
20. Richardson DJ, Grant EG: Scanning techniques and normal anatomy, in Grant GE (ed): Neurosonography of the Pre-Term Neonate. New York, Springer-Verlag, 1986, pp 1–24.
21. Grant EG, Schellinger D, Borts FT, et al: Real-time sonography of the neonatal and infant head. AJR 1981;136:265–270.
22. Shuman WP, Rogers JV, Mack, et al: Real-time sonographic sector scanning of the neonatal cranium: technique and normal anatomy. AJNR 2:349–356.
23. Edwards MK, Brown DL, Muller J, et al: Cribside neurosonography: real-time sonography for intracranial investigation of the neonate. AJR 1981;136:271–276.
24. Pigadas A, Thompson JR, Grube GL: Normal infant brain anatomy: correlated real-time sonograms and brain specimens. AJNR 1981;2:339–344.
25. Harwood-Nash DC, Flodmark O: Diagnostic imaging of the neonatal brain: review and protocol. AJNR 1982;3:103–115.
26. Monteagudo A, Reuss ML, Timor-Tritsch IE: Imaging the fetal brain in the second and third trimester using transvaginal sonography. Obstet Gynecol 1991;77:27–32.
27. Chi JG, Dooling EC, Gilles FH: Gyral development of the human brain. Ann Neurol 1977;1:86.
28. Dorovini-Zis K, Dolman CL: Gestational development of brain. Arch Pathol Lab Med 1977;101:192.
29. Moore KL: The Developing Human. Clinically Oriented Embryology, 4th ed. Philadelphia, WB Saunders Company, 1988, pp 364–401.

30. Vergani P, Ghidini A, Sirtori M, et al: Antenatal diagnosis of fetal acrania. J Ultrasound Med 1987;6:715.
31. Cox GG, Rosenthal SJ, Holpsapple JW: Exencephaly: sonography findings and radiologic-patho-logic correlation. Radiology 1985;155:755.
32. Cunningham ME, Walls WJ: Ultrasound in the evaluation of anencephaly. Radiology 1976;118:165.
33. Icenogle DA, Kaplan AM: A review of congenital neurologic malformations. Clin Pediatrics 1981;9:565.
34. Johnson A, Losure TA, Weiner S: Early diagnosis of fetal anencephaly. J Clin Ultrasound 1985;13:503.
35. Pretorius DH, Russ PD, Rumack CM, Manco-Johnson ML: Diagnosis of brain neuropathology in utero. Neuroradiology 1986;28:386.
36. Rottem S, Bronshtein M, Thaler I, Brandes JM: First trimester transvaginal sonographic diagno-sis of fetal anomalies. Lancet 1989;1:444–445.
37. Hidalgo H, Bowie J, Rosenberg ER, et al: In utero sonographic diagnosis of fetal cerebral anomalies. AJR 1982;139:143.
38. Fiske EC, Filly RA: Ultrasound evaluation of the abnormal fetal neural axis. Radiol Clin North Am 1982;20:285.
39. Chevernak FA, Isaacson G, Mohoney MJ, et al: Diagnosis and management of fetal cephalocele. Obstet Gynecol 1984;64:86.
40. Nyberg DA, Mahony BS, Pretorius DH: Diagnostic Ultrasound of Fetal Anomalies Text and Atlas. Littleton, Year Book Medical Publishers, 1990, pp 83–202.
41. Foderaro AE, Abu-Yousef MM, Benda JA, et al: Antenatal ultrasound diagnosis of iniencephaly. J Clin Ultrasound 1987;15:550.
42. Romero R, Pilu G, Jeanty P, et al: Prenatal Diagnosis of Congenital Anomalies. Norwalk, Conn., Appleton & Lange, 1988.
43. Aleksic S, Budzilovich G, Greco MA, et al: Iniencephaly: neuropathologic study. Clin Neuro-pathol 1983;2:55.
44. Jones KL: Smith's Recognizable Patterns of Human Malformation, 4th ed. Philadelphia, WB Saunders Company, 1988, p 548.
45. David TJ, Nixon A: Congenital malformations associated with anencephaly and iniencephaly. J Med Genet 2976;13:263.
46. Shoham (Schwatz) Z, Caspi B, Chemke J, et al: Iniencephaly: prenatal ultrasonographic diagno-sis—a case report. J Perinat Med 1988;16:139.
47. Lemire RJ, Beckwith JB, Shepard TH: Iniencephaly and anencephaly with spinal retrofelxion: a comparative study of eight human specimens. Birth Defects 1987;23:225.
48. Filly RA, Chinn DH, Callen PW: Alobar holoprosencephaly: ultrasonographic prenatal diagno-sis. Radiology 1984;151:455.
49. Babcock DS: Sonography of congenital malformations of the brain. Neuroradiology 1986;28:428.
50. Page LK, Brown SB, Gargano FP, et al: Schizencephaly: a clinical study and review. Childs Brain 1975;1:348.
51. Komarniski CA, Cyr DR, Mack LA, et al: Prenatal diagnosis of schizencephaly. J Ultrasound Med 1990;9:305.
52. Greene MF, Benacerraf B, Crawford JM: Hydranencephaly: US appearance during in utero evolution. Radiology 1985;156:779.
53. Chevernak FA, Jeanty P, Cantrine F, et al: The diagnosis of fetal microcephaly. Am J Obstet Gynecol 1984;49:512.
54. Chevernak FA, Rosenberg J, Brightman RC, et al: A prospective study of the accuracy of ultrasound in predicting fetal microcephaly. Obstet Gynecol 1987;69:908.
55. Tolmie JL, McNay M, Stephenson JBP, Doyle D, et al: Microcephaly: genetic counseling and antenatal diagnosis after birth of an affected child. Am J Med Genet 1987;27:583–594.
56. Bauman ML: Neuroembryology—clinical aspects. Sem Perinatol 1987;11:74–84.
57. Goldstein I, Reece EA, Pilu G, et al: Sonographic assessment of the fetal frontal lobe: a potential tool for prenatal diagnosis of microcephaly. Am J Obstet Gynecol 1988;158:1057.
58. Kurtz AB, Wapner RJ, Rubin CS, et al: Ultrasound criteria for in utero diagnosis of microceph-aly. J Clin Ultrasound 1980;8:11.
59. Kendall BE: Dysgenesis of the corpus callosum. Neuroradiology 1983;25:239.
60. Hernanz-Schulman M, Dohan FC, Jones T, et al: Sonographic appearance of callosal agenesis: correlation with radiologic and pathologic findings. AJNR 1985;6:361.

61. Babcock DS: The normal, absent, and abnormal corpus callosum: sonographic findings. Radiology 1984;151:449.

62. Barkovich AJ, Norman D: Anomalies of the corpus callosum: correlation with further anomalies of the brain. AJR 1988;151:171.

63. Atlas SW, Shkolnik A, Naidich TP: Sonographic recognition of agenesis of the corpus callosum. AJNR 1985;6:369.

64. Bertino RE, Nyberg DA, Cyr DR, et al: Prenatal diagnosis of agenesis of the corpus callosum. J Ultrasound Med 1988;7:251.

65. Gebarski SS, Gebarski KS, Bowerman RA, et al: Agenesis of the corpus callosum: sonographic features. Radiology 1984;151:443.

66. Lockwood CJ, Ghidini A, Aggarwal R, et al: Antenatal diagnosis of partial agenesis of the corpus callosum: a benign cause of ventriculomegaly. Am J Obstet Gynecol 1988;159:184.

67. Vergani P, Ghidini A, Mariani S, et al: Antenatal sonographic findings of agenesis of corpus callosum. Am J Perinatol 1988;5:105.

68. Meizner I, Barki Y, Hertzanu Y: Prenatal sonographic diagnosis of agenesis of corpus callosum. J Clin Ultrasound 1987;15:262.

69. Dobyns WB: Developmental aspects of lissencephaly and the lissencephaly syndromes birth defects 1987;23:225.

70. Dobyns WB, Kirkpatrick JB, Hittner HM, et al: Syndromes with lissencephaly. II: Walker-Warburg and cerebro-oculo-muscular syndromes and a new syndrome with type II lissencephaly. Am J Med Genet 1985;22:157.

71. Habib Z: Genetics and genetic counselling in neonatal hydrocephalus. Obstet Gynecol Surv 1981;36:529.

72. Burton BK: Recurrence risks for congenital hydrocephalus. Clin Genet 1979;16:47.

73. Vintzileos AM, Ingardia CJ, Nochimson DJ: Congenital hydrocephalus: a review and protocol for perinatal management. Obstet Gynecol 1983;62:539.

74. Russ PD, Pretorius DH, Johnson MJ: Dandy-Walker syndrome: a review of fifteen cases evaluated by prenatal sonography. Am J Obstet Gynecol 1989;161:401.

75. Hirsh JF, Pierre-Kahn A, Renier D, et al: The Dandy-Walker malformation. J Neurosurg 1984;61:515.

76. Nyberg DA, Cyr DR, Mack LA, et al: The Dandy-Walker malformation: prenatal sonographic diagnosis and its clinical significance. J Ultrasound Med 1988;7:65.

77. Taylor GA, Sanders RC: Dandy-Walker syndrome: recognition by sonography. AJNR 1983;4:1203.

78. Fileni A, Colosimo C, Mirk P: Dandy-Walker syndrome: diagnosis in utero by means of ultrasound and CT correlations. Neuroradiology 1983;24:233.

79. Kirkinen P, Jouppila P, Valkeakari T, et al: Ultrasonic evaluation of the Dandy-Walker syndrome. Obstet Gynecol 1982;59:18S.

80. London DA, Carroll BA, Enzmann DR: Sonography of ventricular size and germinal matrix hemorrhage in premature infants. AJNR 1980;1:295.

81. Sauerbrei EE, Digney M, Harrison PB, Cooperberg P: Ultrasonic evaluation of neonatal intracranial hemorrhage and its complications. Radiology 1981;139:677.

82. Poland RL, Slovis TL, Shankaran S: Normal values for ventricular sizes as determined by real time sonographic techniques. Pediatr Radiol 1985;15:12.

83. Rumack CM, Johnson ML: Real-time ultrasound evaluation of the neonatal brain. Clin Diagn Ultrasound 1982;10:179.

84. Shackelford GD: Neurosonography of hydrocephalus in infants. Neuroradiology 1986;28:452.

85. Naidich TP, Schott LH, Baron RL: Computed tomography in evaluation of hydrocephalus. Radiol Clin North Am 1982;20:143.

86. Naidich TP, Epstein F, Lin JP, Kricheff II, Hochwald GM: Evaluation of pediatric hydrocephalus by computed tomography. Radiology 1976;119:337.

87. Edwards MK, Brown DL: Hydrocephalus and shunt function. Semin Ultrasound 1982;3:242.

88. Chitkara U, Cogswell C, Norton K, et al: Choroid plexus cysts in the fetus: a benign anatomic variant or pathologic entity? Report of 41 cases and review of the literature. Obstet Gynecol 1988;72:185.

89. Chan L, Hixson JL, Laifer SA, et al: A sonographic and karyotypic study of second-trimester choroid plexus cysts. Obstet Gynecol 1989;73:703.

90. Benacerraf BR, Harlow B, Frigoletto FD: Are choroid plexus cysts an indication for second-trimester amniocentesis? Am J Obstet Gynecol 1990;162:1001.

91. DeRoo TR, Harris RD, Sargent SK, et al: Fetal choroid plexus cysts: prevalence, clinical significance, and sonographic appearance. AJR 1988;151:1179.

92. Shuangshoti S, Netsky MG: Neuroepithelial (colloid) cysts of the nervous system: further observations on pathogenesis, incidence, and histochemistry. Neurology 1966;16:887.

93. Benacerraf BR: Asymptomatic cysts of the fetal choroid plexus in the second trimester. J Ultrasound Med 1987;6:475.

94. Benacerraf BR, Laboda A: Cyst of the fetal choroid plexus: a normal variant? Am J Obstet Gynecol 1989;160:319.

95. Chudleigh P, Pearce JM, Campbell S: The prenatal diagnosis of transient cysts of the fetal choroid plexus. Prenat Diagn 1984;4:135.

96. Hertzberg BS, Kay HH, Bowie JD: Fetal choroid plexus lesions: relationship of antenatal sonographic appearance to clinical outcome. J Ultrasound Med 1989;8:77.

97. Farhood AI, Morris JH, Bieber FR: Transient cysts of the fetal choroid plexus: morphology and histogenesis. Am J Med Genet 1987;27:977.

98. Nicolaides KH, Rodeck CH, Godsen CM: Rapid karyotyping in nonlethal fetal malformations. Lancet 1986;1:286.

99. Fitzsimmons J, Wilson D, Pascoe-Mason J, et al: Choroid plexus cysts in fetuses with trisomy 18. Obstet Gynecol 1989;73:257.

100. Chuang S, Harwood-Nash D: Tumors and cysts. Neuroradiology 1986;28:463.

101. Banna M: Arachnoid cysts on computed tomography. AJR 1976;127:979.

102. Robinson RG: Congenital cysts of the brain: arachnoid malformations. Prog Neurol Surg 1971;4:133.

103. Menezes AH, Bell WE, Perret GE: Arachnoid cysts in children. Arch Neurol 1980;37:168.

104. Vintzileos AM, Eisenfeld LI, Campbell WA, et al: Prenatal ultrasonic diagnosis of arteriovenous malformation of the vein of Galen. Am J Perinatol 1986;3:209.

105. Ordorica SA, Marks F, Frieden FJ, et al: Aneurysm of the vein of Galen: a new cause for Ballantyne syndrome. Am J Obstet Gynecol 1990;162:1166.

106. Reiter AA, Huhta JC, Carpenter RJ, et al: Prenatal diagnosis of arteriovenous malformation of the vein of Galen. J Clin Ultrasound 1986;14:623.

107. Mendelsohn DB, Hertzanu Y, Butterworth A: In utero diagnosis of a vein of Galen aneurysm by ultrasound. Neuroradiology 1984;26:417.

108. Rodemyer CR, Smith WL: Diagnosis of a vein of Galen aneurysm by ultrasound. J Clin Ultrasound 1982;10:297.

109. Diebler C, Dulac O, Dominique R, et al: Aneurysms of the vein of Galen in infants aged 2 to 15 months: diagnosis and natural evolution. Neuroradiology 1981;21:185.

110. Watson DG, Smith RR, Brann AW: Arteriovenous malformation of the vein of Galen. Am J Dis Child 1976;130:520.

111. Gradin WC, Taylon C, Fruin AH: Choroid plexus papilloma of the third ventricle: case report and review of the literature. Neurosurgery 1983;12:217.

112. Hawkins JC: Treatment of choroid plexus papilloma in children: a brief analysis of twenty years' experience. Neurosurgery 1980;6:380.

113. Milhorat TH, Hammock MK, Davis DA, et al: Choroid plexus papilloma. I. Proof of cerebral spinal fluid overproduction. Childs Brain 1976;2:273.

114. Eisenberg HM, McComb JG, Lorenzo AV: Cerebrospinal fluid overproduction and hydrocephalus associated with choroid plexus papilloma. J Neurosurg 1974;40:381.

115. Smith WL, Menezes A, Franken EA: Cranial ultrasound in the diagnosis of malignant brain tumors. J Clin Ultrasound 1983;11:97.

116. Cappe IP, Lam AH: Ultrasound diagnosis of choroid plexus papilloma. J Clin Ultrasound 1985;13:121.

117. Hoff NR, Mackay IM: Prenatal ultrasound diagnosis of intracranial teratoma. J Clin Ultrasound 1980;8:247.

118. Sauerbrei EE, Cooperberg PL: Cystic tumors of the fetal and neonatal cerebrum: ultrasound and computed tomographic evaluation. Radiology 1983;147:689.

119. Snyder JR, Lustig-Gillman I, Milio L, et al: Antenatal ultrasound diagnosis of an intracranial neoplasm (craniopharyngioma). J Clin Ultrasound 1986;14:304.

120. Lipman SP, Pretorius DH, Rumack CM, et al: Fetal intracranial teratoma: US diagnosis of three cases and a review of the literature. Radiology 1985;157:491.

121. Sabbagha RE, Tamura RK, Compo SD, et al: Fetal cranial and craniocervical masses: ultrasound characteristics and differential diagnosis. Am J Obstet Gynecol 1980;138:511.

122. Dolkart LA, Balcom RJ, Eisinger G: Intracranial teratoma: prolonged neonatal survival after prenatal diagnosis. Am J Obstet Gynecol 1990;162:768.

CHAPTER 16

Vaginal Sonographic Puncture Procedures

Ilan Timor-Tritsch, MD
David B. Peisner, MD
Ana Monteagudo, MD

INTRODUCTION

Ultrasonographically guided puncture procedures, such as aspirating, shunting, or draining fluids, are not new to the sonographer or the clinician. These have been done using transabdominal sonography. The percutaneous aspiration of intra-abdominal abscesses was first described by Smith and Bartrum in 1974.[1] Gerzof et al described the use of a percutaneous abdominal catheter placement to drain pus collections.[2] The success rate of such draining procedures, based on multiple series, is 78.5%; the complication rate is 10.4%.[3]

During its short existence, transvaginal sonography (TVS) has been found to be useful for not only imaging, but also for invasive diagnostic techniques and therapeutic procedures. Vaginally performed procedures gained prominence through the introduction of human egg retrieval, which was the pathway through which vaginal sonography entered the world of gynecology and obstetrics in most countries. The aim of this chapter is to present the various puncture procedures done with the guidance of the vaginal probes, and the experience gained.

The *scope* of any ultrasound-guided puncture should be to expose the patient to the least amount of trauma while exercising the most up-to-date clinical improvement. The *reasons* for performing any puncture procedure should be diagnostic in order to gain access to information by simple insertion of a needle, palliative and/or therapeutic. In most cases, it is a combination of the above-mentioned reasons. The advantages of these procedures are: their ease of mastering; accurate needle placement; almost no injury to adjacent organs; versatile location (it is portable); low cost; and speed of administration. The risks involve bleeding, infection, puncture of organs, and, in the case of multifetal reductions, miscarriage—but these are few and rare.

Two issues require discussion: The first is the *slice thickness artifact*. A common mistake made by many is to consider ultrasound imaging as a "perfect," two-dimensional section of a body part, totally lacking the third dimension. However, this third dimension does exist, and because of the physical properties of the sound, it is thinnest at the focal range of the probe and is inversely proportional with the operating frequency of the transducer crystal. The "third dimension" of the image should always be taken into account. One must keep in mind that at times the tip of the needle used for puncture procedures appears to be within the structure at which it is aimed, while in reality it is in front or behind the structure imaged. However, because of the thickness of the "slice," which includes both the structure and the tip of the needle, both are displayed on the same two-dimensional image on the screen.

The second issue deals with the *free-hand* approach to puncture procedures. Therefore, before discussing the procedures themselves, a few words are required to describe the use of the needle guide attached to the shaft/handle of the vaginal probes.

For several years, transabdominal needle guides were used when a needle had to be directed into any part of the body. However, with increasing experience, the "free-hand" approach has been successfully practiced. The operator's "eye-hand" coordination and the ease of handling the needle to be kept in the scanning plane made this technique easy to apply. However, the "free-hand" technique may sometimes image only the transverse section of the needle, excluding the tip. The actual site of the needle tip may be entirely different and not known to the operator (Fig 16.1**A**, **B**). Using the "abdominal approach" a quick "readjustment" of the scanning plane can be done to find the needle tip. However, using the transvaginal approach, limited mobility of the probe and the needle made the "free-hand" needle approach somewhat cumbersome. The needle guide attached to the shaft of the probe makes it easier for the operator to keep the entire length of the needle within the scanning plane (Fig 16.2**A**, **B**) and have perfect control over the exact plane of the tip of the needle. It also frees the second hand to perform other tasks.

MATERIALS AND METHODS

A general guideline for the majority of the procedures is given here, though some punctures follow additional protocols. These will be discussed separately.

The punctures are usually performed with the guidance of 5.0–7.5 MHz vaginal transducer probes through a needle guide attached to the shaft of the probe. Some companies offer disposable needle guides and attachments. A software-generated fixed line, displayed on screen, marks the path of the penetrating needle. Most of these provide the operator with a centimeter scale to measure needle depth. Depending upon the nature of the procedure performed, needles ranging from 21 to 14 gauge are employed. The thinnest possible needle able to perform the desired task should be used.

For better imaging, the "zoom" feature of the equipment should be used as frequently as possible (Fig 16.3).

Patients should be informed about the procedure and asked to sign routinely used consent forms. Specifically worded consent forms are usually used in procedures such as multifetal reductions and salpingocentesis. Analgesia and local anesthesia is achieved in the majority of cases by IV meperidine (usually 25–50 mg) combined with diazepam (5–10 mg) as well as a local injection of 2–3 ml 1% Lidocaine through the needle guide into the vaginal mucosa at the puncture site. This should be injected through the needle guide and probe in their final position. Additional movement and adjustment of the probe should be minimal after the injection.

The procedures should be documented by still images and/or videotape recordings. Following the withdrawal of the needle the pelvic structures and the cul-de-

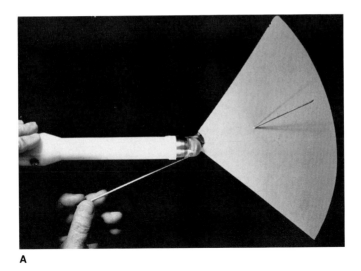

A

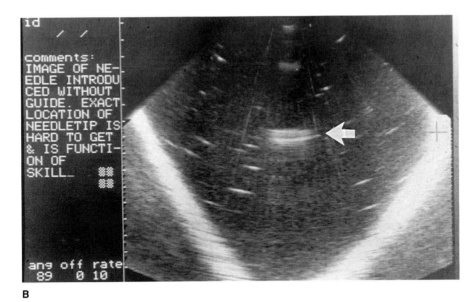

B

Figure 16.1 (**A**) A free-hand puncture procedure is modeled. If the needle is not within the scanning plane (represented by the fan-like plane) only the part of the needle which crosses the scanning plane is imaged. (**B**) The cross-sectional image of the needle is displayed in a water bath (arrow).

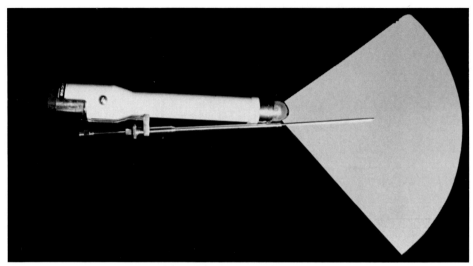

A

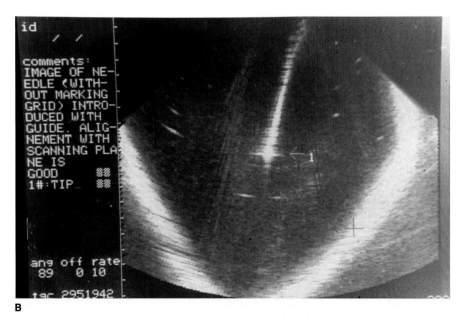

B

Figure 16.2 (A) Use of the needle guide is demonstrated. The needle guide keeps the needle within the scanning plane. **(B)** The image of the needle in the water bath is shown. The entire length of the needle can be seen, including the needle tip.

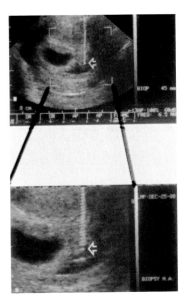

Figure 16.3 The region of interest is enlarged.

sac must be observed for approximately 10 minutes to detect any possible bleeding. The patients are rescanned after a 3-hr observation period for possible complications. A detailed report describing the procedure should be done promptly.

The following puncture procedures guided by transvaginal sonography will be presented:

1. Punctures of ovarian cysts
2. Multifetal reductions
3. Salpingocentesis, treatment of ectopic pregnancies
4. Drainage of pelvic content
5. Culdocentesis

PUNCTURE OF OVARIAN CYSTS

Puncturing an ovarian cyst is probably the simplest of all puncture procedures. It is similar to the most commonly used puncture procedure, the follicular aspiration performed by vaginal sonographic guidance, which is discussed in Chapter 9. Follicular aspiration was the first transvaginally guided puncture procedure introduced in treatment of infertility patients.[4] In these cases, the probe was used to guide a needle into the follicles and aspirate the eggs from the hormonally stimulated ovaries.

Ovarian cysts and symptomatic benign cystic pelvic lesions were punctured successfully.[5,6,7] Ron-El et al performed 30 punctures of ovarian cysts without complications.[8] Technically, aspiration of the cysts is a minor problem. The concern of spilling cells from a potentially malignant ovarian cyst into the abdominal cavity prevented us from using it more frequently. The aspirated fluid was submitted for cytological evaluation with the knowledge that the negative cytological exam may represent a false negative result.

Due to the controversial issue raised in connection with this procedure, at Columbia Presbyterian Medical Center (CPMC) only 4 patients were subjected to ovarian cyst puncture. Patients were rescanned after 3, 6, and 12 months for possible recurrence. All four patients in our small series had relative contraindications for an exploratory laparotomy, favoring a simple puncture procedure. The controversy prompted us to perform a study in which the vaginal sonographic properties and determinants were correlated to the pathological findings in more than 200 ovaries. Some of the results of this study are presented in Chapter 6. However, analysis of the results of that study formed our opinion that an ovarian cyst can safely be punctured if it has a thin wall, it is not of mixed echogenicity, does not demonstrate inner or outer nodularity, and the CA 125 levels are within normal limits (<35 U/ml). We now feel that in a limited number of patients the puncture of a solitary ovarian cyst may be an alternative to a more invasive operative approach. This may be more important in the postmenopausal patient, where an operative intervention carries a relatively high postoperative complication rate.[9]

The final word on the widespread use of ovarian cyst puncture has not been said. More research and evaluation of clinical experience is needed.

REDUCTION OF MULTIFETAL GESTATIONS

The introduction of ovulation-stimulating hormonal drugs, as in vitro fertilization/ embryo-transfer programs, has resulted in an increasing number of multiple gestations. If the number of fetuses is larger than 2 or 3, these pregnancies have a lower chance of a term delivery with healthy neonates than the singleton pregnancy.[10] The burden on the neonatal intensive care units and the costs of care may be high.[11]

Fetal and maternal complication rates for multifetal gestations are high. Mothers of triplets have a 35% risk of postpartum hemorrhage and at least a 20% rate of preeclampsia.[12] An extensive study from Oxford's National Perinatal Epidemiological Unit compared mortality rates among infants born as a result of multifetal gestations between 1975 and 1983. The pertinent statistical numbers are presented in Table 16.1. It is clear that the risk increases almost exponentially after the twin gestations.[13]

TABLE 16.1 Mortality for Single and Multiple Births in England and Wales for 1975–83 (excluding 1981)***[13]

Type of Birth	Stillbirth*	Perinatal*	Neonatal**	Post-Neonatal**	Infant	No. of Births (live and still)
Singleton	7.7	13.8	7.4	4.3	11.7	4,845,382
Twin	25.4	63.2	43.9	9.1	52.9	95,312
Triplet	47.5	164.5	135.0	12.7	147.7	1,812
Quadruplet	30.5	219.5	207.5	12.6	220.1	164
Quintuplet	—	200.0	200.0	—	200.0	20
Sextuplet	—	416.7	500.0	—	500.0	12

* Rates per 1000 total births.
** Rates per 1000 live births.
*** Some numbers were rounded to the closest whole number value.
Source: OPCS series FM1 and DH3 Annual Reference Volumes.

TABLE 16.2 Average Length of Gestation for Pregnancies with Known Time of Ovulation and 20 or More Weeks Gestation

Number of Fetuses	Number of Pregnancies	Weeks Completed*
Singleton	82	39
Twins	21	35
Triplets	5	33
Quadruplets	3	29

* Calculated from 2 weeks before ovulation.
From Caspi et al: Br J Obstet Gynaecol 1976;83:967.[11]

The fact that if the number of fetuses increases, the birthweight decreases is another issue concerning the outcome of multifetal pregnancies. The differences in the mean duration of the gestation is striking: for twins, 260 days (37 weeks), and for triplets, 247 days (35 weeks), compared to 281 days (40 weeks) in singleton gestations.[14] Based on an accurate time of ovulation, the time of delivery was assessed by Caspi et al.[15] The average time of delivery decreased as the number of fetuses increased. That trend is illustrated in Table 16.2.

One of the ways nature deals with the problem of multifetal gestations is that one or more embryos/fetuses ceases developing and expires at very early stages, leaving behind a singleton or twin pregnancy. This, as mentioned before, increases the survival rate of the remaining live fetuses.

After ultrasonography was introduced for imaging and assessing the early pregnancy, the concept of "reducing" the number of fetuses in utero to a desired, lower number was ready to be implemented. The transcervical ultrasound-guided suction procedure was introduced for selectively reducing the number of multifetal gestations.[16]

The transabdominal ultrasound-guided technique was first presented by French physicians[17,18] and adopted by others.[12,19,21,22] With the provision of transvaginal sonography in the guidance of ovum aspiration for in vitro fertilization and embryo transfer, the techniques were attempted and successfully applied in multifetal reduction procedures. A few centers in the world are currently performing this reduction procedure transvaginally. At the time of this writing a total of 95 vaginally performed "fetal reductions" had been reviewed. Relatively few articles on the subject have been published or submitted for publication.[23–28] This information is summarized in Table 16.3.

TABLE 16. 3 Transvaginally Performed Multifetal Reductions Performed at Various Centers*

Author	No. of Cases	No. of Deliveries	No. of "Early Ab"	No. of Late Losses	No. of Ongoing Pregnancies Over 26 Weeks
Itskovitz[23,24,29]	16	11	—	4	2
Gonen[26]	6	3	1	—	2
Shalev[25]	10	8	1	—	1
Timor-Tritsch	63	35	3	4	4
TOTAL	95	56	6 (6.3%)	4 (4.2%)	9

* Data compiled: August 1990.

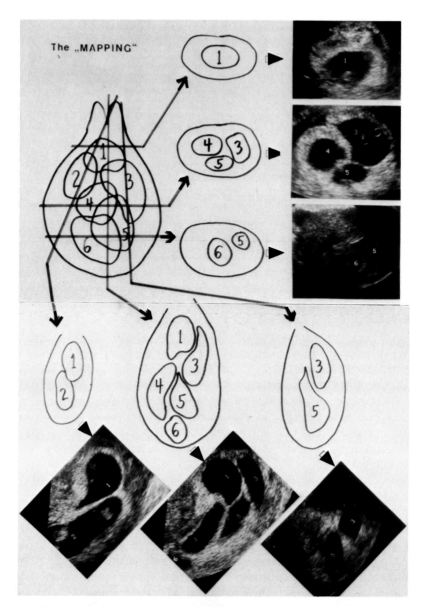

Figure 16.4 The mapping procedure is shown. This was a sextuplet pregnancy. The mapping is performed through parallel horizontal cross-sectional images, seen on the right side of the picture. The almost parallel longitudinal sagittal sections are shown on the lower part of the image. These images show the spatial interrelationships of the gestational sacs.

The technique for the reduction of multifetal gestation employed at Columbia Presbyterian Medical Center and Rambam Medical Center is the following:

After a detailed counseling session, ''baseline'' mapping procedure of the chorionic sacs is performed before the puncture (Fig 16.4). The area of the heartbeats of the targeted fetus is sought, and after the needle tip is placed, $\frac{1}{2}$–1 ml of 2 meq/ml KCl solution is injected through the needle to stop the heart (Figs 16.5 and 16.6). The heartbeat for each injected fetus is observed for 5–10 minutes to ascertain cessation. The patients are rescanned once weekly. If they leave the

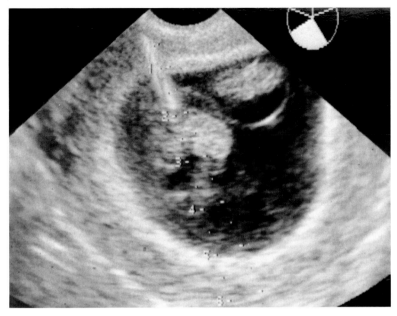

Figure 16.5 Fetal reduction. A 4-to-2 reduction was done on this patient. This illustration depicts two of the four embryos, which were in the same chorionic sac, but were diamniotic. Both were reduced. The tip of the needle is seen in one of the embryos.

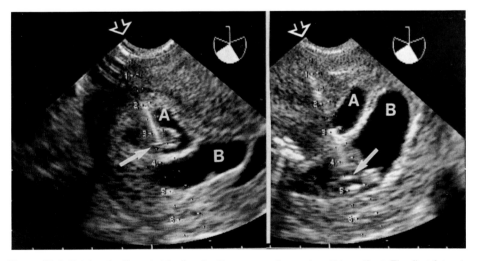

Figure 16.6 Fetal reduction. A 4-to-2 reduction was performed on this patient. The first fetus to be reduced was fetus A. The tip of the needle is seen within the fetus, at the left side. On the right side, the same needle was advanced into fetus B. The advantage of this is that the needle is inserted only once, to minimize maternal morbidity.

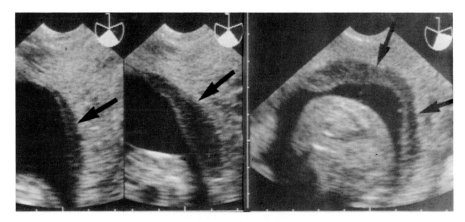

Figure 16.7 From left to right, increasing size of a developing subchorionic bleeding (arrows), following needle insertion for multifetal reduction.

geographical area, they are encouraged to be scanned by the referring physician. The gradual disappearance of the fetal pole and the chorionic sac is monitored. At times a subchorionic hematoma is seen at or around the line of the needle penetration (Fig 16.7). If the placental site of the living fetuses was not involved, no further complication was noted.

If injection of KCl is contemplated, a thin needle (gauge 20–21) is used to minimize bleeding along the needle path. If aspiration of the embryos at 6–7 weeks is planned,[23] a larger gauge needle (gauge 18 or 17) must be considered.

At the Rambam Medical Center in Haifa, Israel, 16 vaginally guided selective multifetal reductions were performed. These are referred to in Table 16.3.

At the Sloane Hospital for Women (Columbia Presbyterian Medical Center), we present the following statistical data:

Seventy-one women were referred for reduction. By the time of the procedure, one of each triplet gestation in two patients showed no more heartbeats; therefore, the patients withdrew. Six sets of twins were not reduced following extensive counseling. Sixty-three reduction procedures were done.

A previously described aspiration-suction technique[23] was used in two 4-to-2 reductions using a 16-gauge needle. The matter aspirated from the sacs was sent for tissue identification.

Twenty-three of the 63 multifetal gestations were the result of in vitro fertilization and embryo transfer. Thirty-six occurred after hormonal stimulation and ovulation induction. Four (three twins and one triplet) occurred ''naturally.''

The gestational ages at which the procedure was performed ranged from 6 weeks and 5 days (in two ''aspiration'' cases) to 13 weeks and 2 days (one case). The remaining 60 cases were between 8 weeks and 0 days, and 10 weeks and 2 days.

The distribution of the initial and final number of embryos can be seen in Table 16.4.

TABLE 16.4 The Initial and Final Number of Embryos (CPMC)

7 to 2	1
6 to 2	1
6 to 3	1
5 to 2	6
4 to 2	21
4 to 1	4
3 to 2	11
3 to 1	12
2 to 1	6
Total	63

Sixteen minutes was the average time to complete the injection of the KCl and ascertain that no more fetal heartbeats were present. Most of this time was spent ascertaining the latter.

Of the 63 patients, 35 delivered. The distribution of the deliveries in this group is shown in Table 16.5.

The antepartum morbidity of these patients is shown in Table 16.6.

Four patients have now passed 26 weeks of their pregnancy. There were seven pregnancy losses. We considered losses up to 3 weeks from the reduction as procedure-related losses and there were three such losses. The detailed information concerning these losses is outlined in Table 16.7. Seventeen patients are continuing their pregnancy but are less than 26 weeks gestation.

The rate of loss can be expressed as the percentage of loss pertinent to the whole series ($7/63 = 11.1\%$). It can also be calculated as the number of losses related to the procedure itself (three) over the total number of already delivered patients plus those having gestations past 26 weeks ($3/46 = 6.5\%$).

The immaturity and prematurity rates are expected to be similar to those of the "nontreated" singletons, twins, and triplets.[30,31] However, the present statistics involve only a few cases; therefore, it is premature to draw final conclusions. Based on the still limited experience with the transvaginally performed multifetal reductions it is unreasonable to compare the efficiency of the transvaginal with the transabdominal method. However, some of the advantages and disadvantages of the vaginal route can be summarized.

The advantage of transvaginal over transabdominal fetal reduction is that the needle path is shorter; it can be done at an earlier gestation; the image is much clearer; a thinner gauge needle can be employed; and at 6–7 weeks, aspiration techniques can be used.

TABLE 16.5 Gestational Age at Delivery by Final Number of Fetuses

Final No.	<32	32–34.5	34.5–36	>37
3 n=1	0	1	0	0
2 n=23	5	3	4	11
1 n=11	0	0	0	11

TABLE 16.6 Pregnancy Complications

	Triplets (n=1)	Twins (n=23)	Singleton (n=11)
Antepartum Hospitalization	–	2	–
Premature Labor	–	8	–
Gestational Diabetes	–	2	–
Preeclampsia	+	2	–
Cesarean Section	+	10	1
Neonatal Hospitalization	–	8	–
Neonatal Death	–	1	–

The disadvantage of transvaginal fetal reduction is that at an earlier gestational age, the number of fetuses is not yet "settled." However, there seems to be very low pregnancy wastage after the fetal heartbeats are established.[31] The fear of "spontaneous reduction" may be the reason for several centers reporting a preference for performing reduction in a two-step procedure—first to three, and then finally to the final number of two or one.[21,22,25,27]

Lately somewhat larger series of multifetal reductions performed through the transabdominal puncture method were produced.[32,33] *What should the final number of fetuses be after the reduction procedure?*

It is clear that a woman carrying four or more fetuses is exposed to a significantly higher fetal loss and maternal risk than one carrying twins. Based on the perinatal outcome for twins, the suggestion that two fetuses be left after a multifetal reduction procedure is reasonable. For the same reasons twin pregnancies should not, as a rule, be offered selective reduction. However, there will always be the case of a woman willing to terminate the entire twin gestation if she cannot be offered the possibility of "reducing" the pregnancy to a singleton gestation with which she feels she and her family can cope. Triplet pregnancies present a unique problem. Statistical data of survival, neonatal mortality, and morbidity have to be included in the patient information together with the risks of the

TABLE 16.7 Results: Fetal Losses

No.	Reduction	Gestational Age at Reduction	Elapsed Time
1	4 to 2	13w 5d	3 weeks
2	3 to 1	11w 3d	11 weeks
3	2 to 1	7w 2d	3 days
4	3 to 2	8w 5d	10 weeks & 13 weeks
5	2 to 1	8w 5d	2 days
6	3 to 1	9w 2d	6.5 weeks
7	3 to 2	14w 3d	10 weeks

puncture procedure. The decision of undergoing a reduction in the event of a triplet pregnancy is a judgmental decision which most of the time is difficult to make.

The Ethical Aspect

There is hardly an article dealing with the subject of multifetal reductions that does not devote thoughtful discussion on the ethical questions involved with this procedure. The confusion surrounding the dilemma of multifetal gestations starts with the multitude of names it is called: (1) selective reduction, (2) selective termination, (3) selective fetocide, (4) selective embryocide, (5) selective abortion, (6) selective birth. Several articles deal just with the nomenclature.[21,35] We agree with Berkowitz et al that the term "reduction of multifetal pregnancy" should be used since this term illustrates the nature of the procedure dissociating it from the "selective" termination of targeted fetuses.[36] The extent to which the ethical issue is discussed may be different; however, the conflicts revolve around two issues: First, the pregnancy is wanted and everything should be done to preserve it. Second, there is the feeling of duty not to destroy human life without ethically justifiable reasons.

Exhaustive and valuable treatises of these moral quandaries are reflected in the works of Evans, Fletcher, et al[21] as well as Hobbins.[36]

The consensus is that this procedure should be offered to patients as a modality to preserve a viable and desired pregnancy. Choosing among the modalities, the physician must advise the one resulting in the least harm and most good for mother and fetus.[37]

SALPINGOCENTESIS

The classic approach to ectopic gestation has always been surgical. The diseased tube or ovary was resected. More conservative approaches such as parenteral or local injection of methotrexate and the simple conservative follow-up have recently gained popularity. All these methods attempt to avoid surgical intervention.

The possibility of diagnosing the different clinical patterns of this disease enabled us to consider different therapeutic approaches to the problem. A nonruptured tubal gestation, which is not bleeding and which demonstrates steady or falling levels of β hCG without a beating fetal heart, may now need only a careful follow-up or the oral administration of methotrexate; whereas a live ectopic pregnancy with positive fetal heart activity may require an operative approach such as laparoscopy or laparotomy.

Since the introduction of transvaginal sonography with a high-frequency probe, a more accurate and faster diagnosis of ectopic pregnancy is feasible.

The use of a needle which is inserted into a tubal embryo under transvaginal ultrasound guidance is just a step away from the combination of the oocyte aspiration and the multifetal pregnancy reduction. It seems indeed logical to use a puncture procedure to treat the ectopic pregnancy, thus saving the patient from a more invasive procedure.

Feichtinger described for the first time the use of the transvaginally guided needle puncture to treat the ectopic tubal gestation.[38] The tube, which was injected with 10 mg of methotrexate in 1 ml solvent, contained a conception without fetal heartbeats.

Since then, several centers began using this modality as an additional tool in the treatment of patients with ectopic pregnancy.[38–40,45] The number of publications on the subject is small. However, we were able to compile published and anecdotal information on about 70–80 such procedures performed in various centers.[38–44] Of these 70–80 cases, only 16 were published. Since the reports are incomplete, it is very hard to compute the success or failure rate of this procedure. It appears, however, that the failure rate of this procedure is about 12–15%.

The procedure should be considered experimental at this time and should be performed under IRB protocol.

The Technique

The technique used was the following. Patients in this group were required to sign a special informed consent form which stated that this was an experimental procedure approved by the Institutional Review Board of our hospital. Needle gauges of 20 and 21 were used. After slight sedation (IV Demerol and Valium) the "tubal ring" containing the ectopic embryo was imaged. Using the machine's software-generated puncture path line, the needle was introduced in the area of the beating heart (Figure 16.8). The automated puncture device described in Chapter 2 facilitated the accurate and virtually painless needle placement. About $\frac{1}{4}$–$\frac{1}{2}$ ml KCl (2 meq/ml) was injected to stop the heart. The area was then watched for 10 minutes. After the procedure, these patients were admitted for an overnight stay to follow their vital signs. The next day, after rescanning the pelvis, they were discharged. Determination of serum βhCG levels and transvaginal sonography were performed twice weekly for three weeks and once weekly thereafter until the βhCG levels reached nonpregnant levels. If surgical intervention followed, the βhCG levels were followed until nonpregnant levels were observed. We performed eight such procedures.

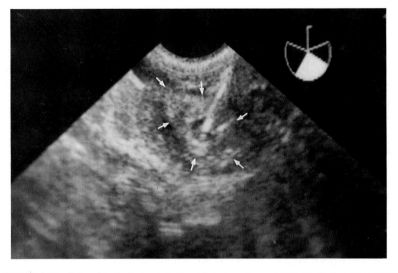

Figure 16.8 The tip of the needle is seen in the gestational sac within the tubal ring, highlighted by small arrows.

TABLE 16.8 Patients Receiving Treatment by Salpingocentesis to Treat a Live Tubal Ectopic Pregnancy

Patient	Initial βhCG MIU/ml (IRP)	Gestational Age at Puncture	Days at Which βhCG Level at Less Than 10 Level	Outcome
H	3,090	6w 6d	82	Normal.
R	77,500	8w 1d	29	Operated because levels increased; tube was not ruptured.
C	25,800	6w 3d	31	Ruptured 4 days after puncture.
P	11,000	6w 4d	58	Normal.
B	8,090	6w 3d	64	Normal. Hysterosalpingogram showed patent tube.
Y	55,000	6w 4d	20	Operated for bleeding from puncture site.
S	3,600	6w 2d	25	Operated after 21 days for complication of a subsequent culdocentesis.
BF	5,370	6w 5d	50	Normal.

Table 16.8 summarizes the gestational ages, initial levels of βhCG, and the time lapse between the procedure and the return of the βhCG to nonpregnant levels in the material at CPMC. The behavior of the serum βhCG levels is depicted in Figure 16.9.

The procedure was successful in 4 patients. In one patient (B), the subsequent hysterosalpingogram showed patency of the only existing tube which had the treated ectopic gestation.

In patient C the tube ruptured 4 days after the procedure. Salpingectomy was performed. Patient R underwent an uneventful procedure, but the levels of the βhCG did not drop for 6–7 days, at which time the managing physician elected to operate and remove the tube. At surgery the tube was not found to be distended and there was no blood in the cul-de-sac. In patient Y, slow but continuous bleeding occurred after extraction at the site of the 20-gauge needle. She was operated on within 30 minutes and had 250 ml blood in the pelvis. The puncture site was still slowly oozing. This was the only procedure-related complication. The last patient (S) had a normal postpartum course. However, after 21 days, she presented to the night emergency service with abdominal pain. A diagnostic culdocentesis was not productive of fluid or blood, and the next day the TVS showed the resolving process. Four days later, fever appeared and surgery was planned for an acute pelvic process. Some trophoblastic tissue and blood clots were found by the pathological examination in the removed tube.

Because of this complication rate (15%), the physician should bear in mind the following: possible bleeding during or immediately following the procedure occurs if the puncture is close to the mesosalpinx. However, it seems impossible to avoid puncturing through this area. One of our cases (Y) was complicated by such

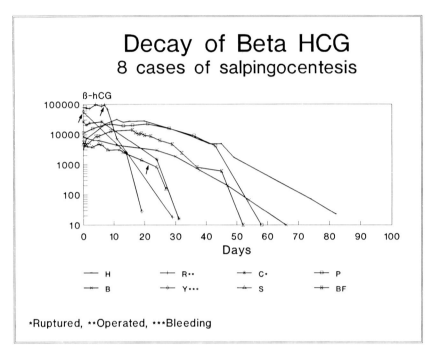

Figure 16.9 Serial determinations showed that in patients who underwent successful salpingo-centesis (H, P, B) the serum levels of βhCG returned to nonpregnant levels between 58 and 82 days, while the levels of those in which the tube was removed by subsequent surgery (R, C, Y) dropped below 10 MIU/ml within 20–31 days. The arrows indicate the time of the laparotomy.

bleeding. Thin needles may reduce this possibility. Late rupture of the tube on subsequent days may occur because of slow but continuous bleeding into the tubal gestational sac, or the continuing growth of the trophoblast in cases of KCl injection. This is witnessed by the elevation or even slowly increasing trends of βhCG levels throughout the first week following the salpingocentesis. This phenomenon could be accounted for in cases R and C.

Obviously, the injected KCl, which stopped the ectopic fetus' heartbeats, did not have any negative feedback to inhibit trophoblastic production of βhCG. Another interesting observation is that the successful cases in our group demonstrated a very slow return of the βhCG to the nonpregnant levels (60–80 days). On the other hand, in the hormonal levels of those patients with salpingectomies the βhCG dropped to nonpregnant levels within two weeks. From the literature it seems that the return of βhCG levels to normal in cases of methotrexate injection in the tube occurs within 3–4 weeks.[45]

To prevent continuing growth of the trophoblast, replacing the KCl by methotrexate is possibly the answer. The question of subsequent tubal patency requires continuing study. One patient (B) underwent hysterosalpingography and her only tube was found to be patent. In the literature, only a limited number of patients treated by salpingocentesis, who underwent hysterosalpingography, have been reported to have patent tubes.[40]

There may be an upper limit of gestational age or tubal size; this would be another area requiring study. After analyzing our failed cases, it appears that ectopic pregnancies of more than 8 completed weeks, or tubes measuring more than 2 cm across their shortest axis, should not undergo such therapy.

In patients it was possible that the infectious course was caused by the diagnostic culdocentesis performed somewhat overzealously in the emergency suite and without first using noninvasive vaginal sonography.

More information is needed to draw the necessary conclusions regarding salpingocentesis as a treatment for live ectopic tubal gestations. The authors stress that at this time the procedure requires adherence to a research protocol.

On the basis of the experience gathered throughout the world, we believe that the transvaginally introduced needle by high-frequency transvaginal sonographic guidance has the potential to become useful in the treatment of an early tubal gestation with a live fetus.

In the future, the treatment of ectopic gestation may fall into one of the following categories:

1. The ruptured or advanced ectopic pregnancy will still necessitate laparotomy or laparoscopy.
2. The unruptured but missed ectopic pregnancy with decreasing levels of βhCG may be safely followed by transvaginal sonography and serial βhCG determinations. Locally or systemically administered methotrexate can be a good alternative in these patients.
3. Selective ectopic pregnancies with a live conceptus may be treated by the transvaginally performed puncture procedure discussed in this chapter.

Early transvaginal sonographic examination of the high-risk population, to identify and classify ectopic gestations, is advisable so that the best therapeutic approach can be selected. The transvaginally performed sonographically directed puncture procedure represents an important addition to the treatment of this widespread complication.

Drainage Procedures

As was mentioned in the introduction, pelvic drainages have a long-lasting tradition in ultrasonography. This invasive procedure was first performed by inserting a needle or a drainage catheter through the vagina, guided by a transabdominal transducer.[47,48]

Transvaginal sonographic imaging of the cul-de-sac is ideal to depict pathological conditions because of their close proximity to the tip of the probe. With the same ease a needle can be directed alongside the shaft of the vaginal transducer into fluid collections. With the needle in place and under continuous observation the fluid can be safely aspirated. Because septations and loculated fluid can accurately be imaged, the needle can subsequently be aimed at the various compartments and they can be aspirated, one pocket after the other.

There are two ways to aspirate or drain pelvic fluid with transvaginal ultrasound guidance. The first technique is the simple aspiration of the contents (Fig 16.10). Extraction of the needle at the end of the aspiration marks the end of the procedure. The second modality is the placement of a plastic catheter, to be left in place for several days to assure continuous drainage. This is particularly useful in the treatment of pelvic abscesses. We developed a catheter placement technique to assure prolonged drainage of the female pelvis. The instrument tray used is shown in Figure 16.11.

The abscesses are first partially drained by the use of a 14-gauge needle (Fig 16.12). A flexible guide-wire is then introduced into the needle (Fig 16.13). After

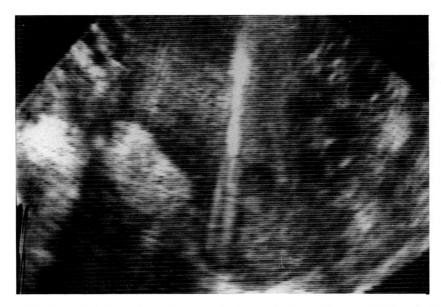

Figure 16.10 The final stage of emptying a pelvic abscess is shown. No more fluid is seen. The tip of the needle dips into a small pocket of fluid.

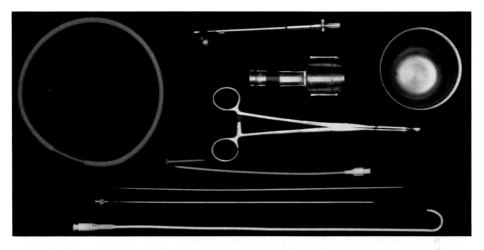

Figure 16.11 A tray used for catheter placement for continuous pelvic abscess drainage. On the left, the curled up wire is seen.

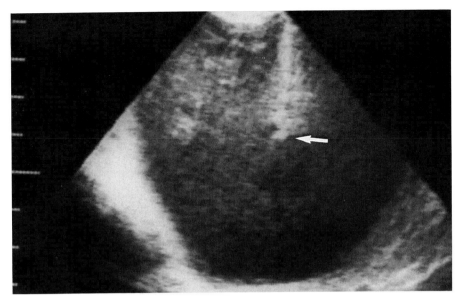

Figure 16.12 The entire length of the needle (arrow) is seen in the pelvic abscess.

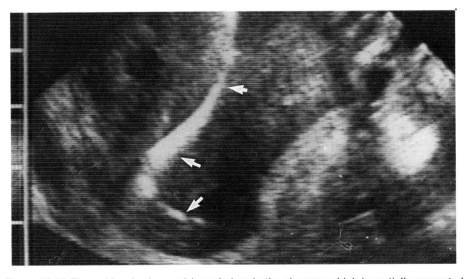

Figure 16.13 The guide-wire (arrows) is curled up in the abscess, which is partially evacuated.

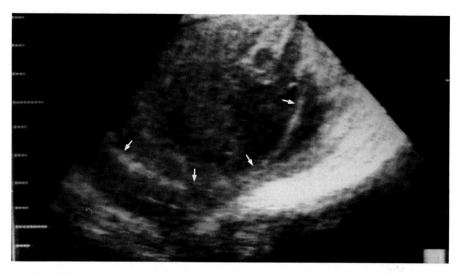

Figure 16.14 The plastic drainage tube is seen within the cavity of the abscess (small arrows).

leaving the wire in place, the needle is extracted. A plastic catheter with multiple perforations is then slid over the guide-wire (Fig 16.14). Finally, the guide-wire is pulled and the indwelling pelvic catheter fixed to the thigh. The patient should be rescanned 2 and 4 days following the procedure and the tube extracted if there is no more drainage of fluid, or no pelvic fluid appears on the scan.

The 18 drainage procedures performed at CPMC are listed and detailed in Table 16.9.

There were five drainage catheter placements for pelvic abscesses as a result of pelvic inflammatory processes, one evacuation of a postoperative pelvic hematoma, and 12 aspirations for postoperative pelvic peritoneal retention cysts. The time from the original operation leading to the fluid retention to the drainage varied from 5 months to one year. Four of the twelve retention cysts reaccumulated, but to a much smaller size, and became asymptomatic. Patients with catheter placements for drainage were discharged in 5–9 days with no need for additional treatment after a follow-up scan confirmed the efficacy of the procedure. No

TABLE 16.9 Patients Treated by Puncture Procedures for Drainage of Pelvic Content

No. of Patients	Remarks	Procedure
Drainage of pelvic abscess with catheter placements	5	Catheter left in place 4–7 days.
Evacuation of pelvic hematoma	1	No catheter was left in place.
Drainage of peritoneal inclusion cysts	12	Amount aspirated was 170–1280 ml. In 3, some reaccumulation was observed.
Total	18	

complications were encountered. In two patients at the time of the procedure the puncture site had to be widened by a #11 surgical blade to accommodate the catheter.

Drainage of pelvic fluid of any origin is an extremely easy procedure with no morbidity and a good patient tolerance. If no catheter is left in place, it can be performed in an office or emergency room setting.

CULDOCENTESIS

Inserting a needle in the cul-de-sac is an accepted diagnostic procedure which can be performed without hospitalization.[48] The technique is simple and it is employed in the evaluation of pelvic fluid. It is mostly performed in the case of a patient suspected of ectopic pregnancy. Fluid-containing fragments of old blood clots, or bloody tinged fluid which does not subsequently clot, gives rise to the possible diagnosis of hemoperitoneum, which is a result of a ruptured ectopic pregnancy. If the blood clots, it may have originated from a perforated blood vessel rather than a ruptured ectopic gestation. One exception can be mentioned: if a brisk bleeding from the site of the ruptured tube occurs, the blood may be aspirated from the cul-de-sac before it has time to clot. However, with such an intense bleeding, culdo-centesis is rarely necessary to obtain the diagnosis. In such instances, the shock resulting from blood loss will be obvious and culdocentesis should be deferred. The culdocentesis may be unsatisfactory in women who had previous inflamma-tory disease of the pelvis with an obliterated cul-de-sac. Therefore, the failure to aspirate blood from the cul-de-sac in no way excludes the diagnosis of hemoperi-toneum and certainly, it is not proof against the presence of an ectopic preg-nancy—either unruptured or ruptured.[50] Recent developments in diagnostic and treatment modalities require the reevaluation of the importance and the role of a blind culdocentesis. The noninvasive techniques, such as a rapid βhCG test or the transvaginal ultrasonography, contributed to a fast and accurate diagnosis without the use of the culdocentesis. Laparoscopy has recently been introduced, not only as a diagnostic, but also a tool through which definitive treatment of ectopic pregnancy can be performed.[49,50]

In previous chapters, the possibility of diagnosing a very small amount of fluid in the cul-de-sac was presented. Most of the time it is possible to distinguish between completely sonolucent pelvic content and particulate matter containing fluid in the pelvis. Despite the wide availability of transvaginal sonography, culdo-centesis continues to be employed in most centers. Recently, the role of culdocen-tesis in the management of ectopic pregnancy was reevaluated by Vermesh et al.[51] Their results reconfirmed previous reports establishing the lack of correlation between the tubal status and the results of culdocentesis. All these studies were in agreement that culdocentesis was of little value beyond the diagnosis of hemoperi-toneum.

The data of this study performed by Vermesh et al reinforce our belief that culdocentesis is an invasive and painful procedure with little value in the clinical setting where transvaginal sonography and rapid pregnancy testing are available. Transvaginal sonography can image the smallest amount of intraperitoneal pelvic fluid, as well as a very early intrauterine pregnancy, which is important for the workup of the patient suspected of ectopic pregnancy. Patients in whom the ectopic gestation could not be ruled out by means of ultrasonography and pregnancy testing are probably best managed by laparoscopy rather than culdocentesis.

As previously mentioned, with the introduction of transvaginal sonography, the need for culdocentesis may be limited. If there is a need to differentiate between clear fluid and blood or pus, the vaginal scanning method should be employed first. If, in conjunction with clinical signs and symptoms, as well as a quick βhCG test, the clinician still requires the information provided by culdocentesis, insertion of the needle can safely and accurately be done by the technically foolproof transvaginal sonographic-guided puncture procedure. Also, if a culdocentesis is performed prior to vaginal sonography, some air can be introduced into the cul-de-sac, and this may act as a sonic curtain in preventing an adequate sonographic study to establish the diagnosis.

At Columbia Presbyterian Medical Center we performed only three culdocenteses by transvaginal sonographic guidance. All of these were performed to rule out purulent content of the cul-de-sac.

It is reasonable to assume that the presence of a sufficiently trained person in transvaginal sonography, and a readily available vaginal probe for the above-mentioned cases, will decrease or perhaps eliminate the need for diagnostic culdocentesis.

OTHER PUNCTURE PROCEDURES

Chorionic Villi Sampling

Ghirardini and Popp suggested the possibility of directing a needle through the vaginal fornix into the chorionic tissue under vaginal sonographic guidance.[52] In a recent article Popp and Girardini[53] reported on the technique and their results in 15 vaginal sonographically guided transmural chorionic biopsies. In all 15 cases, material was successfully obtained.

Early Amniocentesis

Using the transvaginally directed needle it is possible to aspirate amniotic fluid earlier than the clinical 14–18 week span at which this is usually performed. Shalev et al reported on performing this procedure at 9–10 weeks.[54]

SUMMARY

In this chapter, the transvaginally performed puncture procedures have been described, evaluated, and summarized. The advantages of such procedures are their performance under constant real-time imaging, the very low procedure-related complication rate, and the ease and simplicity of the mostly outpatient procedures. In some cases abdominal or vaginal surgery can be avoided.

This experience encourages consideration of this treatment modality in individually evaluated cases. Some of them can be performed in an office or emergency room setting, others in hospitals only under carefully monitored protocols.

REFERENCES

1. Smith EH, Bartrum RJ Jr.: Ultrasonically guided percutaneous aspiration of abscesses. AJR 1974;122:308–312.
2. Gerzof SG, Johnson WC, Robbins AH, Nasbeth DC: Expanded criteria for percutaneous abscess drainage. Arch Surg 1985;120:227–232.
3. Gerzof SG, Johnson WC: Radiologic aspects of diagnosis and treatment of abdominal abscesses. Surg Clin North Am 1984;64:53–65.
4. Dellenbach P, Nisand I, Moreau L, Feger B, Plumere C, Brun B, Gerlinger P, Rumper Y: Transvaginal sonographically controlled ovarian follicle puncture for egg retrieval. Lancet 1984;1:1467.
5. Schwimmer SR, Marik J, Lebovic J: Percutaneous ovarian cyst aspiration using continuous transvaginal ultrasonographic monitoring. J Ultrasound Med 1985;4:259.
6. Fornage BD, O'Keeffe F: Ultrasound-guided transvaginal biopsy of malignant cystic pelvic mass. J Ultrasound Med 1990;9:53–55.
7. Granberg S, Crona N, Enk L, et al: Ultrasound-guided puncture of cystic tumors in the lower pelvis of young women. J Clin Ultrasound 1989;17:107.
8. Ron-El H., Herman A., Weinraub Z., Bukovsky İ, Caspi E: Transvaginal puncture of ovarian cysts. European J Obstet Gynecol (Accepted for publication).
9. Shapiro B: Evaluation of respiratory function in the perioperative period. ASA Refresher Courses 1979;221:1.
10. Walker EM, Patel NB: Mortality and morbidity in infants born between 20 and 28 weeks gestation. Br J Obstet Gynaecol 1987;94:670–674.
11. Caspi E, Ronen J, Schreyer P, Goldberg MD: The outcome of pregnancy after gonadotropin therapy. Br J Obstet Gynaecol 1976;83:967.
12. Syrop CH, Varner MW: Triplet gestation: maternal and neonatal implication. Acata Genet Med Gemellol (Roma) 1985;34:81–88.
13. Botting BJ, Davies IM, Macfarlane AJ: Recent trends in the incidence of multiple births and associated mortality. Arch Dis Child 1987;62:941–950.
14. McKeown T, Record RG: Observations on foetal growth in multiple pregnancy in man. J Endocrinology 1982;5:387.
15. Caspi E, Ronen J, Schreyer P, Goldberg MD: The outcome of the pregnancy after gonadotropin therapy. Br J Obstet Gynaecol 1976;83:967.
16. Dumez Y, Oury JF: Method for first trimester selective abortion in multiple pregnancy. Contrib Gynecol Obstet 1986;15:50–53.
17. Bessis R, Milanese C, Frydman R: Preventive partial termination in multiple pregnancy. The Second International Symposium, the Fetus as a Patient—Diagnosis and Therapy, Jerusalem, Israel, May 26–31, 1985, p 174.
18. Vrijens R, Beckhuizen W, Rombant R: Selective interruption of multiple pregnacy by ultrasonographic guidance. Proceedings of the World Congress of the World Federation of Ultrasound in Medicine and Biology, Sydney, Australia, 1985, p 271.
19. Brandes JM, Itskovits J, Timor-Tritsch IE, Drugan A, Frydman R: Reduction of the number of embryos in multiple pregnancy. Fertil Steril 1987;48:326–327.
20. Berkovitz RL, Lynch L, Chitkara U, Wiikins IA, Mehalek KE, Alvarez E: Selective reduction of multifetal pregnancies in the first trimester. N Engl J Med 1988;318:1042–1047.
21. Evans MI, Fletcher JH, Zador IE, Newton W, et al: Selective first-trimester termination in octuplet and quadruplet pregnancies: clinical and ethical issues. Obstet Gynecol 1988;71:289–296.
22. O'Keane JA, Yuen BH, Farquharson DF, Wittman BD: Endocrine response to selective embryocide in a gonadotropin-induced quintuplet pregnancy. Am J Obstet Gynecol 1988;158:364–367.
23. Itskovitz J, Boldes R, Thaler I, Bronstein M, Erlik Y, Brandes JM: Transvaginal ultrasonography-guided aspiration of gestational sacs for selective abortion in multiple pregnancy. Am J Obstet Gynecol 1989;160:215–217.
24. Itskovits J, Boldes R, Thaler I, Levron Y, Rottem S, Brandes JM: First trimester selective reduction in multiple pregnancy guided by transvaginal sonography. J Clin Ultrasound 1990;18:323–327.
25. Shalev E, Frenkel Y, Goldenberg M, Shalev E: Selective reduction in multiple gestations: pregnancy outcome after transvaginal and transabdominal needle-guided procedures. Fertil Steril 1989;52:416–420.

26. Gonen Y, Blankier J, Casper RF: Transvaginal ultrasound in selective embryo reduction for multiple pregnancy. Obstet Gynecol (in press).
27. Farquharson DF, Wittmann BK, Hansmann M, Ho Yuen B, Bladwin VJ, Lindahl S: Management of quintuplet pregnancy by selective embryocide. Am J Obstet Gynecol 1988;158:413–416.
28. Timor-Tritsch I.E., Peisner D.B., Monteagudo A.: Puncture procedures utilizing transvaginal ultrasonic guidance. Ultrasound Obstet Gynecol 1991;1:144–150.
29. Itskovitz J, Drugan A: Personal communication.
30. Levine MI: Grand multiple pregnancies and demand for neonatal intensive care. Lancet 1986;2:347.
31. Gonen R, Heyman E, Asztalos EV, Ohlson A, Pitson LC, Shennan AT, Milligan JE: The outcome of triplet, quadruplet and quintuplet pregnancies managed in a perinatal unit. Obstetric, neonatal and follow-up data. AJOG 1990;162:454.
32. Birnholz JC, Dmowski WP, Binor Z, Radwanska E: Selective continuation in gonadotropin-induced multiple pregnancy. Fertil Steril 1987;48:873.
33. Tabsh KMA: Transabdominal multifetal pregnancy reduction: report of 40 cases. Obstet Gynecol 1990;75:739–741.
34. Lynch L, Berkowitz RL, Chitkara U, Alvarez M: First trimester transabdominal multifetal pregnancy reduction: a report of 85 cases. Obstet Gynecol 1990;75:735–738.
35. Berkowitz RL, Lynch L: Selective reduction: An unfortuante misnomer. Obstet Gynecol 1990;75:273–274.
36. Hobbins JC: Selective reduction—A perinatal necessity. N Engl J Med 1988;318:1062–1063.
37. McCormick RA: How Brave a New World? Washington, DC, Georgetown University Press, 1981, pp 199–200, 443–444.
38. Feichtinger W, Kemeter P: Conservative treatment of ectopic pregnancy by transvaginal aspiration under sonographic control and methotrexate injection. Lancet 1987;1:381.
39. Timor-Tritsch IE, Baxi L, and Peisner DB: Transvaginal salpingocentesis: A new technique for treating ectopic pregnancy. Am J Obstet Gynecol 1989;160:459–461.
40. Feichtinger W, Kemeter P: Treatment of unruptured ectopic pregnancy by needling of sac and injection of methotrexate or PG E2 under transvaginal sonography control: report of 10 cases. Arch Gynecol Obstet 1989;246:85–89.
41. Popp L: Personal communication, West Germany.
42. Jansen C: Personal communication, The Netherlands.
43. Kurjak A: Personal communication, Yugoslavia.
44. Jeng CJ, Yang YG, Lan CC: Transvaginal ultrasound guided salpingocentesis with methotrexate injection: a minimally invasive treatment for early ectopic pregnancy. Presented at The Third World Congress on Vaginosonography in Gynecology, June 15, 1990, San Antonio, Texas.
45. Menard A, Crequat J, Mandelbrot L, Hauuy JP, Madelanat P: Treatment of unruptured tubal pregnancy by local injection of methotrexate under transvaginal sonographic control. Fertil Steril 1990;54:47–50.
46. Kojima E, Abe YU, Morita M, Ito M, Hirakawa S, Momose K: The treatment of unruptured tubal pregnancy with intratubal methotrexate injection under laparoscopic control. Obstet Gynecol 1990;75:723.
47. McArdle CR, Simon L, Kiejna C: Vaginal drainage of posthysterectomy abscess under direct ultrasonic guidance. Obstet Gynecol 1984;63:908.
48. Nosher JL, Winchman HK, Needell GS: Transvaginal pelvic abscess drainage with ultrasound guidance. Radiology 1987;165:872–873.
49. Williams Obstetrics, edited by F. G. Cunningham, P. C. McDonald, and N. F. Gant, 18th ed. Appleton & Lange, E. Norwalk, CT, 1989, pp 521–522.
50. Pouly JL, Mahnes H, Mage G, Canis M, Bruhat MA: Conservative laparoscopic treatment of 321 ectopic pregnancies. Fertil Steril 1986;46:1093–1097.
51. Vermesh M, Silva PD, Rosen GF, Stein AL, Fossum GT, Sauer MV: Management of unruptured ectopic gestation by linear salpingostomy: a prospective, randomized clinical trial of laparoscopy versus laparotomy. Obstet Gynecol 1989;73:400–404.
52. Girardini G, Popp LW, Gualerzi C, Spreafico L, Fochi F, Agnelli P: Chorionskopische und vaginosonographisch gezielte Trophoglastbiopsie, in Popp LW (ed) Gynäkologisch Endosonographie. Ingo Klemke Verlag, Quickborn 1986, pp 133–141.
53. Popp LW, Girardini A: The role of transvaginal sonography in chorionic villi sampling. J Clin Ultrasound 1990;18:315–322.
54. Shalev E et al.: First trimester transvaginal amniocentesis for genetic evaluation of multiple gestation. Prenatal Diagnosis 1990;10(5):344–345.

CHAPTER 17

Transvaginal Color Doppler Sonography

Asim Kurjak MD, PhD
Ivica Žalud, MD

By using Doppler ultrasound techniques one can gain more information than with the classical morphological ultrasonography.

INTRODUCTION

Transvaginal imaging is achieved with greater resolution and allows closer proximity to the uterus, ovaries, and pelvic vessels compared with transabdominal methods.[1-3] Such an approach is said to be a revolution in gynecologic practice and has grown to widespread use. More information can be obtained using Doppler ultrasound than could previously be gained only by morphological study. Color Doppler indicates direction, velocity, and type of blood flow, whereas pulsed Doppler enables quantification of such flow. However, the combination of high quality B-mode images, pulsed Doppler, and color coded Doppler flow imaging in the same vaginal probe produces a superb simultaneous picture of morphological and blood flow information from the female pelvic circulation. It is the purpose of this chapter to describe our clinical experience with transvaginal color Doppler of the female pelvis (see also Chapter 18).

BASIC PRINCIPLES

Transvaginal color Doppler utilizes an autocorrelating technique, a process for detecting the phase difference between two waves.[4] Blood flow data obtained by the autocorrelation technique must be converted to a form recognizable by the human eye. Since the structures of organs are displayed in black and white on a screen, a different display format must be employed for the imaging of blood flow. A convenient approach is the use of colors. The direction of flow is identified by red and blue, with flows moving toward a probe represented in red, while those moving away are blue. In addition, the two colors are assigned a level of brightness proportional to the blood flow velocity. The remaining color, green, serves to express the turbulence of flow with an increase in color proportionate to the turbulence. In other words, the color of forward flow with turbulence approaches yellow (as a mixture of red and green), and that of a reverse flow with turbulence approaches cyan (as a mixture of blue and green). The more laminar the flow, the more pure the red or blue tone displayed. Thus, the direction, velocity, and turbulence of flow are represented by varying the mixture ratio and brightness of three colors. Such blood flow color data are then superimposed on the anatomical tissue data, which are expressed in black and white and displayed simultaneously.

Although the pulsed Doppler technique has been widely used before in obstetrics, transvaginal application of this method is a recent development. In the pulsed wave Doppler system, pulsive bursts of ultrasonic waves are repeatedly emitted at a predesignated interval. The system permits the acquisition of blood flow data only at a specific depth by collecting the signals at a corresponding time delay from each of the pulses produced. Basically, each vessel imaged by color Doppler can be explored by pulsed Doppler. This is a major advantage when flow is to be studied in specific vessels. Flow can be assessed without interference from other vessels lying distally, or in close proximity to the same axis of investigation and having a different circulatory pattern. Quantification of color flow can be done by pulsed Doppler waveform analysis. The Pourcelot resistance index (RI) is a useful way of expressing blood flow impedance distal to the point of sampling.[5]

$$RI = \frac{A - B}{A}$$

In the above equation, "A" is the highest systolic velocity and "B" is represented by the velocity at the end of diastole. Each separate parameter is angle dependent. But, once they are in proper relation, the resistance index becomes independent of the angle between the investigated vessels and the emitted ultrasound beam. It is believed that the increased value of RI results from increased peripheral vascular resistance.[6]

This type of coupled transvaginal color with pulsed Doppler exploration has been developed recently and we have described its application by studying structures that were not previously reported. Transvaginal color Doppler saves time and increases accuracy of measurement. The most important advantage of this new technique is the display of blood flow across the entire scanning plane of the pelvis. Therefore, pulsed Doppler sample volume can be placed accurately on the area of interest using the guidance of the color flow, and spectral waveform analysis can be done easily. We believe the possibility of adding color Doppler capabilities to the high-resolution transvaginal imaging will become important in selecting the adequate equipment available on the market.

EXAMINATION TECHNIQUE

The procedure has to be explained to the patient and must be done in a relaxed atmosphere. All women should have an empty urinary bladder and should be scanned in the lithotomy position with a slight reverse Trendelenburg tilt to pool free fluid in the cul-de-sac. Women in their reproductive years should be scanned during days 3 to 10 of their menstrual cycle to exclude changes in intraovarian blood flow known to occur during the formation of the corpus luteum.[7,8] The 5 to 10 MHz transvaginal transducers usually produce a sector angle of 90° to 320° allowing a good view of the pelvic organs. Preparing the probe was presented in Chapter 3. The uterus, ovaries, and pelvic vessels are assessed after a systematic evaluation of pelvic anatomy. Sometimes it is difficult to identify the ovaries, especially in postmenopausal women. The internal iliac vessels can be used as a landmark for searching the ovary. After imaging the pelvic anatomy by B-mode, the equipment is switched to color Doppler mode to locate blood flow in normal or newly formed pelvic vessels. The color flow obtained enables detection of a vessel of interest which then could be interrogated with Doppler sample volume until the typical spectral waveform is seen. The angle of the transducer should slowly be adjusted to obtain the maximum waveform amplitude and clarity. The peak-systolic and end-diastolic Doppler frequency shifts can be recorded as well as the A/B ratio. The Pourcelot resistance index or the pulsatility index can be calculated.[9] Five separate cardiac cycles should be examined on each record and their mean value calculated. In experienced hands, the mean duration of a typical examination is usually no longer than 10 minutes. The spatial-peak temporal average intensity of the probe should not exceed 100 mW/cm^2. This is the highest allowed limit of insonation energy recommended by the U.S. Food and Drug Administration for use in fetal medicine.

In continuation, the morphology and sizes of pelvic structures should be reassessed. Subsequently, structures of particular interest should be examined for prominent areas of vascularization. In many cases these reflect neovascularization. These newly formed vessels usually appear as continuously fluctuating color rather than the typical pulsatile color flow seen within normal arteries and veins.

NORMAL PELVIC BLOOD FLOW

Blood flow in the main pelvic vessels can be easily recognized and imaged. The arteries and veins are distinguished according to the pulsation and brightness of the color flow. The external iliac vessels are situated lateral to the ovary, appearing in prominent color due to the high velocity of the blood flow. In all patients examined, the internal iliac vessels can easily be found. The depth of the side wall of the pelvis is close to the ovary (Figs 17.1, 17.2). Both the internal and external iliac arteries produce prominent and pulsating color flow of high velocity with typical reserve flow and very high impedance to the flow. The common iliac vessels can be seen only occasionally because they are usually too far from the tip of the probe. If seen, they present high velocity of blood flow with the most prominent reverse flow during diastole.

The color Doppler signal from the main uterine vessels can be seen in all patients laterally to the cervix at the level of cervicocorporeal junction of the uterus (Fig 17.3). The small branches of the uterine artery can be followed, searching in an ascending fashion along the lateral uterine wall. Even small terminal branches can be depicted in the direction of the ovary or the myometrium. The waveform analysis in these vessels shows a high to moderate velocity. The resistance index depends on the patient's age, part of the menstrual cycle, and special conditions (eg, pregnancy, tumor), and is usually very high.

It is difficult to detect the ovarian vessels, but an experienced operator using modern color Doppler equipment can achieve this in most patients in the lateral upper pole of the ovary. Color flow is usually not prominent; velocity is low, and resistance varies according to the menstrual cycle.

Vascularization of normal ovarian and uterine tissue could not be studied until transvaginal color Doppler was employed. Such small and randomly dispersed vessels present low velocity and moderate resistance blood flow. The ovarian blood flow is a function of the menstrual cycle, and in the proliferative part, the flow usually cannot be detected. Contrary to this, the luteal part is characterized by detectable color. This is due to the physiological angiogenesis in the corpus luteum. These newly formed vessels usually show prominent blood flow detected by transvaginal color Doppler. Such low-impedance and low-velocity flow should not be mistaken for the neovascularization of a tumor which is characterized by low impedance but moderate or high velocity of blood flow.

The Doppler imaging of blood flow in the main pelvic vessels is very important in the study of reproductive physiology and pathophysiology of fertility.[10] Uterine perfusion and cyclic changes of ovarian blood supply can be adequately studied since the typical waveforms of the already mentioned vessels have been established.[11] These will be touched upon in the appropriate section.

NEOVASCULARIZATION

Great interest and studies in recent years have focused on the process of neovascularization (angiogenesis). In males, new blood vessels are not normally produced in postnatal life. In healthy women, new vessels are produced in the vascularization of the corpus luteum each month and, naturally, in pregnancy. This neovascularization allows the functional activity of the ovary to be detected by Doppler technique.

The importance of neovascularization was first recognized by Judah Folkman in 1971, when he proposed the hypothesis that increased cell population must be preceded by the production of new vessels.[12] Folkman's hypothesis has been proven and is now universally accepted. Such abnormal tumor vascular morphology can be used as a valuable marker for tissue characterization. These vessels must be formed very early in the development of the tumor and, therefore, are early markers of the presence of a malignant tumor. New vessels are continually produced at the periphery of the tumor and act as a marker of continued growth and proliferation. The amount and vascularity of the stroma vary greatly in different tumors. In general, rapidly growing tumors, particularly sarcomas, have a highly vascular stroma with little connective tissue. Slow-growing tumors are less well vascularized.

The pathologic features of tumor neovascularity are well recognized. In tumors with peripheral vascularization, the vessels are obviously located primarily at the periphery. The centers of these tumors are usually poorly perfused; hence, penetration of blood-borne substances is difficult. As the tumor grows and invades the surrounding tissue, the vessels proliferate at the periphery. In tumors with central vascularization, vessels proliferate from the center like branches from a tree. In reality, the tumor may have many modules exhibiting one of these two types of idealized vascular patterns. Generally, the tumor vascularity is highly heterogeneous and does not conform to the "standard" normal vascular organization.[13] The vascular morphology of one tumor differs from another and is determined to some extent by the growth pattern of cancer cells. Quantitative morphometric studies in induced animal tumors show that vascular volume, length, and surface area increase during the early stages of tumor growth, and then decrease after the onset of necrosis. Frequency of large-diameter vessels increases in the later stages of growth.[13] New blood vessels and vascular channels in a tumor arise from older, preexisting vessels. Tumor vessels have a relative paucity of smooth muscle in their walls in comparison to their caliber. Since most of the resistance to flow resides at the level of the muscular arterioles, vessels deficient in these muscular elements present diminished resistance to flow, thereby receiving a larger volume of flow than vessels with a high impedance.

Obviously, microcirculation plays an important role in the growth, metastasis, detection, and treatment of tumors. Transabdominal pulsed Doppler imaging offers a view of the surrounding anatomy and evidence of blood flow in major pelvic vessels, but not in the microcirculation.[11,14] Transvaginal color Doppler offers a qualitative picture of blood flow in the vascular system in relation to the surrounding anatomy.[15-24] Unfortunately, most color Doppler machines have been developed for cardiac ultrasound and are insensitive to the detection of neovascular flow. It is not enough to merely demonstrate a vessel in the vicinity of the tumor; the diagnostic features of tumor vascularity are the high velocity and low impedance. Considerable modification in signals processing will very likely be necessary to optimize the color Doppler machines for detecting neovascular flow characteristics. Nevertheless, some of the more sensitive machines already show great potential for this purpose.

Intratumoral blood flow displayed on color Doppler images indicates that the flow is rapid enough to be detected. The presence of arterio-venous communications should be an important factor that produces sufficient velocity above the minimal threshold on color Doppler imaging. When tumoral blood flow is not seen on transvaginal color Doppler examination, the following factors should be taken into consideration:

1. The absence of blood flow is possibly due to lack of newly formed vessels which would be characteristic for a malignant tumor.
2. The velocity of flow may be too slow to exceed the minimal threshold for measurement with the color Doppler system used.
3. Intratumoral blood flow is nonuniform and turbulent, and the detectable blood flow on color Doppler imaging is distributed in certain regions of a tumor. It sometimes requires considerable effort to obtain a good angle of incidence to the target for color flow imaging.

At present, transvaginal color Doppler is not sensitive enough to rule out tumors when blood flow is not demonstrated. However, the technique may be useful in demonstrating pelvic tumors with rapid blood flow and in providing important hemodynamic information. Color Doppler can also depict the hemodynamic characteristic of the tumor, allowing echo sources of the hypoechoic zones to be separated into compartments, vesicles, and the blood pooling or hemorrhage surrounding them. Finally, color Doppler sonography may prove most efficacious in revealing the hemodynamic characteristics of tumors, thereby making ultrasound itself a more reliable procedure.

CLINICAL APPLICATION

Transvaginal color Doppler offers great challenge in scientific work but, equally important, can now be applied in routine clinical practice as well. Early diagnosis of pelvic malignancy, screening programs of ovarian carcinoma, study of uterine and ovarian perfusion in infertile and pregnant women, more accurate diagnosis of early pregnancy failure and ectopic pregnancy, study of embryonal and fetal circulation, etc, are only a few remarkable fields in obstetrics and gynecology that can be improved using this new diagnostic technique. Morphological study is combined directly with functional blood flow study and the combined information allows us better understanding of the nature of health and disease in order to render proper clinical treatment.

Adnexal Masses

Neoplasms of the ovary present an increasing challenge to the physician. Ovarian cancer is the most lethal of the gynecological cancers, presenting late and responding poorly to treatment. Primary ovarian cancer is an insidious and intractable disease, which may originate from different types of cells. Incidence of ovarian cancer is about 13/100,000 but the death rate is 7/100,000.[25] Cumulative risk up to the age of 75 is 1.3%. Five-year survival rate is still about 25%. In general, ovarian cancer represents 4% of all cancers in women and 6% of the death rate. In 1987, there were 18,500 new cases and 12,000 deaths caused by ovarian cancer in the United States. The cost of care per woman with ovarian cancer at stage III is about $100,000.[25] Preinvasive stages of ovarian cancer, such as the stage of cervical cancer, are still an unknown entity. In spite of intensive efforts to improve treatment of the established disease with advances in surgical and chemotherapeutic techniques, the prognosis for ovarian cancer has remained unchanged for 30 years. Attempts to detect early localized ovarian cancer have not yet been successful although many studies of ultrasound scanning with or without the use of CA 125 radioimmunoassay have been performed.[26]

The differentiation between benign and malignant adnexal tumors in vivo still involves many clinical problems. However, there are known features that characterize the difference. Many of them, such as the mitotic index and pleomorphysm, are of histologic nature and not amenable to current imaging methods. One feature of malignancy is the bizarre vascular morphology that characterizes many malignant tumors. Transvaginal color Doppler sonography seems to produce a better characterization of pelvic tumor vascularity than any other currently available diagnostic method. Our own results have shown that it is easy to demonstrate color flow in small vascular branches within tissues in pathological conditions (Figs 17.4–17.7).[15,16] In a group of 162 patients with a clinically and sonographically detected adnexal mass, 27 were histologically proved to be malignant and 135 were benign lesions. The presence of neovascularization was documented preoperatively in malignant ovarian tumors. The characteristic finding was the observation of small vascular channels within the solid part of the tumor. Being very thin and randomly dispersed within the tissue, such vessels are difficult to find unless transvaginal color Doppler is used. Our noncomparative prospective study has shown that tumor vascularity can be successfully used for the characterization of pelvic neoplasia (Table 17.1). Sensitivity, specificity, and accuracy are high within the limitation of the study design, and concern should focus on false negative rather than false positive findings (Table 17.2). Waveform analysis of signals obtained from the "hot" color coded area within masses produced excellent results. All malignant tumors had a resistance index lower than 0.40 and all benign tumors displaying color flow, a resistance index higher than 0.40. In an attempt to avoid normal luteal blood flow, we suggest that patients with an adnexal mass suspected to be malignant or in the screening procedure for ovarian cancer have examination only during days 1 to 10 of their menstrual cycle. It is not possible to see any low-impedance high-velocity blood flow. If during this time in the cycle such flow is detected, this may be characteristic for ovarian malignancy. Further research will undoubtedly develop the criteria for accurate differentiation between normal and abnormal blood flow inside the ovarian tissue. The velocity analysis in each of the above-mentioned situations could play an important role in the final clinical diagnosis.

TABLE 17.1 Transvaginal Color Doppler in the Characterization of Adnexal Masses (N = 162)

PHD	N	Color Flow Present	RI
Simple ovarian cyst	54	12 (22.2%)	0.65 ± 0.08
Endometriosis	27	2 (7.4%)	0.62 ± 0.07
Hydrosalpinx	12	1 (8.3%)	0.70
Dermoid	17	0 (0%)	—
Pseudocyst	1	1 (100%)	0.39
Cystadenoma	24	6 (25%)	0.56 ± 0.10
Cystadenocarcinoma	20	19 (95%)	0.33 ± 0.05
Granulosa cell tumor	3	3 (100%)	0.37 ± 0.02
Metastatic carcinoma	4	3 (75%)	0.29 ± 0.04
Total	162		

RI = resistance index.

The goal of transvaginal color Doppler sonography should be the identification of smaller ovarian tumors. Until now, no one diagnostic method has been successful enough in detecting ovarian cancer at an early stage. Consequently, there was no effective screening program for ovarian cancer and no simple diagnostic and therapeutic approach. Transvaginal color Doppler is a noninvasive method, and its diagnostic sensitivity, specificity, and accuracy seem to be clinically good enough to be used as the potential technique for such screening programs. Color Doppler ultrasound may become a useful diagnostic tool for observing changes in the vascularity of malignant gynecologic tumors before and following treatment.

It is reasonable to believe that women will be attracted to a screening program that indicates the chances of detecting this dreaded disease at its early stages are high. The development of procedures for the early detection of the disease is probably the best approach for achieving a reduction in the mortality. It is our belief that the routine application of transvaginal color Doppler sonography will enable the identification of those women with hydrosalpinx, tumor-like conditions, or benign tumors and save unnecessary operations. The application of this new technique to a larger number of cases, and collaboration of pathologist and geneticist, will enable the tumorigenic sequence of cellular and molecular events in the ovaries to be defined more precisely. The assessment of vascular changes and the resistance to blood flow may reduce the number of conventional ultrasono-

TABLE 17.2 Sensitivity, Specificity, and Accuracy of Transvaginal Color Doppler in the Detection of Ovarian Malignancy (N = 162)

Color Flow and RI	Pathological Diagnosis		
	Malignant	Benign	Total
Malignant	25	1	26
Benign	2	134	136
Total	27	135	162

RI = resistance index; PPV (positive predictive value) = 96.1%; NPV (negative predictive value) = 98.5%; sensitivity = 92.6%; specificity = 99.2%; accuracy = 98.1%.

graphic scans required to give definitive screening results. The ideal screening test for ovarian cancer would detect the disease in a premalignant phase, and thus provide a method for prevention of invasive disease. Unfortunately, there is as yet no reported precancerous lesion of the ovary analogous to cervical intraepithelial neoplasia or atypical endometrial hyperplasia. Perhaps early vascular changes inside the ovarian tissue could help in such an early diagnosis of ovarian malignancy. Current efforts to improve survival rates for ovarian cancer by screening are, therefore, directed toward the detection of early stage disease.[26] It is reasonable to hypothesize that a survival benefit would accrue from a screening program using a test with sufficient sensitivity to permit the diagnosis of a greater proportion of ovarian cancer cases at an early stage. Furthermore, the natural history of ovarian malignancy, particularly the length of preclinical phase is unclear. If the preclinical phase is short, the screening interval would have to be more frequent, maybe too frequent to be acceptable in clinical practice. Ultimately, a randomized controlled multicentric study will be required in order to assess the validity of the hypothesis. Such a prospective study is now in progress at institutes in Zagreb, New York, and London.

Uterine Masses

The presence of uterine tumor is often associated with hypervascularity as is also the case with hypervascular ovarian masses (Figs 17.8–17.10). Transvaginal color Doppler can be helpful in the diagnosis of uterine malignancy. Patients with suspected uterine tumors have been examined using 5 MHz transvaginal color Doppler. Color flow inside the endometrium and myometrium has been detected in all of 6 cases with endometrial carcinoma. The peripheral impedance was very low (RI = 0.34 ± 0.06).[15] In 5 cases of carcinoma in situ of the uterine cervix, no abnormality was found. We surmised that newly formed vessels are too small, and velocity and volume flow are below the resolution power of the equipment. In several uterine fibroids, color flow was detected in the border of the tumor. However, when peripheral impedance was compared in cases of myoma uteri and carcinoma endometrii, a significantly lower resistance index was obtained in the latter. Transvaginal color Doppler offers an acceptable sensitivity, specificity, and accuracy in the diagnosis of uterine malignancy.

Infertility

Transvaginal color Doppler measurements in the arteries of the pelvis can be used to study the changes of the blood flow during the spontaneous and stimulated ovarian cycle. The Doppler waveform classification of these arteries is based on absence or presence and duration of diastolic flow.[10] It was noted that diastolic and/or end-diastolic flow were not present in every infertile patient. While continuous diastolic flow was found in the recordings of all 154 healthy volunteers in our institute, it was not found in 19 of 66 infertile women. The preliminary data from an ongoing study suggest that the poor uterine perfusion response to endogenous hormones may be a cause of infertility. It is also postulated that a blood flow around a normal dominant follicle may also be an important hemodynamic parameter of its maturation, ovulation, and development of corpus luteum during spontaneous and stimulated cycles.

The technique of transvaginal color Doppler measurement offers the possibility

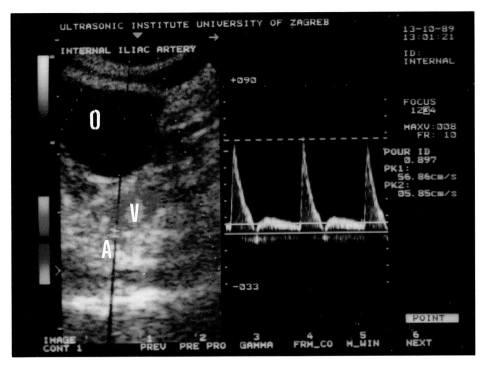

Figure 17.1 Transvaginal color Doppler of the internal iliac vessels. Waveform analysis (right) of the internal iliac artery presented high velocity and resistance of blood flow. Typical reverse flow was noted. A = internal iliac artery; V = internal iliac vein; O = ovary.

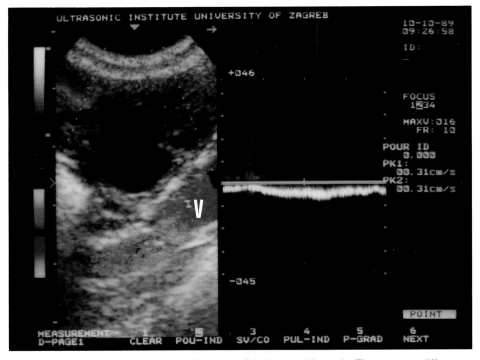

Figure 17.2 Color Doppler and pulsed Doppler of the internal iliac vein. There was no difference between systolic and diastolic flow. Typical finding for the venous blood flow. V = internal iliac vein.

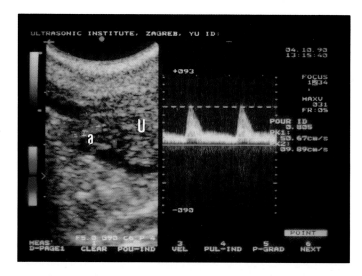

Figure 17.3 Color Doppler of the uterine artery. Pulsed Doppler analysis showed high velocity and resistance of blood flow. Typical normal finding. a = uterine artery; U = uterus.

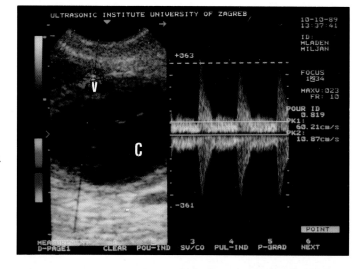

Figure 17.4 Cystic adnexal mass. Transvaginal color Doppler showed blood flow on the border of the cyst. Pulsed Doppler analysis (right) revealed normal high-resistance flow. Benign tumor was the diagnosis. C = ovarian cyst; v = tumor vessel.

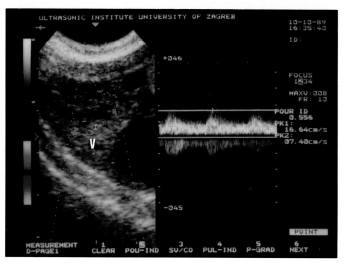

Figure 17.5 Mixed ovarian tumor. Color flow detected in the solid part of the tumor. Decreased resistance of flow indicated borderline case. v = tumor vessels.

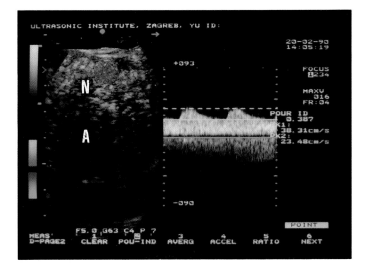

Figure 17.6 Dominantly solid adnexal mass. Neo-vascularization of the tumor was detected. Very low resistance of blood flow is specific for ovarian malignancy. N = neovascularization; A = adnexal mass.

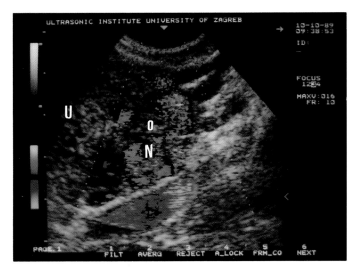

Figure 17.7 Abundant color flow in the case of ovarian malignancy. N = neo-vascularization; o = ovary; U = uterus.

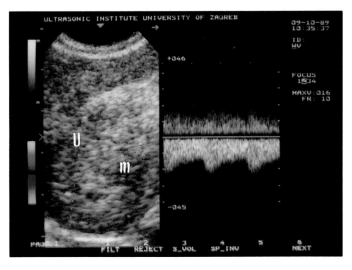

Figure 17.8 Myoma uteri. Color and pulsed Doppler indicated a benign uterine mass. Increased diastolic flow was obvious. U = uterus; m = myoma.

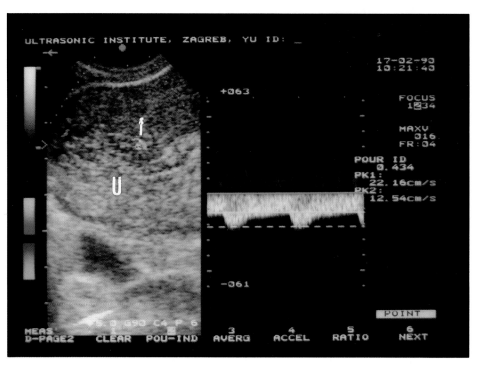

Figure 17.9 Borderline Doppler finding of the uterine mass. Low resistance index was obtained. U = uterus; f = blood flow.

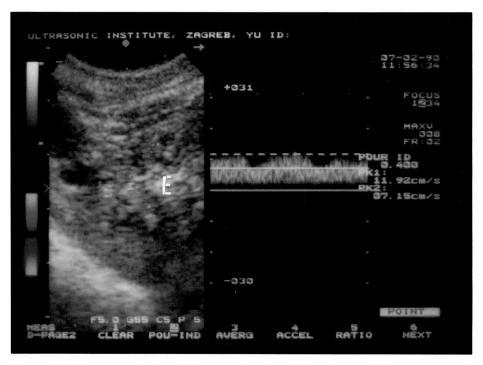

Figure 17.10 Neo-vascularization in the case of endometrial carcinoma. Malignant pattern of blood flow as assessed preoperatively. E = endometrium.

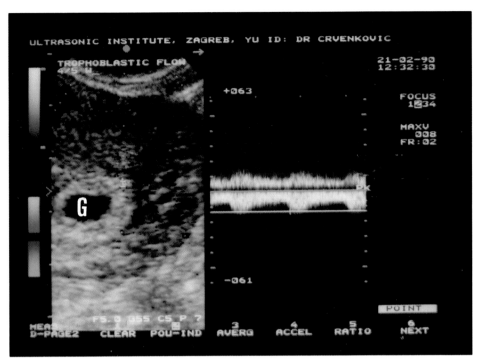

Figure 17.11 Trophoblast blood flow detected at 4 weeks and 5 days of amenorrhea. Doppler signal (right) indicated very low resistance of flow. G = gestational sac.

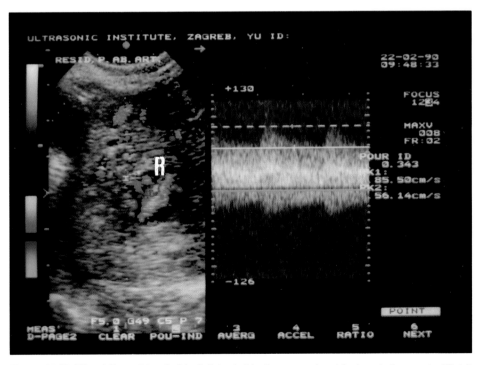

Figure 17.12 Blood flow of trophoblast detected in the case of residual gestation postartificial abortion. R = residual gestation.

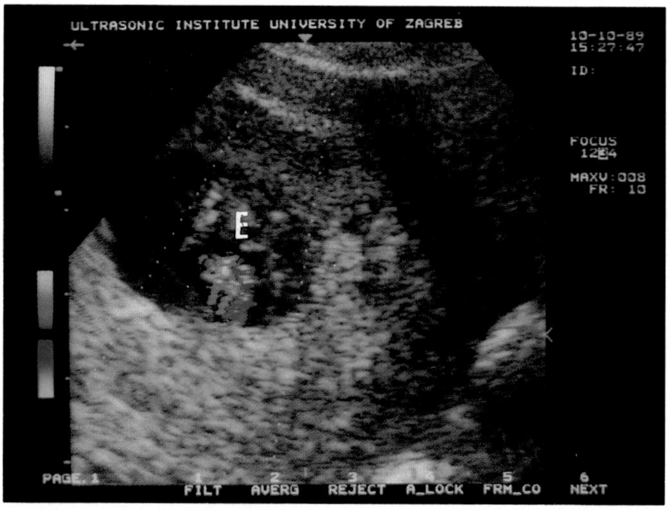

Figure 17.13 Umbilical blood flow imaged by transvaginal color Doppler at 7 weeks of gestation. E = embryo.

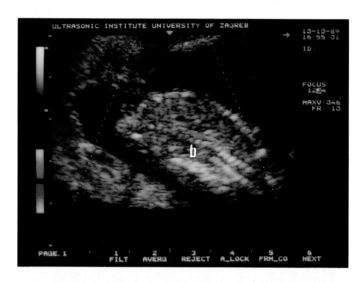

Figure 17.14 Imaging of color flow in the fetal aorta at 12 weeks of gestation. b = fetal body.

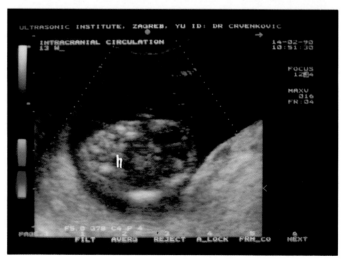

Figure 17.15 Intracranial circulation detected at 13 weeks of gestation. h = fetal head.

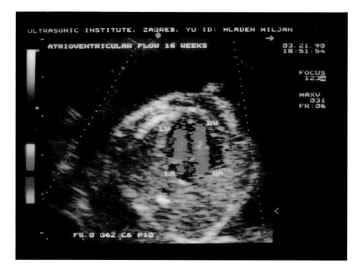

Figure 17.16 Four-chamber view of the fetal heart in sixteenth week of pregnancy. Atrioventricular flow during ventricular diastole is coded in red color. LA = left atrium; LV = left ventricle; RA = right atrium; RV = right ventricle.

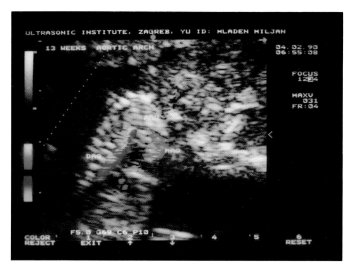

Figure 17.17 Blood flow in ascending (red) aortic arch and descending aorta (blue) detected by transvaginal probe in a fetus at 13 weeks of gestational age. AAo = ascending aorta; AAr = aortic arch; DAo = descending aorta.

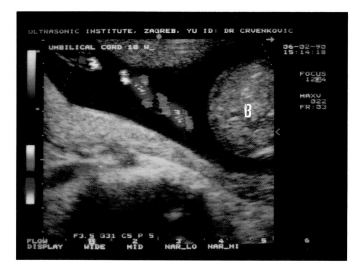

Figure 17.18 Umbilical cord seen by transvaginal color Doppler at 18 weeks of gestation. B = fetal body.

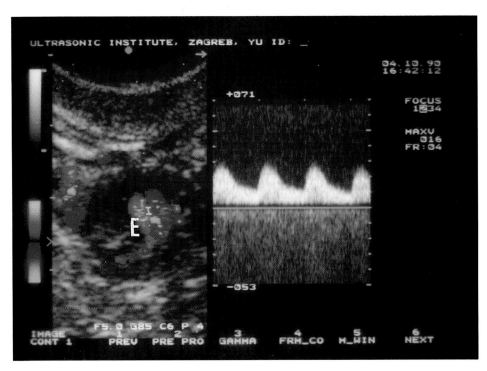

Figure 17.19 Extrauterine pregnancy. Ectopic trophoblast inside a solid adnexal mass detected by color and pulsed Doppler. E = ectopic pregnancy.

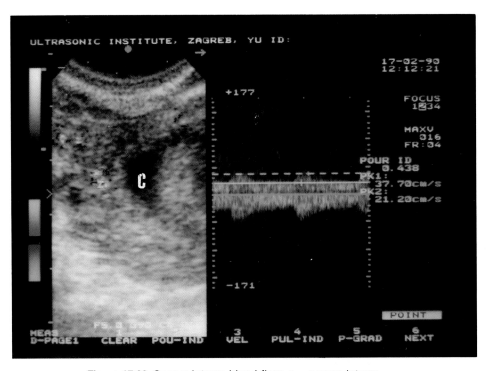

Figure 17.20 Corpus luteum blood flow. c = corpus luteum.

TABLE 17.3 Imaging Rate of Color Doppler Signal of Trophoblast, Umbilical Artery, Fetal Aorta, and Brain in Normal Early Pregnancy (N = 117)

Weeks	N	Trophoblast	A. Umbilicalis	Aorta	Brain
5	10	4 (40%)	0	0	0
6	17	9 (53%)	5 (29%)	0	0
7	25	100%	100%	6 (24%)	0
8	14	100%	100%	13 (93%)	0
9	5	100%	100%	100%	0
10	7	100%	100%	100%	0
11	3	100%	100%	100%	1 (33%)
12	3	100%	100%	100%	2 (67%)

of studying the changes of the ovarian and uterine blood flow under physiologic and pathophysiologic conditions. This method can also be used in an in vitro fertilization program (IVF) in order to evaluate the blood pattern and correlate it with the overall success rate of IVF therapy.

Early Pregnancy

The role of fetal and uteroplacental blood flow study is now well established in the management of the obstetrical patient, but until now there has been no reliable way to noninvasive blood flow measurements in the embryonal period. Transvaginal color Doppler enables a close look at early embryonic development and blood flow studies in embryonal and fetal vessels. Color Doppler studies could contribute to imaging the blood flow in the trophoblast, umbilical cord, and vessels of the embryo (Figs 17.11–17.15; Table 17.3).[20,21] In the future, such information could play an important role in the diagnosis of normal early pregnancies or pregnancy failures. We are unaware of any evidence that Doppler investigation of fetal and material vessels is advisable as a screening procedure.

Transvaginal color Doppler seems to detect luteal flow easily and accurately in normal and abnormal early pregnancy. It is reasonable to expect that further investigation would prove transvaginal color imaging as a valid diagnostic tool for evaluation of normal morphological and functional features of the ovary in the first trimester of pregnancy, since the integrity of luteal flow might play a notable role in predicting pregnancy outcome.[8,27]

The Second and Third Trimesters of Pregnancy

From the twelfth week on, the fetal cardiovascular system can be almost entirely seen. Despite the fact that fetal heart and great vessels are of small dimensions, by zooming the observed structure, its picture magnifies significantly, allowing recognition of cardiac morphology. Superposition of color Doppler on two-dimensional scan gives additional data about intracardiac flow. The success rate of intracardiac and great vessels blood flow imaging increases with gestational age. It was found that the optimal period for transvaginal color Doppler examination of the fetal heart is between the thirteenth and sixteenth weeks of pregnancy. In that gestational age, fetal heart and great vessels as well as blood flow through them are clearly imaged (Figs 17.16, 17.17). In the same period even a carotid artery and jugular vein are seen, and blood flow can be detected. Thus, the transvaginal approach in evaluation of fetal heart and morphology of the great vessels and their hemodynamics gives new perspectives to fetal echocardiography. Similar data, which could be obtained from the sixteenth to the eighteenth week by transabdominal approach, can now be achieved 4 weeks earlier. Athough we have not had the opportunity to test the possibilities of transvaginal echocardiography in detecting congenital heart defects, our experience in evaluating the normal fetal heart and the great vessels lead us to believe that this could be feasible.

Blood flow in the descending aorta as well as in the iliac arteries and veins may be seen even earlier, in the late first trimester of pregnancy, but their imaging in the second trimester becomes easier. Another important area of fetal circulation in which the transvaginal probe offers new possibilities is the visualization of intracranial circulation. Although intracranial blood flow is already visible from the tenth week of pregnancy, in the second trimester its demonstration becomes easier and more accurate. The anterior and posterior arteria cerebri media can be clearly distinguished from the fourteenth or fifteenth week on, and their blood flow studied.

As previously described, the trophoblastic circulation is the first to be detected in pregnancy. Later, different parts of chorion frondosum are depicted and from the ninth week, the placenta becomes more pronounced. In the early second trimester, blood flow in the lacunar spaces situated between the placenta and the endometrial tissue, as well as a prominent flow in the vessels located between the endometrium and the myometrium, are seen. Blood flow in umbilical vessels may be easily viewed later in pregnancy (Fig 17.18).

Ectopic Pregnancy

The diagnosis of ectopic pregnancy continues to be one of the major problems in gynecological emergency. Sonographic examination has become the most reliable instrument in the diagnosis of abnormal intrauterine pregnancy, but it has not reached this level of success in the diagnosis of ectopic pregnancy. Many ectopic pregnancies do not develop an embryo so that these specific ultrasonic findings are not seen and, therefore, the presence of an adnexal mass may be ambiguous.

Transvaginal color and pulsed Doppler can help to characterize the nature of the adnexal mass, thus permitting preoperative diagnosis when the ectopic embryo and its characteristic heartbeat cannot be seen (Figure 17.19). We have studied the value of transvaginal color Doppler in the blood flow detection of ectopic trophoblast.[28] Trophoblastic flow was defined as ectopic color flow, usually very prominent and randomly dispersed inside the solid part of the adnexal mass. It is clearly separated from the ovarian tissue and corpus luteum. Pulsed Doppler waveform analysis showed a very low impedance signal and calculated RI was always below 0.40 due to increased end-diastolic flow. Taylor et al hypothesized that the low-impedance flow around ectopic gestations resulted from the peculiar hemodynamics of early placentation.[27]

For diagnosing of ectopic pregnancy, the results obtained by transvaginal color Doppler have been good enough to justify its clinical application (Table 17.4). We examined 148 patients with suspected ectopic pregnancy. Nine false negative findings were observed in cases of tubal abortion. Color flow could not be appreciated due to an inactive trophoblast. In these patients serum βhCG was measured and found to be decreased. The highest value was 720 mIU/ml (IRP) and the lowest, 80 mIU/ml. Two false positive findings were obtained in the case of cor-

TABLE 17.4 Transvaginal Color Doppier in the Detection of Ectopic Pregnancy (N = 148)

Color Flow and RI	Ectopic Pregnancy		Total
	Yes	No	
Ectopic	64	9	73
Non-ectopic	2	73	75
Total	66	82	148

PPV = 87.7%; NPV = 97.3%; sensitivity = 97.0%; specificity = 89.0%; accuracy = 92.6%.

pus luteum cysts. Our current policy is to expectantly manage the patients without ectopic trophoblastic flow in amenorrheic patients. The hypothesis is that the absence of color flow within the trophoblast and the corpus luteum may indicate that the ectopic pregnancy is no longer active. On the contrary, if there is color flow in the adnexal region with a resistance index of < 0.40, the patients are scheduled for laparoscopy regardless of clinical signs.

Certain overlap between luteal blood flow and color flow in the case of ectopic pregnancy or ovarian malignancy can be expected (Figure 17.20).[8,27,28] Using high-quality B-mode transvaginal sonography and superimposed color Doppler flow, it is possible to distinguish the luteal and ectopic trophoblast blood flow. Only ovarian pregnancy can produce a real diagnostic challenge; however, this condition is extremely rare.

SUMMARY

Each vessel imaged by color Doppler can be explored by pulsed Doppler. This is a major advantage when flow is to be studied in specific vessels. Flow can be assessed without interference from other vessels, which may lie distally or proximally in the same axis or plane of investigation, having a different circulatory pattern. Transvaginal color Doppler saves time during pulsed Doppler examination and increases measurement accuracy. The most important advantage of this new technique is the display of blood flow across the whole scanning plane of the pelvis. Therefore, the pulsed Doppler sample volume can be placed precisely on the color flow of interest and spectral waveform analysis can be done easily.

Early diagnosis of pelvic malignancy, screening programs of ovarian carcinoma, the study of uterine and ovarian perfusion in infertile and pregnant women, more accurate diagnosis of early pregnancy failure and ectopic pregnancy, and the study of embryonal and fetal circulation are only a few remarkable fields in obstetrics and gynecology that can be improved upon using this new diagnostic technique. Our current experience has shown that ultrasound examination of pelvic circulation by a transvaginal probe combined with color and pulsed Doppler assessment may increase the reliability of ultrasound diagnosis in certain pathological pelvic conditions. The opportunity to analyze flow characteristics in pelvic vessels will undoubtedly provide new data on the physiology and pathophysiology of pelvic circulation. We think that the possibility of adding color Doppler capabilities to the superb transvaginal imaging will become important when selecting from the devices currently available on the market.

REFERENCES

1. Fleischer AC, Gordon AN, Entman S: Transabdominal and transvaginal sonography of pelvic masses. Ultrasound Med Biol 1989;15:529–533.
2. Andolf E, Jorgensen C: A prospective comparison of transabdominal and transvaginal ultrasound with surgical findings in gynecologic disease. J Ultrasound Med 1990;9:71–75.
3. Coleman BG, Arger PH, Grumbach K, et al: Transvaginal and transabdominal sonography: prospective comparison. Radiology 1988;166:325–329.
4. Omoto R, Kasai C: Physics and instrumentation of Doppler color flow mapping. Echocardiography 1987;4:467–482.
5. Pourcelot L: Applications cliniques de l'examen Doppler transcutane, in Peronneaoue P (Ed): Velocimetrie Ultrasonore Doppler. Seminare INSERM, Paris, 1975, p 213.
6. Kurjak A, Alfirevic Z, Miljan M: Conventional and color Doppler in the assessment of fetal and maternal circulation. Ultrasound Med Biol 1988;14:337–343.
7. Campbell S, Bhan V, Royston P, Whitehead MI, Collins WP: Transabdominal ultrasound screening for early ovarian cancer. BMJ 1989;299:1363–1367.
8. Zalud I, Kurjak A: The assessment of luteal blood flow in pregnant and non-pregnant women by transvaginal color Doppler. J Perinat Med 1990;18:215–221.
9. Thompson RS, Trudinger BJ, Cook CM: Doppler ultrasound waveform indices: A/B ratio, pulsatility and Pourcelot ratio. Br J Obstet Gynaecol 1988;95:581–588.
10. Goswamy RK, Steptoe PC: Doppler ultrasound studies of the uterine artery in spontaneous ovarian cycles. Human Reproduction 1988;3:721–725.
11. Taylor KJW, Burns PN, Wells PNI, Conway DI: Ultrasound Doppler flow studies of the ovarian and uterine arteries. Brit J Obstet Gynaecol 1985;92:240–246.
12. Folkman J: Anti-angiogenesis: new concept for therapy of solid tumors. Ann Surg 1972;175–183.
13. Jain RK, Ward-Hartley KA: Dynamics of cancer cell interaction with microvasculature and interstitium. Biorheology 1987;24:117–125.
14. Long MG, Boulbee JE, Hanson ME, Begent RHJ: Doppler time velocity waveform studies of the uterine artery and uterus. Br J Obstet Gynaecol, 1989;96:588–593.
15. Kurjak A, Zalud I, Jurkovic D, Alfirevic Z, Miljan M: Transvaginal color Doppler for the assessment of pelvic circulation. Acta Obstet Gynecol Scand 1989;68:131–135.
16. Kurjak A, Zalud I: Early diagnosis of ovarian tumors: transvaginal color Doppler ultrasound, in ECO Italia, Napoli, 1989, p 189.
17. Kurjak A, Zalud I: Transvaginal colour flow imaging and ovarian cancer. BMJ 1990;300:330.
18. Kurjak A, Zalud I, Alfirevic Z, Jurkovic D: The assessment of abnormal pelvic blood flow by transvaginal color Doppler. Ultrasound Med Biol 1990;16:437–442.
19. Kurjak A, Jurkovic D, Alfirevic Z, Zalud I: Transvaginal color Doppler. J Clin Ultrasound, 1990;18:227–234.
20. Kurjak A, Zalud I, Crvenkovic G: Transvaginal color Doppler in the assessment of maternal and fetal circulation, in Proceedings of International Symposium: Transvaginal Sonography, Rotterdam, 1989, pp 93–98.
21. Kurjak A, Miljan M, Jurkovic D, Alfirevic Z, Zalud I: Color Doppler in the assessment of fetomaternal circulation. Rech Gynecol 1989;1:269–275.
22. Alfirevic Z, Kurjak A: Transvaginal color and pulsed wave Doppler in the assessment of blood flow in the first trimester of pregnancy. J Perinat Med 1990;18:173–180.
23. Kurjak A: Transvaginal color Doppler in the assessment of pelvic circulation. Jap J Med Ultrasound 1989;16(supp 2):1.
24. Kurjak A, Jurkovic D: Transvaginal color Doppler in the assessment of pelvic masses, in Proceedings of Sixth World Congress In Vitro Fertilization and Alternate Assisted Reproduction, Jerusalem, 1989, p 26.
25. Jacobs IJ, Bast RC: The CA 125 tumor associated antigen: a review of the literature. Human Reprod 1989;4:1–12.
26. Campbell S, Collins WP, Royston P, Bourbe TH, Bhan V, Whitehead MI: Developments in ultrasound screening for early ovarian cancer, in Sharp F, Mason WP, Leake RE (eds): Ovarian cancer. London, Chapman and Hall Medical, 1990, pp 217–228.
27. Taylor KJW, Ramos IM, Feyock AL, Snower DP, Carter D, Shapiro BS, Meyer WR, DeCherney AH: Ectopic pregnancy: duplex Doppler evaluation. Radiology 1989;173:93–97.
28. Kurjak A, Schulman H, Zalud I: Transvaginal color Doppler: new technique for the diagnosis of ectopic pregnancy (submitted for publication, 1991).

CHAPTER 18

The Transvaginal Image-Directed Pulsed Doppler System— Methodology and Clinical Applications

Israel Thaler, MD
Zeev Weiner, MD
Joseph Itskovitz, MD, DSc
Dorit Manor, MD

INTRODUCTION

Recent technological advances in ultrasound imaging have contributed greatly to patient care in the fields of obstetrics and gynecology. Of particular importance was the recent development of high-frequency transvaginal sonography, which is emphasized by its extensive application in the various fields of obstetrics and gynecology. Such applications include monitoring of follicular development, follicle aspiration and various puncture procedures, and scanning of the endometrium, the ovaries, and other normal and abnormal pelvic structures. Another important area is scanning in early pregnancy, which enables the monitoring of embryonic development and the detection of developmental abnormalities from as early as the first and early second trimesters.

A new and exciting development has emerged with the introduction of the transvaginal image-directed pulsed Doppler system (or pulsed-duplex Doppler system). This is obtained by incorporating a pulsed, range-gated Doppler into the transvaginal two-dimensional B-mode real-time scanner, transforming it into a high-quality "flow probe," which offers a novel approach to the noninvasive hemodynamic evaluation of the female pelvis, in both the pregnant and the nonpregnant situation.

In this chapter the methodology of transvaginal Doppler sonography will be described, followed by a description of the clinical applications and clinical potential of this diagnostic tool.

PHYSICAL CONSIDERATIONS OF TRANSVAGINAL IMAGE-DIRECTED DOPPLER SONOGRAPHY

A duplex Doppler system (ie, image-directed Doppler system) is one that enables two-dimensional real-time scanning to guide the appropriate placement of an ultrasonic Doppler beam. In this way, the blood vessel from which the Doppler signals originate can be identified. The first part of the duplex scanning always begins with a real-time imaging so that the operator can get an anatomical image and identify the sites for Doppler studies. When applying the endovaginal ultrasonic probe, the full advantage of this imaging modality can be exploited. The

463

physical principles upon which image formation and image-directed Doppler flow measurements are based will be discussed very briefly, emphasizing the special features of the transvaginal probe. A comprehensive review on this subject is given in Chapter 1 and in reference 1 and 2.

Imaging of Pelvic Structures

The female pelvis contains various soft tissue structures which have a similar acoustic impedance, and are therefore poor reflectors. The main advantage of using the transvaginal probe is the short distance between it and the scanned organs. This proximity to the transducer makes it possible to increase its frequency, typically between 5 and 7 MHz, while attenuation is still acceptable at these distance ranges. As the vagina is rather an elastic organ, the probe can be manipulated to bring it as close to the scanned organ as possible, thereby placing it in the focal region of the transducer. The net result is a significant increase in image resolution, obtained by the high frequency of the transducer and by the application of a stronger focus. When a transvaginal duplex system is applied, the use of a high-frequency transducer that is placed near the vessel of interest generates high-quality images, reflecting an axial resolution of 0.5 mm and a lateral resolution of 1.3 mm. Under such conditions, even a vessel as small as 1–2 mm can be picked up. Another important feature is the ability to greatly magnify the image ("zooming"), which, albeit at the cost of a somewhat decreased resolution, highlights small anatomical structures such as blood vessels.[3]

Doppler Blood Flow Measurements

The proximity of the probe to the pelvic vessels also permits the application of a higher frequency Doppler transducer, thereby obtaining higher Doppler shifts at any given angle of insonation. Moreover, when high flow velocities are encountered, the limitations of the range-velocity product are largely overcome.[4] With the transvaginal approach, Doppler flow measurements of some pelvic vessels can be obtained at a smaller angle of insonation, thereby increasing the accuracy of measurement.[4] Transvaginal Doppler flow measurements are performed with an empty bladder, which is an important advantage over the transabdominal approach, where the bladder is fully distended. This causes ovarian and uterine displacement and can modify the impedance to flow in the vessels supplying these organs. All these properties turn the transvaginal Doppler duplex system into a versatile, accurate, and convenient tool for measuring blood flow characteristics in the female pelvis.

METHODOLOGY

All the measurements which will be described were taken with an Elscint ESI 2000 Doppler duplex system employing a 6.5 MHz mechanical sector probe, especially designed for convenient intravaginal insertion and manipulation. A 5 MHz pulsed Doppler transducer is incorporated into the imaging probe and for this purpose the imaging transducer itself is used. The duplex transducer probe arrangement is such that it can be servo-controlled to the desired stationary position for Doppler measurements. This arrangement provides for a line, representing the desired eventual servo-controlled direction of the ultrasonic Doppler beam, to be superimposed on the real-time image to allow appropriate orientation and positioning of the sample volume. The transducer crystal is housed in a rounded spherical acoustic window, which enables good tissue contact.[3]

During the examination the patient is lying in the supine position on a gynecological examination table. This makes it possible for the examiner to manipulate the vaginal probe at different angles, applying the push-pull technique,[3] and to locate the vessels under study.[5] A coupling gel is applied to the vaginal probe, which is then introduced into a rubber glove. The probe is then introduced into the vaginal fornix and a real-time image of the vessel is obtained. The line of insonation of the Doppler beam is adjusted (by manipulating the probe) so that it crosses the long axis of the vessel at as small an angle as possible. The sample volume is then placed to cover the entire cross-sectional area of the vessel.[5] At this stage the system is switched to the dual-mode operation, in which the two-dimensional scanning and the range-gated pulsed Doppler operate in a quasi-simultaneous fashion. The flow velocity waveforms are displayed on the lower half of the screen after spectral analysis in real-time (Fig 18.1). Once a good quality signal is obtained, based on audio recognition, visual waveform recognition, and maximum measured velocity, the image is frozen, including at least 3 waveform signals. A thump filter between 100 and 200 Hz is used to eliminate signals originating from vessel wall movements. At this point the following calculations can be performed:

1. The ratio between peak-systolic and end-diastolic flow velocity—commonly termed S/D ratio.
2. The difference between peak-systolic and end-diastolic flow velocity, divided by the maximum velocity of flow during systole. This parameter is also termed the resistance index (RI).

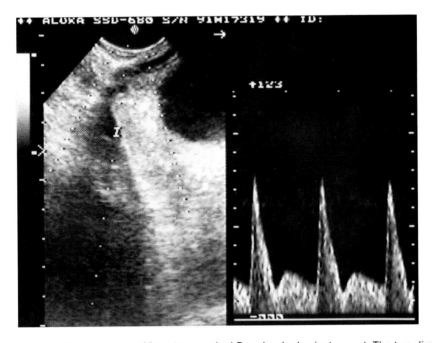

Figure 18.1 An image generated by a transvaginal Doppler duplex instrument. The two-dimensional real-time scan displaying the vessel under study is shown on the left side. The user can manipulate the sample volume, measure vessel diameter, and determine the angle of insonation. When switching to the Doppler mode, a sonogram is displayed (right half of the figure), showing the Doppler frequency shift (ie, the velocity of flow) on the time axis. This is also referred to as flow velocity waveforms.

3. Volume flow rate—this measurement is based on the product of the mean velocity and the cross-sectional area of the vessel. The latter is calculated from the vessel diameter (determined as the distance between two electronic calipers which are positioned over the vessel walls). The instantaneous flow rate is then integrated over time, to give the minute volume flow, expressed as milliliters per minute.

While the first two measurements are not angle dependent, the latter one is. This angle of insonation is determined by the user as the angle between the line of insonation (which is projected on the video screen) and the long axis of the vessel that is being measured. The calculations and analyses are displayed on an ancillary video display unit and can also be recorded on a video recorder. An immediate hard copy can also be obtained using a video printer.

ANATOMICAL CONSIDERATIONS

A schematic representation of the transvaginal probe in relation to the pelvic vessels is shown in Fig 18.2.

The main pelvic vessels that can be studied by the transvaginal Doppler duplex system are:

1. The uterine vessels.
2. The ovarian vessels.

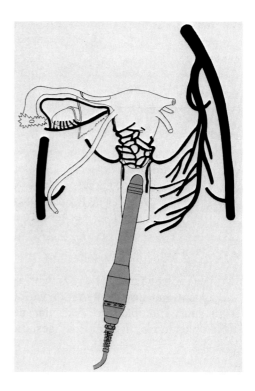

Figure 18.2 A schematic presentation of the transvaginal probe in relation to the female pelvic vessels. (Reprinted with permission from Thaler et al).[2]

3. The hypogastric artery.
4. The arcuate artery.
5. Fetal vessels.

The Uterine Artery

The ascending branch of the uterine artery is located in the parametrial region, at the level of the internal cervical os. The latter can be readily visualized, adjacent to the cervical canal. During diastole, relatively high flow rates are maintained, particularly in the luteal phase and in pregnancy.[5] This "attenuates" the pulsatility of the vessel, making it more difficult for the examiner to detect the arterial pattern which is so common in high-resistance vessels (eg, the hypogastric and the internal iliac artery). While the direction of flow is generally away from the transducer (negative velocity), it is possible in many instances to identify flow toward it, originating from the cervical branch of the uterine artery.

The Ovarian Artery

The ovarian artery originates from the aorta and reaches the ovary via the infundibulo-pelvic ligament. It can usually be detected lateral to the ovary in the inferior aspect (ie, closer to the vaginal probe and in the direction of the pelvic wall). As the uterine artery forms anastomoses with the ovarian artery medial to the ovary and on the inferior border of the fallopian tube, this approach eliminates erroneous measurements of signals originating from the distal branches of the uterine artery. Care should also be exercised so as to avoid sampling the hypogastric arteries, which are located adjacent to the lateral ovarian border. Fortunately, signals originating from these vessels demonstrate a distinct pattern that is different from those of the ovarian artery.[5] Flow velocity signals can also be elicited from within the ovary itself, demonstrating a much lower impedance (reflected by the substantially higher flow velocity during diastole). However, it is usually impossible to image these small intraovarian arterial branches, and to measure their diameter.

Fetal Vessels

With the transvaginal approach it is possible to sample the umbilical artery from as early as the first trimester. Doppler measurements of other fetal vessels (eg, aorta, umbilical vein, vessels of the lower limb) can already be obtained at the late first trimester. Doppler measurements of fetal intracranial vessels can be obtained conveniently from mid-trimester to term when the vertex is presenting.

Complex Vascular Beds

With the introduction of the transvaginal color flow mapping, the geometric arrangement and flow patterns of various vascular beds can be studied in detail. Two such examples are vascular nets in the ovarian stroma and the peritrophoblastic plexuses in early gestation.

TRANSVAGINAL DOPPLER MEASUREMENTS IN NONPREGNANT PATIENTS

Normal Menstrual Cycle

The feasibility of transvaginal Doppler measurements of the ovarian and uterine arteries was demonstrated in earlier reports.[6,7] It was shown that the pulsatility index (PI) was lower in the artery supplying the ovary carrying the dominant follicle or the corpus luteum, indicating increased blood flow to the "dominant" ovary.[6] We have also observed such differences between the two ovaries[5,8] (Fig 18.3). When measurements were obtained from within the ovarian stroma (intraovarian branches of the ovarian artery), a much lower impedance to flow was observed, reflecting high rates of flow to the functioning ovary. The rich blood supply to the ovary is required for optimal production and secretion of progesterone from the corpus luteum, as has been demonstrated in animal experiments.[9–11] Changes in flow patterns in the uterine arteries are also observed during the menstrual cycle. A preovulatory increase in systolic blood flow in the uterine artery was described.[7] We have observed an overall decrease in the impedance to flow throughout the normal ovarian cycle (Fig 18.4). In another transvaginal Doppler study, a significantly lower ovarian artery PI was found on the side of the ovary bearing the corpus luteum, suggesting a reduced downstream impedance.[12] Contrary to earlier reports, a continuous forward end-diastolic flow velocity was documented in 74% of the ovarian artery and in nearly all of the uterine artery flow

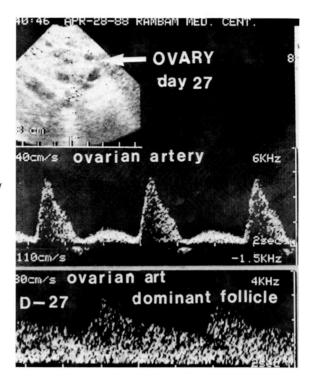

Figure 18.3 Flow velocity waveforms in the ovarian artery at day 27 of a normal menstrual cycle. There is a substantially higher diastolic flow velocity in the artery supplying the ovary carrying the corpus luteum than in the contralateral ovary. This signifies decreased resistance to flow in the "dominant" ovary.

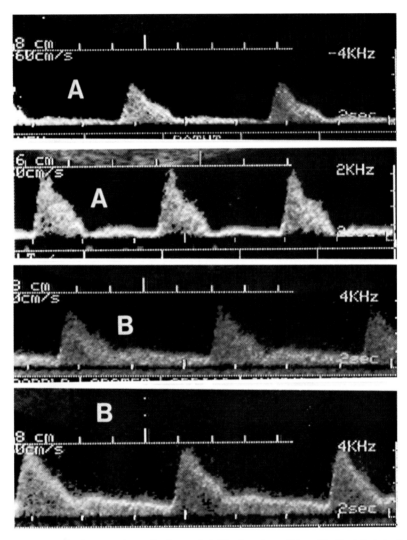

Figure 18.4 Flow velocity waveforms in the early follicular phase (**A**) and in the late luteal phase (**B**) of a normal ovulatory cycle. Notice the increase in diastolic flow velocity throughout the cycle.

velocity waveforms.[12] We have obtained similar observations. The PI from the uterine artery only seemed marginally involved in the observed impedance changes during the luteal phase of the menstrual cycle. Recently, a transvaginal color pulsed ultrasound was used to study uterine arterial blood flow during the ovarian and menstrual cycles.[13] The peak mean PI values occurred on day 1 of menses, the day of plasma estradiol peak, and the day of the LH peak plus 3. The lowest mean PI values occurred on the day of the LH peak minus 6 and the day of the LH peak plus 9. These periods of least impedance to blood flow represent the time of the rapid follicular growth and the time of peak luteal function (around the presumed time when implantation might occur), respectively. There were no significant differences in the PI values between the left and right uterine arteries. These studies demonstrate that there are complex temporal relationships between uterine and ovarian blood flow, concentrations of ovarian hormones in peripheral venous plasma, and morphological changes of the ovary and endometrium throughout the normal ovulatory cycle. Undoubtedly, many vasoactive substances (eg, prostaglandins) play a mediating role in regulating uterine and ovarian blood flow throughout the menstrual cycle. Ovarian steroids have been shown to alter α-1 adrenergic receptors number in periarterial sympathic nerves and cause marked changes in uterine blood flow in gilts.[14] Injections of E_2 to nonpregnant sheep caused an increase in pelvic arterial blood flow.[15] Recently an estrogen receptor–related protein was identified in the muscularis layer of major vessels of the female.[16] This makes it possible for a direct effect of estrogens on arterial status through a conventional sex-hormone receptor mechanism.

Another issue that is yet unresolved is the relationship between uterine and ovarian blood flow. These two vascular systems form anastomoses with each other (Fig 18.2) and could have a reciprocal relationship. In the cow, 20–40% of the total ovarian blood flow is supplied by the uterine artery during peak ovarian flow in the oestrous cycle.[17] Throughout the estrous cycle, ovarian blood flow was positively correlated with systemic concentrations of progesterone and negatively correlated with systemic concentrations of E_2, while uterine blood flow demonstrated an inverse relationship to these hormones.[17] We have observed a decline in uterine blood flow from the beginning of the cycle to midcycle (ovulation day). Thereafter there was a rapid increase in volume flow rates (Fig 18.5). The impedance to flow during the first half of the menstrual cycle did not change or fell slightly in the patients studied. Following ovulation there was a rapid decline in the impedance to flow throughout the luteal phase.

Studies in Infertile Patients

It is tempting to speculate that a decreased uterine or ovarian perfusion may be associated with infertility. Preliminary studies support this possibility,[18,19] but further investigation is required in this field.

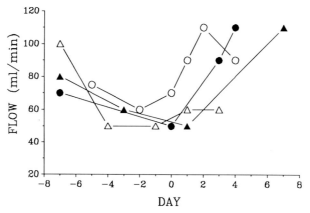

Figure 18.5 Volume flow rates in the uterine artery of 3 patients during a normal ovulatory cycle. There is a gradual decline in the rate of flow until midcycle. Following ovulation, a rapid increase in flow rates is observed. (Reprinted with permission from Thaler et al).[2]

Studies in Patients with Ovarian Failure

We have studied the effect of estrogen and progesterone replacement in patients with premature ovarian failure, immitating the normal menstrual cycle. The initial RI values in the uterine arteries were markedly increased, usually to the point of absent or partial diastolic flow velocity in flow velocity waveforms. During estrogen administration, there was a small increase in diastolic flow velocity, with a concomitant fall in RI. When progesterone was given to these patients after sufficient endometrial response, a substantial decrease in RI values was observed. When only progesterone was administered to patients with premature ovarian failure (without estrogen replacement) a decline in uterine artery resistance index was measured.

In a preliminary report, ten healthy postmenopausal women were treated with continuous transdermal oestradiol and sequential oral norethisterone acetate.[20] The pulsatility index in the uterine arteries was measured with a transvaginal ultrasound probe and pulsed Doppler, before treatment and after at least 6 weeks of therapy. A 50% reduction in the PI occurred within 6–10 weeks of treatment. Endometrial thickness increased by 55% over the same period. Further work is required to learn about other hemodynamic effects of estrogen replacement therapy.

Blood Flow in the Uterine and Ovarian Arteries During Cycle Stimulation and After Follicle Puncture and Embryo Transfer

Flow measurements of the uterine and ovarian arteries were obtained from 10 in vitro fertilization embryo transfer IVF-ET protocol patients who were treated with gonadotropins. In the menstrual cycle that preceded the treatment cycle, no treatment was given. The Doppler studies were performed every 2–3 days, starting from the third day of the cycle, prior to treatment. The day of hCG administration was marked as day 0 and all measurements were expressed in relation to this time (eg, the first day of treatment was usually marked as day −9 to −7, and ET was performed on day +2). Daily measurements of serum E_2, progesterone, and follicular growth were obtained in each patient.

The resistance index in the uterine artery before treatment was relatively low and demonstrated a gradual increase until the day of follicle aspiration. There was a short-lasting decrease in RI in day −5. A rapid decline occurred shortly following hCG administration which continued throughout the luteal phase (Fig 18.6). Blood flow in the uterine artery during the treatment cycle is shown in Fig 18.7. Increased volume flow rates were measured prior to treatment. Blood flow then decreased gradually, reaching the lowest levels at about day 0. Within 24 hours of the administration of hCG, there was a sharp increase in flow rates in this vessel throughout the luteal phase.

The periovulatory increase in RI and the decrease in volume flow rates coincided with the decrease in E_2 levels at midcycle. The subsequent increase in flow rates and the rapid decline in RI were associated with the exponential increase in progesterone levels in the luteal phase. The lower RI and the increased volume flow at the beginning of the cycle may express the situation in the late luteal phase of the preceding cycle (which was always untreated in this group of patients). The changes observed in the follicular phase reflect a "readjustment" of uterine blood flow in the current treated cycle.

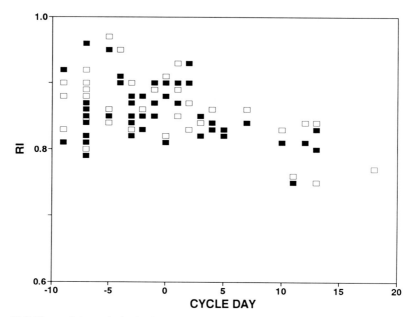

Figure 18.6 The resistance index in the uterine artery throughout an IVF-ET treatment cycle. The filled and open squares represent the right and the left uterine arteries, respectively. (Reprinted with permission from Thaler et al).[2]

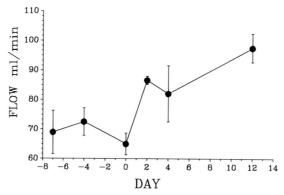

Figure 18.7 Volume flow rates in the uterine artery during an IVF-ET treatment cycle. In flow rates is observed. (Reprinted with permission from Thaler et al).[2]

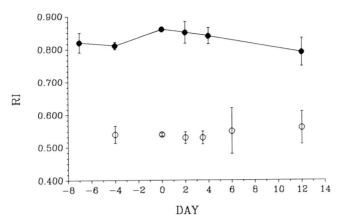

Figure 18.8 The resistance index in the ovarian artery during an IVF-ET treatment cycle. The upper trace demonstrates the main ovarian artery. The RI in an intraovarian artery is shown in the lower trace. The Ri is much lower than the resistance in the main artery, and changes very little throughout the cycle. (Reprinted with permission from Thaler et al).[2]

Changes in the resistance index of the ovarian artery are shown in Fig 18.8. A midfollicular decline in the impedance to flow was observed, with a subsequent rise in day 0. A gradual steady decline in the RI occurred in the luteal phase. The flow profile was also obtained from within the ovarian substance itself as described above. The resistance index in this ''luteal artery'' is shown in the lower part of Fig 18.8. There were no significant changes in this vessel throughout the treatment cycle, although the values displayed an increased variability in the luteal phase. Volume flow in the ovarian artery increased from 40 ml/min prior to treatment to 70 ml/min in midcycle and 90–100 ml/min in the late luteal phase. Within the treatment cycle then, the ovarian flow more than doubled itself. No significant difference was found between the left and the right side for any of the measured variables, which could be expected in a situation where both ovaries are stimulated to ovulate by gonadotropins. The changes in flow volume throughout the treatment cycle demonstrate, similar to the uterine artery, an association with estrogen and particularly with progesterone levels.

In another study, pulsed Doppler measurement of blood flow velocity in the ovarian artery was performed during cycle stimulation and after follicle puncture.[21] The pulsatility index was high 4 days before follicle puncture (ie, day −2). It decreased markedly toward the day of embryo transfer. The impedance to flow was significantly lower in patients with high endocrine response compared to those with low endocrine response (ie, E_2 levels below 200 pg/follicle>15 mm on the day of ovulation induction). All patients in the latter study were treated with a long-acting gonadotropin-releasing hormone (GnRH) agonist prior to cycle stimulation. Doppler flow measurements were not performed following embryo replacement. The decline in vessel resistance as one moves from the ovarian artery to the ''luteal artery'' (about 40%) is more striking than when one moves from the ascending uterine artery to the radial or arcuate artery, and reflects the relatively high flow volume to the corpus luteum. In the rabbit, blood flow to the corpora lutea was sevenfold higher than to the ovarian stroma and follicles.[9] There was a positive correlation between blood flow to the corpus luteum and the rate of

ovarian progesterone secretion. Lowering of blood pressure caused a marked
decline in luteal blood flow and in ovarian venous progesterone concentration.
This suggests that high blood flow rate is necessary for an optimal secretion of
progesterone from the fully developed corpus luteum.

The association between hemodynamic parameters and successful implantation was also investigated.[22] In a group of 12 patients who became pregnant after
embryo transfer, the vascular resistance of the uterine arteries was significantly
lower on the day of follicular aspiration than in a group of 33 patients who did not
conceive. No differences could be detected in the ovarian vessels. This suggests
that the receptivity of the endometrium can be evaluated on the basis of not only
morphological but also hemodynamic parameters.

Pelvic Tumors

Recently it has been demonstrated that uterine and ovarian tumors are associated
with distinct hemodynamic changes to these organs. We shall deal separately with
the uterus and ovaries.

Uterine Fibroids

It was demonstrated that uterine fibroids are associated with a marked reduction
in the resistance to flow in the uterine arteries.[23] In 8 patients with large uterine
fibroids who were treated with the GnRH agonist Buserelin, there was an increase
in the mean RI values which became significant after 4 months of treatment. These
changes were associated with a decrease in the mean total uterine volume, in the
mean individual fibroid volume, and in the mean serum E_2 levels. This study,
which was first to describe such hemodynamic changes in patients with uterine
fibroids, was performed with a transabdominal pulsed wave duplex system.

We have studied 10 patients with large uterine fibroids before and following
treatment with the GnRH agonist Buserelin (administered either intramuscularly
or transnasally). Doppler measurements were performed with a transvaginal image-directed pulsed Doppler system. The results are described in Table 18.1. After
discontinuation of treatment, regrowth of the fibroids was observed in some of the
patients, with a decrease in the resistance to flow. These observations again
support the hemodynamic effect of estrogen on the uterus as described above. It is
possible that the reduction in uterine and fibroid volume could be in part related to
the induced changes in uterine blood flow.

**TABLE 18.1 Mean S/D Ratio in the Uterine Artery, Uterine Volume, and Volume
of Largest Myoma in Patients with Uterine Fibroids Before and After Treatment
with the GnRH Agonist Buserelin**

	Uterine Artery S/D Ratio	Uterine Volume	Myoma Volume
Pretreatment	3.85 ±0.4	296 ±55	135 ±44
After 2 months of treatment with GnRH agonist	5.22 ±1.7	130 ±29	66 ±46

Using a transvaginal color Doppler imaging, neovascularization (ie, the formation of new blood vessels—angiogenesis) could be demonstrated in 6 out of 10 patients with uterine fibroma.[24] This was characterized by the presence of flow in very thin vessels within the tumor with low impedance and low velocity waveform characteristics on pulsed Doppler evaluation.

Ovarian Tumors

An important development in this area was the observation that in patients with malignant ovarian tumors there is a clear evidence of neovascularization and a very low pulsatility index.[24,25] Patients with morphologically normal ovaries (either premenopausal or postmenopausal) did not demonstrate areas of neovascularization and the PI of the ovarian vessels was relatively high.[25] Patients with nonmalignant masses also did not demonstrate new growth of blood vessels (excluding one case, in which bilateral dermoid cysts, containing nests of thyroid-like cells were found. In this patient signs of neovascularization and low PI were detected, similar to the group with malignant tumors). The size of the malignant tumor probably affects the ability to detect it by this method, since one patient with intraepithelial serous cystadenocarcinoma in a small ovary had no signs of any vascular changes and the PI was high.[25] The results of these studies show that the absence of intratumoral neovascularization and a high pulsatility index can be used to exclude the presence of primary ovarian cancer. This feature could be particularly useful in large-scale screening procedures by reducing the rate of false positive results. By identifying the benign nature of the ovarian pathology, it should also be possible to prevent unnecessary operations. Further investigation is required before these data may be used in routine clinical work.

TRANSVAGINAL DOPPLER MEASUREMENTS IN PREGNANT PATIENTS

Normal Pregnancy

Throughout pregnancy, profound changes in uterine blood flow are observed. These changes are related to a marked decrease in the resistance to flow and to an increase in vessel diameter.[26] The most striking changes occur in the first half of gestation, as was measured by a transvaginal image-directed pulsed Doppler system.[2,26,27] Figure 18.9 demonstrates flow velocity waveforms in the ascending uterine artery before pregnancy and at various stages of gestation. The samples were obtained from a segment of the ascending uterine artery at the level of the internal os. It can be seen that diastolic flow increases gradually until term. Some of the samples were obtained from the arcuate vessels (at 14 and at 19 weeks). The difference between the two vessels is readily recognized, with the arcuate vessels having a much lower impedance to flow than the main branch of the uterine artery. A post-systolic notch was found in most patients until the end of the second trimester. This notch reflects a momentary decrease in the velocity of flow just following systole, with a rapid "recovery" following. The resistance to flow, expressed as the peak-systolic to end-diastolic flow velocity ratio, declines rapidly over the first half of gestation and then continues to decline at a much lower rate (Fig 18.10). Overall, the S/D ratio declined from a mean of 5.3 in the nonpregnant state (luteal phase) to 2.3 near term. These data were obtained from 24 patients in a longitudinal manner.[26] Such changes in the resistance to flow during pregnancy were previously described by using a continuous wave Doppler,[28,29] a transabdom-

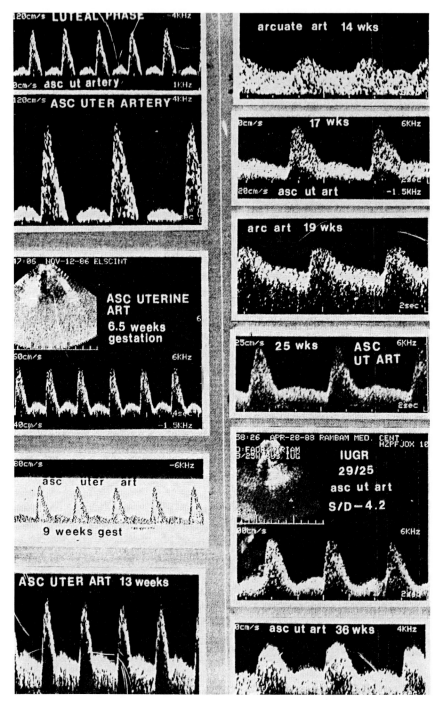

Figure 18.9 Flow velocity waveforms in the ascending uterine artery and the arcuate vessels before and at various stages of gestation. (Reprinted with permission from Thaler et al).[5]

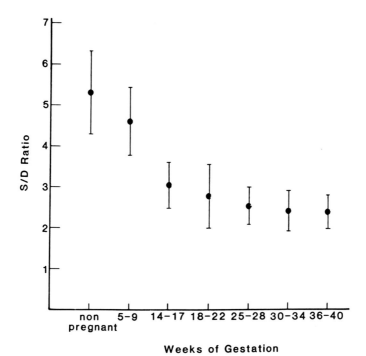

Figure 18.10 Changes in the S/D ratio of the uterine artery throughout normal pregnancy. (Reprinted with permission from Thaler et al).[26]

inal image-directed pulsed wave Doppler,[30] or a transvaginal pulsed Doppler transducer.[27] Similar to the latter study, we did not find a significant difference in the mean S/D ratio between the left and the right uterine artery throughout pregnancy (Fig 18.11), although individual differences were observed. This period of rapid decline in uterine arterial resistance extends from the time of implantation to midgestation and is reflective of placental growth and development of new blood vessels. The trophoblast invades the inner third of the myometrium and migrates through the entire length of the spiral arteries, which supply the intervillous

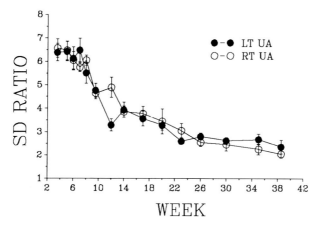

Figure 18.11 Changes in the S/D ratio in both uterine arteries during pregnancy. There is no significant difference between the two sides.

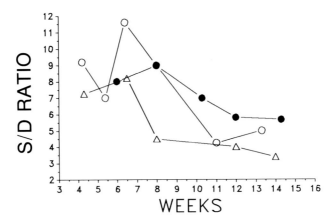

Figure 18.12 Systolic/diastolic flow velocity ratio in the uterine artery in the first trimester of pregnancy in 3 patients following IVF-ET. (Reprinted with permission from Thaler et al).[2]

space.[31] The spiral artery is stripped of its musculoelastic coat and loses its capacity to react to vasoactive substances. Using color Doppler imaging, trophoblastic blood flow could be observed from the sixth week, and Doppler examination showed characteristics of low impedance with RI values significantly lower than in waveforms obtained from the uterine artery.[24]

Prominant changes already occur in the first trimester. A rapid decline in the S/D ratio occurs over this period (Fig 18.12). These patients were studied longitudinally every 2 to 3 weeks, starting as soon as pregnancy was confirmed by serum βhCG. A substantial increase in volume flow rates was observed in the same period (Fig 18.13). The mean diameter of the uterine artery increased from 1.6 mm in the nonpregnant state to 3.7 mm near term (Fig 18.14). These changes are attributed to hypertrophy of the vascular smooth muscle accompanied by a decrease in the collagen fraction of the uterine arterial tree[32] and to vasodilation of the uteroplacental vascular bed.[33] The decrease in vascular resistance and the increase in the cross-sectional area of the uterine vascular bed may account for

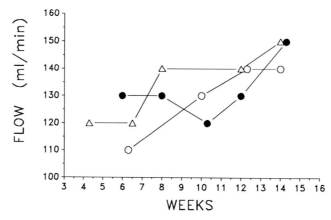

Figure 18.13 Volume flow in the uterine artery in the first trimester of pregnancy as measured in 3 different patients. (Reprinted with permission from Thaler et al).[2]

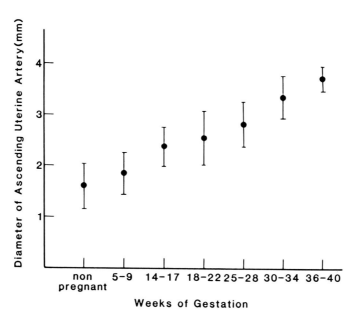

Figure 18.14 Changes in the diameter of the uterine artery during pregnancy. (Reprinted with permission from Thaler et al).[26]

the almost linear increase in volume flow rates in the uterine arteries during pregnancy.[26] This is demonstrated in Fig 18.15. Unilateral uterine blood flow increased from 95 ml/min in the luteal phase to 342 ml/min near term. No significant difference was measured between the left and the right side (Fig 18.16), so that these flow values can be doubled to represent the contribution of the ascending uterine arteries to the total blood flow. Most of this flow (80–90%) is distributed to the placenta to accommodate for fetal growth.[34,35] Based on the values obtained, the fraction of the cardiac output distributed to the uterine vessels is 3% in early pregnancy, rising to 12% near term.[26]

Striking changes in ovarian blood flow were also observed during the first trimester in the vessels supplying the ovary. The resistance index in the ovarian artery decreased rapidly over the first 12 weeks (Fig 18.17). The RI in the intraovarian branches of the ovarian artery remained low (around 0.5) and did not change significantly over this period. A typical flow velocity waveform is shown in Fig 18.18, demonstrating a substantial increase in diastolic velocity compared to that observed during the menstrual cycle (Fig 18.3). Volume flow rates increased by more than 50% (Fig 18.19). The rate of rise of ovarian artery flow volume is higher during the first trimester compared to the uterine artery. Although the actual flow expressed in ml/min is similar in both arteries during this time period, the uterus is much heavier than the ovary, and therefore the ovary receives a very large blood supply per unit of weight (Fig 18.19). It is not completely understood why the ovary has such rich blood supply. In the rabbit, a rapid increase in ovarian blood flow is observed until midgestation.[36] The corpus luteum receives exceptionally high blood supply, similar to the carotid body.[36] A similar trend was observed in the rat ovary.[37] It was suggested that large ovarian flow is necessary for adequate steroidogenesis which is required for the maintenance of pregnancy.[36,37] It is also possible that local concentrations of ovarian hormones result

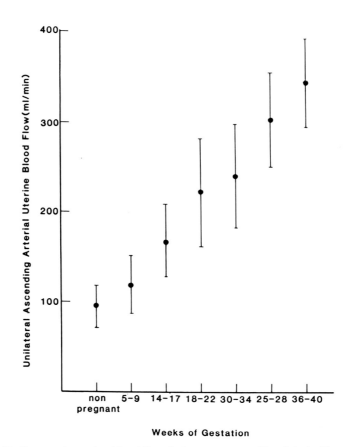

Figure 18.15 Changes in uterine blood flow during pregnancy. (Reprinted with permission from Thaler et al).[26]

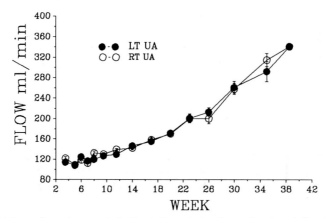

Figure 18.16 Volume flow changes in both uterine arteries throughout gestation. There were no significant differences between the two sides.

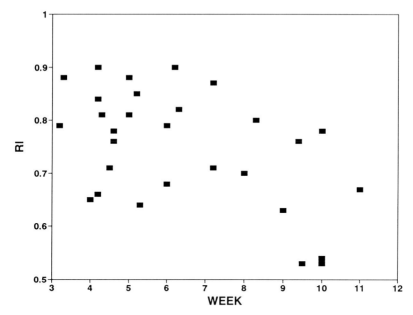

Figure 18.17 Changes in the resistance index of the ovarian artery throughout the first trimester. (Reprinted with permission from Thaler et al).[2]

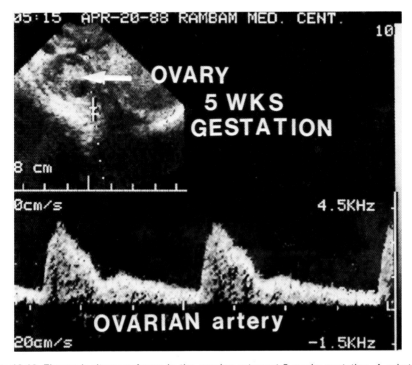

Figure 18.18 Flow velocity waveforms in the ovarian artery at 5 weeks gestation. A substantial increase in diastolic flow velocity is noted compared to that measured in the menstrual cycle. (Reprinted with permission from Thaler et al).[2]

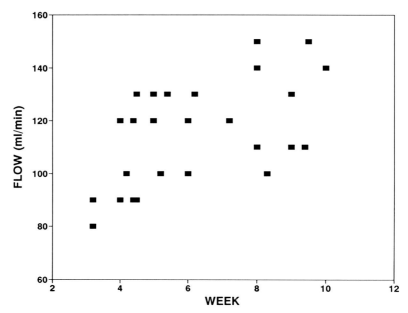

Figure 18.19 Changes in volume flow in the ovarian artery throughout the first trimester. (Reprinted with permission from Thaler et al).[2]

in vasodilation, a low vascular resistance, and high flow rates.[36] This is also supported by the observation that the "luteal" artery has a much lower impedance to flow compared to the main ovarian artery as was discussed earlier.

Using color Doppler imaging, trophoblastic flow could be observed in normal and extrauterine pregnancies.[24] Blood flow in the fetal vessels, specifically the fetal aorta and umbilical arteries, could be assessed from as early as 6 weeks of gestation. This relatively new imaging modality carries a significant potential for Doppler studies in early gestation.

Studies of the Uterine Artery in Pregnancy Hypertension

Fetal growth has been shown to be directly related to the incremental increase in uterine blood flow.[34,35] Any long-term alterations in the normal incremental increase of this flow could disrupt oxygen and nutrient supply to the growing conceptus and result in abnormal growth of the fetus and the placenta.[34] The high-frequency transvaginal image-directed pulsed Doppler system offers a novel approach for investigating the perfusion characteristics of the uteroplacental circulation. It has an obvious potential for studying hemodynamic alterations in a wide variety of disorders. Perhaps the most common complication in pregnancy, which is associated with altered perfusion of the uteroplacental circulation, is hypertension. Placental ischemia was postulated to be present in patients with preeclampsia.[38] Adverse outcome of pregnancy has been described in hypertensive pregnant patients[39,40] and this has been attributed to vascular lesions in the uteroplacental circulation, with resultant decrease in blood flow, leading to hypoxic complications of the fetus.[41] Indeed, changes in flow velocity waveforms have been described in hypertensive pregnant patients, using Doppler velocimetry.[42–44] In these and subsequent studies, Doppler flow patterns indicative of increased impedance in the uterine vasculature in pregnancies complicated by preeclampsia and fetal growth retardation were observed. This pattern was associated with adverse pregnancy outcome, and a classification of hypertension in pregnancy was proposed based on Doppler velocimetry of the uterine and the umbilical circulations.[45] The mechanism that may be responsible for these changes may be failure of trophoblast cells to invade the intima and media of uterine spiral arteries. The vessels thus retain vasomotor tone and remain constricted.[46] Uteroplacental velocimetry has also been used for predicting preeclampsia and fetal compromise (eg, IUGR and fetal asphyxia).[47]

Most investigators of the uteroplacental circulation reported the use of a continuous wave Doppler system. Others have used a transabdominal pulsed-duplex Doppler device. With these methods, the Doppler signals have been collected from different locations in the uteroplacental circulation, namely the uterine artery, the arcuate artery, and arteries in the placental bed. It may be impossible to define vessel location with certainty with these methods and to repeat the test in the same vessel during follow-up examinations. In addition, when using continuous wave Doppler, the ultrasonic beam "samples" the velocity profiles of all the vessels it crosses. This may present a serious problem if one considers the rich network of venous plexuses surrounding the proximal uterine artery and its branches.[48] These limitations are reflected in the wide range of interobserver and intraobserver variability reported in the literature by investigators employing such techniques.

The transvaginal pulsed-duplex Doppler method can overcome many of these problems for reasons that were previously discussed. We have used this approach to study flow patterns in the uterine artery in hypertensive pregnant patients and to investigate whether there is any relationship between these patterns and adverse pregnancy outcome.

We studied 140 hypertensive pregnant patients in a cross-sectional manner. They were divided according to the type of hypertension (chronic, pregnancy-induced hypertension—PIH, and preeclamptic toxemia—PET), its severity (systolic/diastolic blood pressure greater than or equal to 160/110 or values below this), and the presence or absence of intrauterine growth retardation (IUGR). The cutoff level for the ratio between peak-systolic and end-diastolic flow velocity was set to 2.8. The S/D ratio was increased near term in all groups. Between 32 and 36 weeks it was significantly higher in the PIH/PET group than in the chronic hypertensives group, where the values were in the upper limit of the normal or just above it (Fig 18.20). In the PIH/PET group the S/D ratio was above the cutoff level regardless of the severity of hypertension. However, it was higher in the group with severe hypertension compared to the other group (Fig 18.21). A similar observation was found in the group with chronic hypertension. In the PIH/PET group the proportion of patients who had an S/D ratio >3 was substantially higher compared to the chronic hypertensive group (Fig 18.22). The resistance to flow was significantly higher in patients with IUGR compared to those with average for gestational age fetuses for all the groups studied (Fig 18.23). Volume flow rates were decreased in patients with severe hypertension in all groups (Fig 18.24). The site of placentation influenced the resistance to flow so that if the placenta was lateral, the resistance to flow on that side was lower compared to the other side. This is demonstrated in Fig 18.25, where the effect of right placental insertion is shown.

An interesting observation was the frequent occurrence of a diastolic notch in

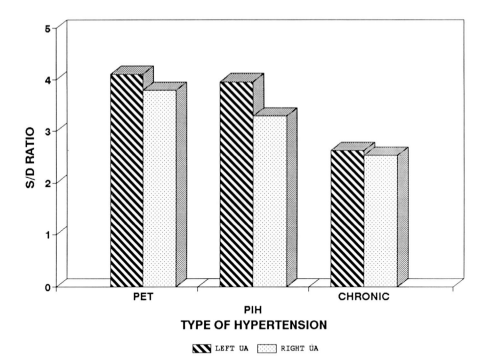

Figure 18.20 Mean S/D ratio in the uterine arteries between 32 and 36 weeks gestation according to the types of hypertension.

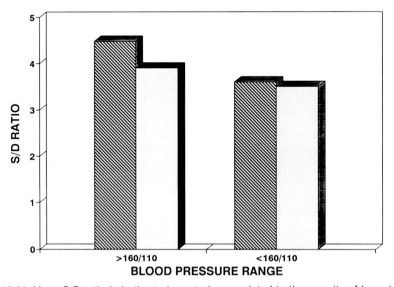

Figure 18.21 Mean S/D ratio in both uterine arteries as related to the severity of hypertension.

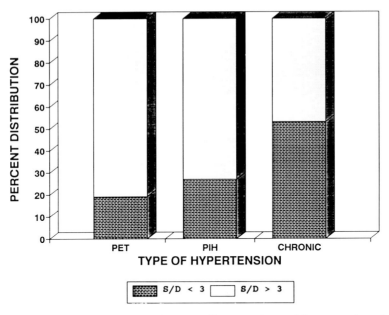

Figure 18.22 The relationship between the type of hypertension and the proportion of patients with a uterine artery S/D ratio >3.

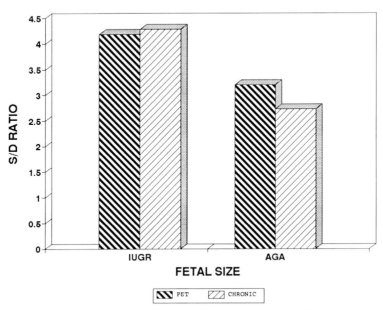

Figure 18.23 The relationship between S/D ratio in both uterine arteries and patterns of fetal growth during the third trimester.

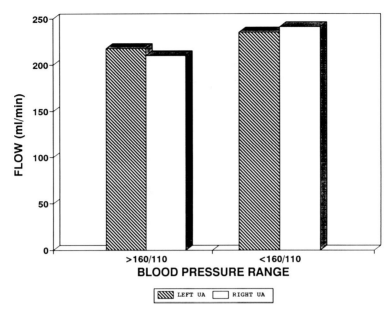

Figure 18.24 Volume flow rates in the uterine arteries according to the severity of hypertension.

RIGHT PLACENTAL INSERTION

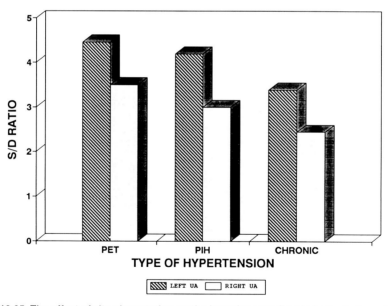

Figure 18.25 The effect of site placentation on the impedance to flow in both uterine arteries. In this example, all patients with right placental insertion were studied. The S/D ratio in the uterine artery on the side of the placental insertion (ie, right side) was substantially lower than in the opposite side, regardless of the type of hypertension.

the uterine artery flow velocity waveform (FVW), with or without a systolic notch. Examples of the two types of notches are shown in Fig 18.26. Diastolic notch was more frequent than systolic notch and the incidence of both was higher in the group with severe hypertension (Fig 18.27). This pattern was observed almost exclusively in patients with PIH/PET. Diastolic notch in the uterine artery was reported in hypertensive pregnant patients.[44,49] If a notch was present and the resistance to flow was increased, the pregnancy suffered the consequences of inadequate nutrition and oxygenation.[44]

We examined the relationship between the presence of systolic or diastolic notch in uterine artery flow velocity waveforms and pregnancy outcome in the hypertensive group. Parameters of outcome included: perinatal mortality rates, rates of IUGR, cesarian section rates, rates of induction of labor, the incidence of low Apgar scores (5 minutes Apgar score < 7), admission to the neonatal intensive care unit (NICU) for more than 48 hours, abnormal NST or biophysical profile score, birth weight, and gestational age at delivery.

One hundred one patients had no notch in the uterine artery FVW, 39 patients only had a diastolic notch, and 14 patients had a systolic notch (that was always associated with a diastolic notch). One hundred twenty-six patients did not have a systolic notch (in 101 no notch was present and in 25 a diastolic notch was detected). Table 18.2 summarizes the outcome of pregnancy in those patients. The presence of notch—either systolic or diastolic—was associated with a significant increase in low Apgar scores, in the rate of IUGR, in cesarian section rates, and in the number of days spent in the NICU. Abnormal FHR patterns during labor were much more frequent in patients who had a notch in the uterine artery FVW. The presence of notch was also associated with a significantly lower mean birth weight and earlier deliveries.

We also examined the relationship between perinatal outcome and the presence of systolic and diastolic notch in patients with different flow velocity waveform patterns in the uterine and the umbilical arteries. Table 18.3 demonstrates the outcome of pregnancy in these patients. When both the uterine and the umbilical arteries reflected an increased resistance to flow (13 patients) the outcome was worse than in patients in whom only the uterine artery demonstrated this pattern (11 patients). When a notch was present in the uterine artery FVW despite normal

TABLE 18.2 The Relationship Between the Presence or Absence of Diastolic and Systolic Notch in the Uterine Artery and Pregnancy Outcome

No.	DN− 101	DN+ 39	SN− 126	SN+ 14
Apgar 5 min (%)	6.9	25.6**	11.9	14.3
IUGR (%)	12.9	64.1***	23.0	64.3**
Induction (%)	49.5	59.0	50.8	64.3
Cesarian section (%)	29.7	51.3*	32.5	64.3*
NICU >2 days (%)	16.8	53.8***	22.2	71.5***
NND (%)	5.0	12.5	6.3	14.3
NST (in labor) (%)	13.9	25.6	14.3	42.9*
Delivery	37.2	33.8***	36.6	33.8**
Birth weight	2820	1753***	2610	1789***

DN+ = presence of diastolic notch. ND− = absence of diastolic notch. SN+ = presence of systolic notch. SN− = absence of systolic notch. IUGR = intrauterine growth retardation. NICU = neonatal intensive care unit. NND = neonatal death.
*p < 0.05.
**p < 0.01.
***p < 0.001.

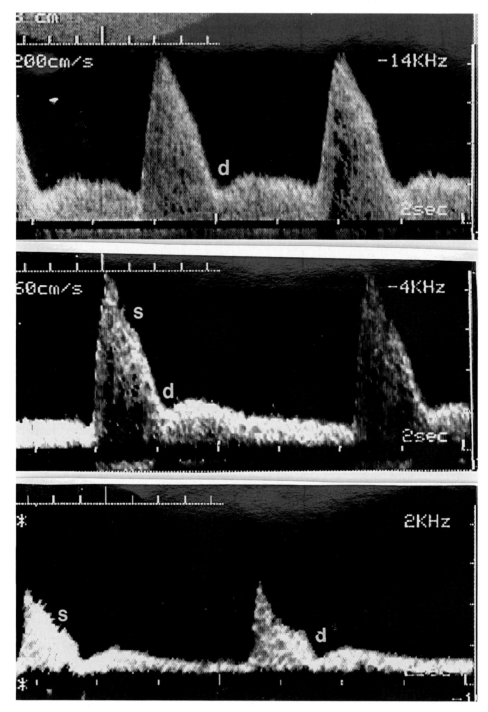

Figure 18.26 Flow velocity waveforms in the uterine arteries demonstrating systolic (s) and diastolic (d) notch.

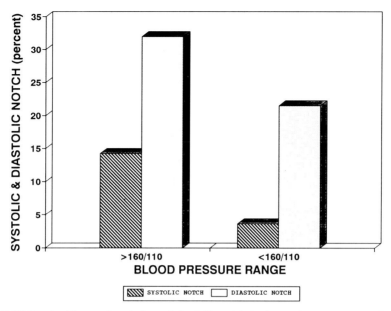

Figure 18.27 The incidence of systolic and diastolic notch in the uterine artery according to the severity of hypertension.

TABLE 18.3 The Relationship Between FVW in the Uterine and the Umbilical Arteries and Pregnancy Outcome

No.	HUt 11	HUtN 8	HUtUmb 13	HUtUmbN 19
Apgar 5 min (%)	0	37.5*	7.7	21.1
IUGR (%)	0	62.5**	15.4	73.7**
Induction (%)	54.5	62.5	61.5	52.6
Cesarian section (%)	27.3	50.0	46.2	52.6
NICU >2 days (%)	0	62.5**	30.8	63.2
NND (%)	0	12.5	0	21.1
Abnormal FHR patterns (%)	0	37.5*	23.1	36.8
Delivery	38.2	33.6	36.1	33.5
Birth weight	2975	2131*	2503	1662**
Lt. Uterine S/D Ratio	3.65	5.39*	4.42	5.59
Rt. Uterine S/D Ratio	3.67	5.37*	3.70	4.22
Umbilical S/D Ratio	2.41	2.62	4.35	5.31

HUt = elevated uterine S/D ratio without notch. HUtN = elevated uterine S/D ratio with notch. HUtUmb = elevated uterine and umbilical S/D ratio without notch. HUtUmbN = elevated uterine and umbilical S/D ratio with notch. IUGR = intrauterine growth retardation. NICU = neonatal intensive care unit. NND = neonatal death.

*$p < 0.05$.
**$p < 0.01$.
***$p < 0.001$.

umbilical S/D ratio (8 patients) or when there was an abnormal S/D ration in both vessels with a notch in the uterine artery (19 patients) the outcome was worse. The latter group had the highest rates of IUGR and the lowest mean birth weight. The S/D ratios in the uterine and umbilical arteries in this group of patients are shown in Fig 18.28.

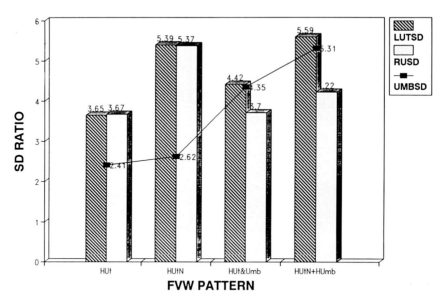

Figure 18.28 Mean S/D ratios in the uterine and the umbilical arteries in the group of 51 hypertensive patients that are described in Table 18.3.

CONCLUSION

The high-frequency transvaginal Doppler duplex system offers a novel approach for the investigation of perfusion characteristics in the uterine and ovarian circulation. It is more accurate and convenient than the transabdominal route, and is ideal for monitoring blood flow patterns in patients undergoing ovarian stimulation, infertility workup, and various hormonal therapies. It also has an obvious potential for studying hemodynamic alterations in normal and abnormal pregnancies from the very early stages of gestation and for monitoring the effect of drugs and medications on uterine blood flow during pregnancy. An important development in this area is the application of color Doppler imaging, which facilitates vessel recognition and localization. It is particularly useful for studying complex vascular beds, and its prospects in the screening and diagnosis of pelvic tumors seem promising. Further studies in these areas and new technological advances in the field of ultrasound imaging and in Doppler signal acquisition and analysis will undoubtedly turn this noninvasive "flow probe" into a useful clinical tool in the daily routine.

REFERENCES

1. Thaler I, Manor D: Transvaginal imaging: applied physical principles and terms. J Clin Ultrasound 1990;18:235.
2. Thaler I, Manor D, Brandes JM, et al: Basic principles and clinical applications of the transvaginal Doppler duplex system in reproductive medicine. J In Vitro Fertil Embryo Transfer 1990;7:74.
3. Timor-Tritsch IE, Thaler I, Rottem S: Review of transvaginal ultrasonography: a description with clinical application. Ultrasound Quart 1988;6:1.

4. Eik-Nes SH, Marsal K, Kristofferssen K: Methodology and basic problems related to blood flow studies in the human fetus. Ultrasound Med Biol 1984;10:329.
5. Thaler I, Manor D, Rottem S, et al: Hemodynamic evaluation of the female pelvic vessels using a high-frequency transvaginal image-directed Doppler system. J Clin Ultrasound 1990;18:364.
6. Taylor KJW, Burns PN, Wells PNT, et al: Ultrasound Doppler flow studies of the ovarian and uterine arteries. Br J Obstet Gynaecol 1985;92:240.
7. Feichtinger W, Putz M, Kemeter P: Transvaginale Doppler-Sonography zur Blutflussmessung im kleinen becken. Ultraschall Med 1988;9:30.
8. Thaler I, Manor D, Rottem S: Hemodynamic study of the female pelvic vessels by a transvaginal Doppler duplex system, in Chervenak F, Isaacson G, Campbell S (eds): Textbook of Ultrasound in Obstetrics and Gynecology. Boston, Little, Brown, 1990 (in press).
9. Janson PO, Damber JE, Axen C: Luteal blood flow and progesterone secretion in pseudopregnant rabbits. J Reprod Fert 1981;63:491.
10. Niswender GD, Dickman MA, Nett TM, et al: Relative blood flow to the ovaries of cycling and pregnant ewes. Biol Reprod 1973;9:87.
11. Janson PO, Albrecht AI: Methodological aspects of blood flow measurements in ovaries containing corpora lutea. J Apl Physiol 1975;38:288.
12. Scholtes MCW, Wladimiroff JW, van Rijen HJM, et al: Uterine and ovarian flow velocity waveforms in the normal menstrual cycle: a transvaginal Doppler study. Fertil Steril 1989;52:981.
13. Steer CV, Campbell S, Pampiglione JS, et al: Transvaginal colour flow imaging of the uterine arteries during the ovarian and menstrual cycles. Hum Reprod 1990;5:377.
14. Ford SP, Reynolds LP, Farley DB: Interaction of ovarian steroids and periarterial alpha-adrenergic receptors in altering uterine blood flow during the estrous cycle of gilts. Am J Obstet Gynecol 1984;150:480.
15. Randall NJ, Beard RW, Sutherland IA, et al: Validation of thermal techniques for measurement of pelvic organ blood flow in the nonpregnant sheep: comparison with transit-time ultrasonic and microsphere measurements of blood flow. Am J Obstet Gynecol 1988;158:651.
16. Padwick ML, Whitehead MI, Coffer A, et al: Demonstration of estrogen receptor related protein in female tissues, in Studd JWW, Whitehead MI (eds): The Menopause. Oxford, Blackwell, 1989;227.
17. Ford SP, Chenault JR: Blood flow to the corpus luteum-bearing ovary and ipsilateral uterine horn of cows during the oestrous cycle and early pregnancy. L Reprod Fert 1981;62:555.
18. Goswamy RK, Williams G, Steptoe PC: Decreased uterine perfusion—a cause of infertility. Hum Reprod 1988;3:955.
19. Steer C, Campbell S, Mills C, et al: Transvaginal colour flow Doppler of the uterine arteries. Presented at the Sixth World Congress of In Vitro Fertilization and Alternate Assisted Reproduction, Jerusalem, Israel, April 2–7, 1989.
20. Bourne T, Hillard TC, Whitehead MI, et al: Oestrogens, arterial status, and postmenopausal women. Lancet 1990;335:1470–1471.
21. Deutinger J, Reinthaller A, Bernascheck G: Transvaginal pulsed Doppler measurements of uterine blood flow velocity in the ovarian arteries during cycle stimulation and after follicle puncture. Fertil Steril 1989;51:466.
22. Sterzik K, Grab D, Sasse V, et al: Doppler sonographic findings and their correlation with implantation in an in vitro fertilization program. Fertil Steril 1989;52:825.
23. Matta WHM, Stabile I, Shaw RW, et al: Doppler assessment of uterine blood flow changes in patients with fibroids receiving the gonadotropin-releasing hormone agonist Buserelin. Fertil Steril 1988;49:1083.
24. Kurjak A, Jurkovic D, Alfirevic Z, et al: Transvaginal color Doppler imaging. J Clin Ultrasound 1990;24:227.
25. Bourne T, Campbell S, Steer C, et al: Transvaginal colour flow imaging: a possible new screening technique for ovarian cancer. BMJ 1989;299:1367.
26. Thaler I, Manor D, Itskovitz J, et al: Changes in uterine blood flow during human pregnancy. Am J Obstet Gynecol 1990;161:121.
27. Deutinger J, Rudelstorfer R, Bernascheck G: Vaginosonographic velocimetry of both main uterine arteries by visual vessel recognition and pulsed Doppler method during pregnancy. Am J Obstet Gynecol 1988;159:1031.
28. Schulman H, Fleischer A, Farmakides G, et al: Development of uterine artery compliance in pregnancy as detected by Doppler ultrasound. Am J Obstet Gynecol 1986;155:1031.
29. Trudinger BJ, Giles WB, Cook CM: Uteroplacental blood velocity-time waveforms in normal and complicated pregnancy. Br J Obstet Gynecol 1985;92:39.

30. Cohen-Overbeek TE, Pearce JM, Campbell S: The antenatal assessment of uteroplacental and fetoplacental blood flow using Doppler ultrasound. Ultrasound Med Biol 1985;2:329.
31. Pijneborg R, Dixon G, Robertson WB, et al: Trophoblastic invasion of human decidua from 8 to 18 weeks of pregnancy. Placenta 1980;1:3.
32. Griendling KK, Fuller EO, Cox RH: Pregnancy induced changes in sheep uterine and carotid arteries. Am J Physiol 1985;248:H658.
33. Greiss FC Jr: Pressure-flow relationship in the gravid uterine vascular bed. Am J Obstet Gynecol 1966;96:41.
34. Clapp JF, McLaughlin MK, Larrow R, et al: The uterine hemodynamic response to repetitive unilateral vascular embolization in the pregnant ewe. Am J Obstet Gynecol 1982;144:309.
35. Rosenfeld CR, Morris FH, Makowski EL, et al: Circulatory changes in the reproductive tissues of ewes during pregnancy. Gynecol Invest 1974;5:252.
36. Abdul-Karim RW, Bruce N: Blood flow to the ovary and corpus luteum at different stages of gestation in the rabbit. Fertil Steril 1973;24:44.
37. Niswender GD, Reimers TJ, Dickman MA, et al: Blood flow: a mediator ovarian function. Biol Reprod 1976;14:64.
38. Chesley LC: Hypertensive disorders in pregnancy. New York, Appleton-Century-Crofts, 1978.
39. Lin CC, Lindheimer MD, River P, et al: Fetal outcome in hypertensive disorders of pregnancy. Am J Obstet Gynecol 1982;142:255.
40. Naeye RL, Friedman EA: Causes of perinatal death associated with gestational hypertension and proteinuria. Am J Obstet Gynecol 1979;133:8.
41. Khong TV, DeWolf F, Robertson WB, et al: Inadequate maternal vascular response to placentation in pregnancies complicated by preeclampsia and by small-for-gestational age infants. Br J Obstet Gynaecol 1986;93:1049.
42. Campbell S, Griffin DR, Pearce JM, et al: New Doppler technique for assessing uteroplacental blood flow. Lancet 1983;1:675.
43. Trudinger BJ, Giles WB, Cook CM: Uteroplacental blood flow velocity-time waveforms in normal and complicated pregnancy. Br J Obstet Gynaecol 1985;92:39.
44. Fleischer A, Schulman H, Farmakides G, et al: Uterine artery Doppler velocimetry in pregnant women with hypertension. Am J Obstet Gynecol 1986;154:806.
45. Ducey J, Schulman H, Farmakides G, et al: A classification of hypertension in pregnancy based on Doppler velocimetry. Am J Obstet Gynecol 1987;157:680.
46. Brosens I, Robertson WB, Dixon HG: The role of the spiral arteries in the pathogenesis of pre-eclampsia. Obstet Gynecol Ann 1972;1:177.
47. Campbell S, Pearce JM, Hackett G, et al: Qualitative assessment of utero-placental blood flow: early screening test for high risk pregnancies. Obstet Gynecol 1986;68:649.
48. Bieniarz J, Crottogin JJ, Curuchet E, et al: Aortocaval compression by the uterus in late human pregnancy. II. An arteriographic study. Am J Obstet Gynecol 1968;100:203.
49. Cohen-Overbeek TE, Pearce JM, Campbell S: The antenatal assessment of utero-placental and feto-placental blood flow using Doppler ultrasound. Ultrasound Med Biol 1985;11:329.

CHAPTER **19**

Office and Emergency Room Use of Transvaginal Sonography

Ilan E. Timor-Tritsch, MD

I am asked frequently why anyone should be enthusiastic about transvaginal sonography (TVS); why anyone would purchase a machine to use in an office practice. Administrators ask why they should invest in dedicated ultrasound equipment to be used only part of the time in an emergency room.

The answer is simple, short, and expresses in a concise manner all that has to be said to give the most appropriate answer: *because it is good!* This answer will suffice for those obstetricians and gynecologists who have already been exposed to this scanning technique. This laconic answer, however, will not convince the uninitiated.

This chapter is directed to the large group of obstetricians and gynecologists, as well as emergency room physicians, who rightfully expect a more scientific answer—an answer that is based on experience, data, and facts rather than subjective enthusiasm. Before presenting the literature and lining up statistical data to support the message, I would like to employ the tarnished and overused cliche, "one picture is worth a thousand words." This saying could not be more applicable than in this case. One glance at the pictures on the monitor at the examination table will convert more skeptics than reading articles or listening to lectures.

WHY IS TRANSVAGINAL SONOGRAPHY GOOD?

Picture Quality

The answer is: the clarity of the images. Through clear images a quick, accurate diagnosis can be made at an early stage of the disease or the pregnancy. This in turn facilitates an adequate therapeutic approach or is reassuring to the healthy patient.

The basic physical properties of the probe make all of the above possible. Chapter 1 was devoted to explaining the physics of sound and how one may harness its properties to be incorporated and used in the vaginal probe. The key is the use of higher frequencies with better resolutions, which yield clear pictures. These high-resolution images are not affected by magnification. The term "sonomicroscopy," used by Goldstein,[1] may sound pretentious; however, a 6.5 or 7.5 MHz vaginal probe can definitely be compared to the power of a good "dissecting microscope."

The clear picture of the ventricular system in the brain, the neural tube (spine) at nine menstrual weeks, or the bony structure of the fingers at 11 weeks effectively support the claim. Furthermore, the detection of the embryonic heartbeat just about 5 days after it began (at 21 days) in a 3–4 mm fetal pole, and the adjacent 4 mm extremely thin-walled yolk sac are so striking that one must be impressed by the power and abilities of this new scanning method. The detection of an intrauterine gestational sac during the fifth week, the potential for imaging several milliliters of pelvic fluid with great accuracy, and, finally, the early and reliable diagnosis of a tubal gestation leave no alternative but to believe in the high-resolution picture generated by TVS.

Dynamic Use

The answer to our initial question is not complete without mentioning its use of TVS in detecting the origin of pelvic pain. Structures and organs can be gently pushed by the tip of the probe so that the site of pain can literally be "seen."

The abdominal hand may add valuable information by moving structures in and out of the "eyesight" of the probe. In fact, the entire examination is performed as if the examiner had an eye on the examining finger.

One can also test for the free movement and motion of organs in relation to the pelvic wall or to each other. This was reported by our group as the "sliding organs sign."[2] Adhesions and "frozen organs" can be detected by exerting a push–pull motion with the probe. The same tugging of the probe can reveal the floating motion of debris; hence the nature of the fluid-filled structures. It is almost impossible to chart all the above-mentioned dynamic "tests" that can be done with an abdominal probe.

Ease of Operation and Learning

Previous experience using an abdominal transducer has its obvious advantages if the learning of transvaginal sonography is considered. However, the speed with which residents in obstetrics and gynecological services get used to, and become at first reasonably proficient and later "dependent" on, the technique (without previous abdominal scanning experience), is truly amazing. The training factor will be expanded on later.

In short, there is a very brief learning period because the transvaginal probe is extremely operator "friendly."

The Use in Obese or "Guarding" Patients

Transvaginal sonography is a good adjunct to, but will probably never completely replace, the thorough bimanual pelvic examination of most patients. However, most of the time vaginal sonography can replace an *inadequate bimanual examination*. This is particularly so in a patient who tenses the abdominal muscles to guard a tender pelvis, or in a patient who is simply obese. Many healthy patients do not lend themselves to a meaningful palpatory pelvic examination. The vaginal ultrasonographic examination furnishes information in the vast majority of cases in which the lack of tactility in the pelvis cannot be overcome even by other more expensive laboratory tools.

WHY IS TRANSVAGINAL SONOGRAPHY USEFUL IN THE OFFICE?

In responding to this question, the articles reviewed and the impression gained from personal experience all came into play.[1,3-5,8] The "ingredients" for the usefulness of TVS in the office are its easy availability, good quality machines, and a mounting data base on the subject.

Availability of the Equipment

Portable machines equipped with the vaginal probe can be easily set up at the side of the examining table in the office to be used when the patient is still on the examining table. As such it has the ability to confirm or rule out the most commonly encountered diagnoses. The bulk of the problems raised throughout morning or afternoon sessions in the office are simple ones: early pregnancy—yes or no: embryonic/fetal heart beats present or absent. Is the pregnancy in the uterus? Is it a singleton pregnancy? Is the uterus enlarged (fibroids?) or is it an ovary? Is there fluid in the pelvis? Is the cervix dilated (short? effaced?)? What is the size of the follicle? Is there a cyst in the adnexa? Did the previously detected cystic structure change in size or disappear? The answer to all of these commonly occurring questions becomes exceptionally simple by inserting the vaginal probe *immediately following* the bimanual pelvic examination. The sonographic images of all the above-mentioned entities are clear and obvious.

The ultrasonographic examination follows the previously used palpating fingers and is directed exactly at the site of the finding, while the "abdominal hand" stabilizes the structures. This imaging modality suddenly improves the physician's ability to evaluate the pelvis, thus enhancing the quality and speed of the diagnosis. Unnecessary patient anxiety and precious time can be saved and appropriate treatment instituted without delay.

Good Quality, "User Friendly" Equipment, Information, and Backup Consults

There has never been a better time than as part of the examination to incorporate the vaginal scan with the bimanual examination of the pelvis.[3] All components for its successful adaptation to routine office procedure are existent, for instance:

1. They are relatively inexpensive, simple to operate ("user friendly"), and portable machines equipped with both abdominal and vaginal probes.
2. Educational courses are widespread and held frequently throughout the world, including hands-on courses offered by many laboratories.
3. Numerous medical centers have added vaginal sonography as an additional means of pelvic sonography, providing resources for a backup scan or a consult.
4. Books and manuals, and an increasing number of articles in journals on vaginal sonography, are widely published. These represent a reference source for all those performing office scans.

Only limited information on the office use of transvaginal sonography is available in spite of the fact that an increasingly large number of private offices are using it at the present time.

A study on the use of the vaginal probe in a private office is reviewed first. This study presents the results of routine office use in 535 patients from the sixth to the thirteenth week[4]: 56 patients (11%) were scanned for vaginal bleeding and 479 (89%) were asymptomatic. Twenty-six of the 56 bleeding patients had nonviable pregnancies (missed abortion: 12, incomplete abortion: 6, complete abortion: 4, ectopic pregnancy: 3, anembryonic gestation: 1). Thirty of the 56 patients with vaginal bleeding had fetuses with heartbeats but had various pathologies (ie, subchorionic bleeding: 7, fibroids: 7, twin gestation: 1; however, no pathology was seen in 15).

The asymptomatic patients (a = 479) showed normal findings in 53% of the cases, but the surprising findings in the rest of the cases were: no pathology but size and date discrepancies of more than one week in 67 (14%), fibroids larger than 4 cm and/or a corpus luteum larger than 2.5 cm resulting in size and date discrepancies in 25 (1.25%), twin gestation in 10 (2.1%), and other pathologies in 19 (3.5%).

The conclusion of the study indicated that about one-third of the asymptomatic patients had clinically significant findings, most important of these being the need for correction of the expected date of delivery (in 20%) and a more viable gestation (5% of asymptomatic patients). A reassuring follow-up could be offered to over 50% of bleeding first-trimester patients who went on to have a favorable outcome.

The experience of utilizing transvaginal ultrasonography in another private group practice is mentioned here.[6]

A busy private practice in New York consisting of three obstetrician gynecologists scans about 170 patients monthly. Three-quarters of these are usually new obstetrical patients, whereas 25% consist of suspected first-trimester pathology. Ninety-five percent of their obstetrical population is scanned. Forty-seven percent of the scans performed in the office were done transvaginally. At present, this ob–gyn group does not employ sonographers in their practice. They scan the patients themselves. One partner in this group had extensive previous experience with abdominal sonography, and the two other partners had some limited experience with obstetrical ultrasonography in the delivery room during their residency year. After a learning curve of several months, they summarized their experience in the following manner.

1. There was no disruption of patient flow during their office hours.
2. There was wide patient acceptance of the immediate and concomitant scans. This acceptance was greater than during a previous period when a sonographer was employed, or when an outside referral was sought.
3. There was the opportunity of inside consultation on special findings.
4. There was increased patient confidence in the group.
5. There was a reduction in the level of patient anxiety normally attributed to the delay in reporting time when there is an outside referral.

This group considered the office scanning in general and the addition of the transvaginal probe in particular an important professional achievement of their practice.

To summarize, the use of transvaginal scanning in private offices in the United States is increasing at an astonishing rate. Data generated by the ultrasound manufacturing companies attest to this matter.[7]

WHY IS TRANSVAGINAL SONOGRAPHY USEFUL IN THE EMERGENCY ROOM?

A significant number of articles were published and reviewed about the use of transabdominal scanning in the emergency suite.[8-14]

Shea et al[8] reported the efficacy of abdominal and pelvic ultrasound in the emergency department. They assessed the diagnostic value of abdominal and pelvic ultrasound to the emergency room physician by following 43 patients who required ultrasound out of 1010 patients presenting to the emergency suite with abdominal pain and/or vaginal bleeding. Ultrasound confirmed the preliminary diagnosis in 12 patients, supported the preliminary diagnosis in 8 patients, and ruled out the preliminary diagnosis in 23 patients. Ultrasound shortened the evaluation process by narrowing the differential diagnosis or by excluding potentially serious conditions, thus eliminating the need for additional testing and frequently allowing for *safe discharge* of the patient. This group found the use of ultrasound in the emergency room to be not only helpful, but also cost-effective in certain patients with abdominal and/or vaginal bleeding in whom an emergency department evaluation without ultrasound could not exclude the condition necessitating admission or urgent surgery.

In 1986, Grumbach et al performed a study following which they concluded that ultrasound plays an important role in the evaluation of patients presenting with pain or bleeding during pregnancy. Ultrasound was found to be important as an imaging modality in the workup of many patients treated by the emergency room physician.[9]

In a review published by Trott in 1987,[10] the author expressed his views on the gynecologic emergencies as an integral part of the practice of an emergency physician; the diagnostic modalities available to this emergency physician, particularly serologic pregnancy testing and ultrasonography, have kept pace by undergoing tremendous technology improvements that allowed more rapid and accurate diagnosis of these potentially life-threatening diseases. The above-mentioned tools enabled him to make the statement that the emergency physician "has never been in a better position to cope with the distressed gynecological patient."

In 624 women referred to an emergency gynecological ultrasound clinic, with a provisional diagnosis of threatened miscarriage based on history of amenorrhea and vaginal bleeding with or without abdominal pain, Stabile et al made interesting observations.[11] Fetal size and viability as well as uterine and placental size were examined to identify features that might indicate impending fetal death. In 158 women there was no evidence of pregnancy and 60 women had an ectopic pregnancy. In the remaining 406 patients, the ultrasound examination correctly identified the underlying cause of vaginal bleeding at first presentation in all but the 6 who subsequently aborted. In this study, 3.9% of the patients had a second empty sac, and 5.4% had an intrauterine hematoma. None of these women subsequently aborted. Two patients had early onset oligohydramnios, and spontaneous abortion occurred in both. This article clearly expresses the need for available emergency room ultrasound equipment.

Further observations on the use of a transabdominal ultrasound machine in the emergency room were presented by Gilling-Smith et al[12] in 1988. The necessity for using an ultrasound machine in the emergency room was stressed by the fact that during the 6-month prestudy period, 179 patients were complaining of bleeding from pregnancies of less than 20 weeks gestation. After this observation, the use of an ultrasound machine dramatically changed the incidence of admission, which fell from the previously experienced 28% to 12%, and the use of gynecologists on call, which was reduced from 44% to 22%. The rescan rates fell from 15% to 4%. All these changes were significant at a level of $p < 0.05$. In 1989 a feasibility study was done by Jehle et al.[13] This was a retrospective study conducted to examine whether emergency physicians can perform accurate ultrasonography, influencing the diagnosis and treatment of selected disorders in the emergency department. These physicians acquired a moderate level of expertise in sonography using a series of practical demonstrations and lectures. Accuracy of the positive sonographic findings was assessed by confirmatory testing formerly reviewed, or a confirmatory clinical course. The study concluded that the emergency physicians were able to diagnose correctly the presence or absence of intrauterine pregnancy in patients with lower abdominal/pelvic complaint and the position of intrauterine devices in patients with suspected uterine perforation among other conditions. It was further concluded that reliable sonography, which influences diagnosis and therapy, can be performed by emergency physicians and that sonography should become a standard procedure in emergency rooms. It should be noted that in this last study, the emergency physicians were not gynecologists–obstetricians. However, they performed at an above-expected level of expertise in handling the ultrasound equipment. Other pertinent articles supported the usefulness of employing ultrasound equipment as an adjunct in emergencies.[14-15]

After reviewing the pertinent literature, we would like to reiterate the obvious advantages for using an ultrasound machine in the emergency suite: (1) it shortens the time to reach a diagnosis leading to therapeutic decision making; (2) relatively high accuracy of diagnosis is made; (3) there is a higher turnover of patients in a highly congested area; and (4) last but not least, it allows periods of well-needed rest to those emergency physicians who are overwhelmed in many places.

The prerequisite for operating the dedicated ultrasound scanner in such a setting requires a financial investment, but more importantly, the adequate training of the residents performing the scans. The presumption is that in the case of a gynecological emergency room, the transvaginal scans are performed by the residents on call at the time of the pelvic bimanual examination of the patient. The obstetrical emergencies are usually different from the scanning of the gynecological patients. The gynecological patients present themselves to the general emergency room, while the obstetrical emergencies are encountered usually in the obstetrical labor and delivery suites. In spite of the fact that an increasing number of residency programs train their residents to perform emergency obstetrical scanning, unfortunately, in many places, residents use this imaging modality in the delivery suite at night, on their own, without proper supervision and teaching. This is still the way many residents "train" in abdominal sonography. "Teaching" is done by a senior resident who, at best, has been introduced to the "mysteries" of this laboratory tool in a similarly informal manner. The routine use of the transabdominal linear scanners is now an indispensable diagnostic tool in almost all labor and delivery suites. They found their way into the caring hands of the residents, not as the result of extensive studies to prove their efficacy and cost effectiveness, but simply because the images were easy to evaluate, accurate, and shortened the time to render appropriate patient care. There are only a few studies to prove the usefulness of transabdominal ultrasound in the obstetrical suite.[16]

Several departments employ a policy of liberal and immediate availability of transvaginal scans for emergency use. However, there are no published evaluations on the use of the transvaginal probe in the gynecological emergency room.

At the Sloane Hospital for Women (Columbia Presbyterian Medical Center), a study was devised to determine the feasibility and the effectiveness of an ultrasound machine equipped with a 5 MHz vaginal probe operated by the residents on call. Two years prior to this project, the first-year residents started to rotate formally through the ultrasound unit of the department, receiving formal training in the use of ultrasound in obstetrics and gynecology, including the use of the transvaginal probe. The "Emergency Room study" was preceded by circulating a questionnaire to all 20 residents during their residency program. Sixteen responded to the questionnaire; five residents out of the 20 did not have formal ultrasound training, (mostly third- and fourth-year residents). However, most of these 5 residents had some exposure to handling the vaginal probe. All thought that vaginal ultrasound could be introduced in the everyday office procedure. All expressed the opinion that ultrasound should be done by the "generalist" ob–gyn practitioner after proper training, and more than half of the responses expressed the feeling that vaginal ultrasound in the emergency room could help in 50% to 70% of the cases. Fifteen of the 16 felt that the average time to work up a patient would be decreased, and 15 out of 16 wanted to have the probe in the emergency room. Encouraged by the responses, the program was begun. The efficacy and feasibility of the use of the transvaginal probe in the emergency room was assessed with a comparison of the pre- and postscan diagnosis by measuring the time elapsed from the patients arrival to the time of the decision making. Finally, the residents expressed their objective feelings toward the scanner and the help given by the scan in the management of the patient. "Scanning days" alternated with "no scanning days." On the "no scanning days" the times the patients arrived and the decision-making time was noted. However, the patients were scanned the usual way by referring them to the ultrasound unit situated in a different geographical area in the building. The documentation was performed by means of a written report and images recorded on a thermal paper printout, which were then attached to the patient's files. The results of the study were as follows:

One hundred twenty-six patients were scanned (study group) and 35 patients, who presented on nonscan days, constituted the control group. There were 124 cases with completed data forms. Sixty-two had follow-up confirming the diagnosis and 82 patients were not readmitted at our hospital. The correct diagnosis was made in 56 of the 62 cases (90%). There were 6 misdiagnoses (10%). As to the type of scan, there were 15 abdominal scans, 86 vaginal scans, and 13 in which both abdominal and vaginal scanning was used. The length of the scan was less than 5 minutes in 23 cases; 5–15 minutes in 81 cases; and less than 15 minutes in 9 cases. Fifty-eight patients were scanned during the day and 55 patients were scanned during the night.

The time to the diagnosis in the emergency room of the 124 cases was an average of 38 minutes, ranging between 7 and 120 minutes. The diagnosis in the 35 patients who had to be referred out on nonscan days was made in an average of 4 hours and 50 minutes and the range was between 15 minutes and 19 hours. We measured the efficacy in the management of the patients. Fifty-one patients went home sooner, 9 went to surgery sooner, 9 were admitted faster, and 1 went home later due to the ultrasound scan. In the rest of the 63 patients, the residents indicated that there was no change in the speed and efficacy of the case management.

We charted the residents' confidence in their scanning process. Seventy-eight residents expressed high confidence, 26 intermediate confidence, and 6 low confidence. In 7 patients this question was not answered. We tried to estimate the time to the diagnosis on which the treatment was based. In 85 patients the residents felt that it was faster than usual. In 5 cases it took longer and in 23 cases it took about the same time as it would have taken without ultrasound. The subjective assessment of this scan was found to be easy in 87 cases, about the same as without ultrasonography in 20 cases, and harder in 4 cases. The following misdiagnoses occurred:

1. A molar pregnancy was diagnosed as missed intrauterine pregnancy.
2. An incomplete abortion was diagnosed as a complete abortion.
3. A right adnexal mass was diagnosed in a case of appendiceal abscess.
4. An ectopic pregnancy was diagnosed as a complete abortion.
5. An ectopic pregnancy was missed, after a positive βhCG. A rescan established the diagnosis.
6. A missed abortion was diagnosed and subsequently an ectopic pregnancy was found.

It should be stated that none of the cases of ectopic pregnancy were discharged home before the correct diagnosis was made.

In conclusion, there was a significant decrease in time required for the diagnosis of patients presenting to the emergency room when the emergency room sonography was available. Residents trained in sonography had a high level of confidence in its use and made correct diagnoses at least 90% of the time.

1. The residents were able to operate the vaginal probe and obtain the necessary information to correctly manage the overwhelming majority of the cases.
2. The patients spent less time for workup on "scanning days" than on the "control" days. A decision for treatment, admission, surgery, or discharge was made quicker with an immediate scanning than with a same-day ultrasound referral (control days) or a subsequent later appointment to the ultrasound unit. It was our impression (this was not coded) that the number of appointments and rescans decreased as a result of the emergency room scan performed on the "scanning days."
3. Finally, the residents expressed their confidence in TVS as a complementary tool to their bimanual vaginal examination and unanimously requested that a machine with a vaginal probe for permanent use be placed in the emergency room area.

THE NECESSITY OF TRAINING

It can never be overemphasized that training in the use of the vaginal probe is essential. Several issues should be considered regarding the training.

Theoretical Versus Practical Courses

Theoretical courses are important to attend; however, they are not sufficient to enable the immediate use of a probe. Theoretical courses are a basis and have to precede practical training. *Hands-on experience is necessary*. This hands-on experience is even more important if the user has no previous abdominal sonographic experience.

The Length of Practical Experience

The ultimate purpose of practical experience is to give the scanner a clear orientation of the pelvis in order to recognize the normal organs within the pelvis, and, of course to recognize abnormalities.

There are no clear length-of-time requirements for such practical training experience. The Royal College of Radiology in the United Kingdom requires 300 hours of supervised training in an approved center, a completed logbook of 50 cases to show experience, and attendance at an approved educational course.

Where to Train

Postresidency training is feasible and possible through courses and joining an established laboratory. After purchasing a machine, one can scan patients for some time without using the obtained information clinically. At the same time, the patients should be sent, as in the days prior to owning a machine, to the ultrasound laboratory employed before. After the results and the diagnosis match, or are increasingly consistent with the results obtained by the "formal" laboratory used, the clinical use of the machine can start.

The residency programs are the most natural opportunities in which to learn ultrasonography in general, and vaginal scanning in particular. Sonographic imaging should be an integral part of obstetric–gynecologic residency training. It is time to consider ultrasonography as an integral part of the diagnostic algorithm and elevate it from its clandestine and dilettante use to its rightful place as the right hand of most subspecialties of obstetrics and gynecology departments. As such, it has to be taught formally.

Heads of obstetrics and gynecology departments and directors of ultrasound units as well as coordinators of obstetrics and gynecology residency and fellowship programs have to provide their residents with a proper and formal teaching of ultrasonography and, of course, vaginal scanning in particular.

The residents and fellows have to be receptive and open-minded to acquire proficiency in this exceptional diagnostic modality as part of their clinical diagnostic skill during the residency years. Once these residency years pass, it becomes increasingly difficult and expensive to catch up and attend 2- to 3-day courses followed by hands-on experience, to become acquainted with this procedure.

To summarize the ease of training to the users of the probe, I have this quote: "Given a general familiarity with real-time pelvic sonography, the technique of vaginal sonography was *easily adopted and basically self-taught*."[23]

OFFICE-BASED ULTRASOUND SCREENING FOR OVARIAN CANCER

In the minds of most clinicians who were convinced by the crisp and clear pictures obtained by transvaginal ultrasonography, the natural question arose: Could this outstanding device be used in screening for ovarian cancer? As a matter of fact, this is probably the question that is voiced by participants of ultrasound courses in the whole world.

This question is addressed in great detail in Chapter 7. However, because of the importance of the topic, some of its aspects will be raised here in the context of office use of the vaginal probes.

It should be stated at the beginning that no studies using the transvaginal probe as a screening tool in the early detection of ovarian cancer have been published. The two major studies addressing this question were prepared by using the transabdominal scans.[17,18,19] The two studies[17,19] included 5479 and 805 women, respectively, who were screened by transabdominal sonography. Women with positive results on screening were referred in both studies for laparoscopy and laparotomy. Outcome measures in both were the findings of the abnormal ovaries at surgery and pathology. In Campbell's study, 326 of the 5479 patients had positive screens; in Andolf's study, 50 of the 805 patients had positive screens (5.9% and 6.2%, respectively). In Campbell's study, 4 cases of stage 1A diseases, one case of stage 1B disease and 4 metastatic ovarian cancers were detected. Of the 326 patients with positive screening, 50% had tumor-like conditions, 37% had benign epithelial tumors, 9% had sex-cord, or germ cell, tumors, 11% had unclassified nonmalignant lesions, 18% resolved and were not ovarian, and 3.7% (12 women) had no disease at surgery. Three of the patients with primary and one with metastatic ovarian cancer had normal initial scans and an abnormal second scan. In the study performed by Andolf, two borderline ovarian cancers, one stage 3 disease, 23 benign epithelial tumors, one cancer of the rectum, and, finally, 4 cases that had no disease at surgery were reported. It is important to stress that in this study none of the three ovarian cancers were discovered on pelvic examination.

The following important aspects were learned from these two studies of transabdominal screening:

1. Ultrasound screening detected ovarian cancers missed on bimanual exam.
2. A large number of scans must be done to detect one ovarian cancer (1096 and 402, respectively).
3. A large number of patients will undergo surgical procedures in order to detect a small number of ovarian cancers. In Campbell's series only 9 of the 326 women who underwent surgery had ovarian cancer.
4. Since three of the cases of ovarian cancer in Campbell's series were detected at the second, not the first, yearly screening, one could imply that perhaps a yearly screening is more beneficial.
5. Morphologic characteristics detected by transabdominal ultrasound could not be used to distinguish between benign and malignant lesions.

The Use of Transvaginal Sonography and Color Flow Doppler Studies

In spite of the fact that this subject, at this time, seems to be still remote from being adapted as an office-based scanning technique, it will be mentioned briefly. A speculation that is shared by others is that it will take no longer than several years until the color coding Doppler capability will be used in the office and emergency setting. Transvaginal sonography is expected to answer the problem of not only detecting small lesions or small ovaries, but also to characterize these ovarian lesions in order to distinguish between benign and malignant lesions. This will then decrease the unnecessary surgical interventions that were done in the previous studies for benign ovarian lesions, which can be followed up by the same means: transvaginal sonography.

One of the promising tools that, as said before, will certainly gain importance in the future is the transvaginal color Doppler flow imaging which holds great promise for distinguishing between benign and malignant lesions (see Chapter 17). Recent reports by Bourne et al[21] and Kurjak et al[22] showed that malignant tumors, compared to benign tumors, have an increased intraovarian vasculature due to new developing blood vessels, which is associated with the growth and progression of the tumor, and have a decreased vascular impedance. To avoid false positive results, premenopausal women should, therefore, be examined in the early follicular phase of the menstrual cycle only, since characteristics of angiogenesis of tumors may be similar to that of the normally occurring corpus luteum.

The two above-mentioned studies dealing with transvaginal color Doppler flow to screen for ovarian cancer have a low number of patients; however, using the model they developed one could speculate on the future importance of this method.

Three of the 35 malignant lesions—2 studies—were not correctly identified using color flow Doppler. This low sensitivity for the detection of this lethal disease seems less than optimal. If one looks at the false positive results, these were low. Of the 145 patients, only two were described as malignant by ultrasound criteria. The only false positive case in Campbell's series was a dermoid cyst with nests of thyroid cells, which showed increased vascularity.

To summarize the importance of the color flow addition to the vaginal scanning for ovarian malignancy, one should express the desire for more information. However, the high sensitivity and specificity of these procedures are promising.

Obviously we should know more about the natural history of the disease, such as the length of time the ovarian cancer remains in stage I. What is the nature of the time of borderline tumors? What is the natural history of a benign disease? And do benign epithelial tumors have an increased propensity to undergo neoplastic changes or to become symptomatic? If this is true, their detection should not be considered a cost but rather a part of the effectiveness of the screening program.

And lastly, the question arises as to whether laparotomy can be avoided in the evaluation of positive scans. Perhaps by using laparoscopic techniques one could avoid a laparotomy which would then decrease the burden of false positive results.

To conclude the subject of office screening for ovarian cancer, one should state clearly that as more and more gynecologists gain in experience and purchase equipment for their offices, transvaginal sonography will increasingly be used to extend the bimanual examination of women. For the postmenopausal woman, a priority at the annual checkup is cancer screening. After examining the breasts, looking for blood in the stool, and taking a Pap smear, is it really reasonable to screen for an enlarged ovary by palpation alone when the ultrasound machine with the vaginal probe is situated next to the examining table?

We have been screening and continue to screen for ovarian cancer using the bimanual examination, a technique which we know to be unreliable, inadequate, and inferior to transvaginal ultrasound for the detection of an ovarian enlargement.[19,20] For the present, if we are doing office screening for ovarian enlargement, and we have transvaginal sonography available, it seems utterly logical that one would use this tool. Regarding color flow Doppler, we need more information. However, this interesting technology will undoubtedly prove beneficial in the future.

LEGAL ASPECTS

Most people who object and warn against the office and emergency room use of sonography in general and the vaginal probe in particular raise many issues, but the first one always is the legal issues. The potential liability for performing TVS is not higher than doing laser surgery, hysteroscopy, or a simple cesarean section. If someone is trained in TVS in a similar way, she/he is trained for other procedures performed in obstetrics and gynecology, and there is no need to be upset by the legality of this diagnostic and therapeutic tool. It is illogical to think that by *adding* a diagnostic tool to the low-yield bimanual examination, making it more accurate or more reliable, one *increases* the liability by missing structures and diagnoses. *Au contraire!* Logic dictates that this will *decrease liability* by increasing the reliability of the bimanual examination and providing better definition of structures.

Considering the achievement of TVS and the fact it can be taught in a formal way in postgraduate courses as well as throughout residency training programs, it is logical that the office use and the emergency room use of vaginal sonography is feasible, inevitable, and will not result in an increased liability. To reiterate our dictum: adequate training is the key. Obstetricians and gynecologists are able to master much more complex skills. Transvaginal sonography is among the easy skills to learn.

Anecdotal conversations with residents and ob–gyn practitioners have reassured us of the user-friendliness of TVS. After a certain period of adjustment and learning, they come to be dependent on vaginal sonography to the extent that they could not again practice without it. Its use, according to the above group of doctors, was particularly effective in the triage of patients requiring prompt attention in emergency situations.

To conclude the topic of "legal issues" in TVS, our belief is that the time is fast approaching when failure to use the vaginal probe to complement the bimanual examination will be considered inadequate clinical practice. All involved in resident education and in policy-making should strive to construct, implement, and supervise appropriate and sensible rules and regulations for adequate education and training within residency or postgraduate programs rather than warn against misuse and liability! If the residents are properly trained, they will become part of the solution and not part of the problem.[1]

Skeptics will voice concern about office scanning by saying that imaging is not the specialty of gynecologists, and one should not compete with the imaging laboratory. The answer to these arguments is easy: true gynecologists are not imaging specialists, but after a bimanual examination of the pelvis (which gynecologists know how to do well), a unique opportunity is given to the examiner and this is: to "look" at the palpated structure at the time of the examination. This modified or advanced pelvic examination is in no way a competition to the specialized imaging laboratory. It merely completes the physical and pelvic examination of the patient. Women with doubtful findings and unexplained images will and *should* always be sent to the imaging specialist. "Knowing one's limitation, that is, when to obtain consultation, has always been the sign of a good physician."[1]

The last argument is: it will take more time for the patient's office examination. This may be true; however, after the initial training period, the additional time to scan a patient may not be more than 1–3 minutes.[1] Even if 5 minutes were added to the average time spent in the office, the patient would be likely to emerge with a faster, better diagnosis and, in most cases, with a proper diagnosis-related treatment. In most cases a second visit (after the trip to the imaging or biochemistry laboratory) will be spared.

WHICH EQUIPMENT TO BUY?

The answer once again is the machine displaying the most clear, crisp diagnostic quality image enabling the scrutiny (by "zooming in") of the on-screen image. The best investment for an office or for an emergency ward is good-quality equipment. Don't compromise by comparing prices. Compare performance in light of the individual office needs. A world champion in tennis or skiing will outperform anyone using inferior quality equipment. However, the average tennis player or skier can improve on performance with good-quality equipment. Similarly, the office-based gynecologist–obstetrician should purchase the machine with the best performance and the highest resolution available—which is not necessarily the most expensive machine—to enhance her or his understanding of the picture by a high-quality image on the screen.

For detailed information on equipment, including vaginal probes, the interested reader is referred to Chapter 2.

As a rule, one should never buy or lease equipment not tested or intensively looked at before the final deal. One of the best investments for the ob–gyn office and for a busy emergency room is a good-quality ultrasound unit with a transvaginal probe, capable of producing high-resolution images for instantaneous evaluation.

CONCLUSION

Among the most important advances in obstetrics and gynecology in the last twenty years is ultrasonography. The introduction of the high-frequency, high-resolution vaginal probe is the "icing on the cake," because its simplicity and ease of operation is changing the office practice of gynecology and obstetrics.

The author firmly believes, and this belief is now shared by many others, that in the near future *every ob–gyn practitioner* will operate one or several transvaginal ultrasound probes in the office and in the emergency room. *But remember— formal training on its use is mandatory.*

REFERENCES

1. Goldstein SR: Incorporating endovaginal ultrasonography into the overall gynecologic examination. Am J Obstet Gynecol 1990;162:625–633.
2. Timor-Tritsch IE, Bar-Yam Y, Elgali S, Rottem S: The technique of transvaginal sonography with the use of a 6.5 MHz probe. Am J Obstet Gynecol 1988;158:1019–1024.
3. Timor-Tritsch IE: Is office use of vaginal sonography feasible. Am J Obstet Gynecol 1990;162:983–985.
4. Weiss RR, Khulpathea T, Lau GK: Transvaginal ultrasonography screening in early gestation. Presented at the Third World Conference on Vaginosonography Gynecology, June 14–17, 1990, San Antonio, Tex.

5. Copel JA: Diagnostic ultrasound in the obstetrician's office: what should the obstetrician do and expect? Obstetrics Gynecology Forum 1989;3(6):3–5.

6. Kerenyi TD: Office use of transvaginal sonography—the "real life" in the practitioner's office. Presented at The Third International Conference on Transvaginal Sonography, September 14–15, 1990, New York.

7. Dowden M: Should you equip for vaginal scanning? OBG Management, March, 1990 pp 49–56. Publ: N. Minicucci Jr. Dowden Publ. Corp, Inc.

8. Shea DJ, Aghababian RV: The efficacy of abdominal and pelvic ultrasound in the emergency department. Ann Emerg Med 1984;13:311–316.

9. Grumbadi K, Mechlin MB, and Mintz MC: Computed sonography and ultrasound of the traumatized and acutely ill patient. Emerg Med Clin North Am 1985;3:607–624.

10. Trott A: Diagnostic modalities in gynecologic and obstetric emergencies. Emerg Med Clin North Am 1987;5:405–423.

11. Stabile I, Campbell S, and Grudzinskas JG: Ultrasonic assessment of complications during first trimester of pregnancy. Lancet 1987;2:1237–1240.

12. Gilling-Smith C, Zelin J, Touquet R, Steer P: Management of early pregnancy bleeding in the accident and emergency department. Arch Emerg Med 1988;5:133–138.

13. Jehle D, Davis E, Evans T, Marchelroad F, Martin M, Zaizer K, Lucid J: Emergency department sonography by emergency physicians. Am J Emerg Med 1989;7:605–611.

14. Davis RO, Brumfield CG: The use of real-time ultrasound in the management of obstetrics emergencies. Clin Obstet Gynecol 1984;27:68–77.

15. Stabile I, Campbell S, Grudzinskas JG: Can ultrasound reliably diagnose ectopic pregnancy? Br J Obstct Gynaccol 1988;95:1247–1252.

16. Vournal KA, Reed KL: The use of ultrasound in a labor and delivery unit. Presented at the Thirty-fourth Annual Meeting of the AIUM, March 4–7, 1990, New Orleans.

17. Campbell S, Bhan V, Royston P, Whitehead MI, Collins WP: Transabdominal screening for early ovarian cancer. BMJ 1989;229:1363–1367.

18. Goswamy RK, Campbell S, Whitehead MI: Screening for ovarian cancer. Clin Obstet Gynecol 1983;621–626.

19. Andolf E, Svalenius E, Astedt B: Ultrasonography for early detection of ovarian carcinoma. Br J Obstet Gynaecol, 1986;93:1286–1289.

20. Granberg S, Wilkland M: A comparison between ultrasound and gynecologic examination for detection of enlarged ovaries in a group of women at risk for ovarian cancer. J Ultrasound Med 1988;7:59–64.

21. Bourne T, Campbell S, Steer C, Whitehead MI, Collins WP: Transvaginal color flow imaging: a possible new screening technique for ovarian cancer. BMJ 1989;299:1367.

22. Kurjak A, Zalud I, Alfirevic Z, Jurkovic D: Transvaginal color Doppler in the assessment of pelvic tumors. Ultrasound Med Biol (in press).

23. Bateman BG, Nunley WC, Kolt LS, Kitchin JD, Felder R: Vaginal sonography findings and hCG dynamics of early intrauterine and tubal pregnancies. Obstet Gynecol 1990;75:421–427.

Index

A

Abcesses
    drainage of, 88
    pelvic, 138, 443, 444f–446f
    tubo-ovarian, 97f
Abdomen, fetal, 263f, 270f
Abdominal cysts, fetal, 349–350, 350f
Abdominal pregnancy, 389–390
Abdominal sonography
    frequency for, 31
    linear transducers in, 30
Abdominal wall, fetal anomalies of, 345–346, 346f,
        347, 347f–348f, 349, 349f, 350, 350f–351f
Abortion
    holoprosencephaly and, 410
    incomplete, 299
    inevitable, 299
    missed, 238, 299–300, 314, 316, 321
    recurrent, 299
    selective, 439
    spontaneous, 299–300, 306f, 315f, 320, 322f–323f
    therapeutic, 342, 343f
    threatened, 299, 308, 321
    tubal, 379
Abruptio placenta, 214
Absorption, 4
Acoustic Imaging machines
    financial considerations for, 56–57
    operational considerations for, 44–48
    physical considerations for, 38–43
    transducer probes by, 49–55
Acoustic impedance, 4
Acoustic shadow, 4
Acquired immune deficiency syndrome (AIDS), 215
Acrania, 331–332, 332f–333f, 408
Acuson machines
    financial considerations for, 56–57
    operational considerations for, 44–48
    physical considerations for, 38–43
    transducer probes by, 49–55
Adenocarcinoma
    ovarian, 146, 158f, 167
    tubal, 143
Adenomyoma, uterine, 125

Adenomyomatosis, uterine, 129f
Adenomyosis, uterine, 125
Adenovirus type 2, disinfectants against, 64
Adnexa
    in infertility, 200
    scanning routine and, 67
    transabdominal ultrasonography and, 80f, 88, 95
    transvaginal ultrasonography and, 80f
Adnexal mass
    in ectopic pregnancy, 99, 104
    endometrial thickening and, 121
    fallopian tube, 131
    ovarian, 88, 90f–91f, 96f–97f
    transvaginal color Doppler sonography and, 456–
        458
ADR/ATL machines
    financial considerations for, 56–57
    operational considerations for, 44–48
    physical considerations for, 38–43
    transducer probes by, 49–55
AFP, *see* α-Fetoprotein
Age
    conceptual, 232
    gestational, 232–233
    menstrual, 233
Agenesis, disorders of, 336–338, 408, 412–413
Agyria, 408
AIDS, *see* Acquired immune deficiency syndrome
Air
    acoustic impedances of ultrasound in, 4
    half-intensity depth of in different frequency ranges,
        5
    ultrasound velocity in, 3
Aliasing, 23
Allantoid cysts, 353, 354f
Aloka machines
    financial considerations for, 56–57
    operational considerations for, 44–48
    physical considerations for, 38–43
    transducer probes by, 49–55
Alternative data input, 35–36
Amniocentesis, early, 448
Amnion, 229, 245, 245f, 258, 266f
Amniotic fluid, 229